Those who devote their careers, even their lives, to advancing reproductive self-determination are often characterized, even caricaturized, as devoid of basic human compassion. None have been more vilified than Warren Hern. Nevertheless, his enduring and unyielding service, on the front lines of one of the most intense social, political, ethnic and economic conflicts in American history, is undaunted by his personal vulnerability and often professional isolation. Warren's revelations unveil the foundation and fiber on which he has amassed admiration as a public health visionary and medical practitioner. The most powerful lessons are the insights gained from his human journey, a path lighted by exceptional life experiences and undaunted determination not to return women to the dangers and injustices of 17th Century servitude.

Faye Wattleton, *President/CEO, Planned Parenthood*
Federation of America, 1978–1992

There is no one in the United States who knows more about abortion practice and politics than Dr. Warren Hern. And there is no one who writes more cogently and trenchantly about these matters. Dr. Hern has lived through and in the midst of every phase of the abortion wars, building a unique practice and dedicating his life to (and risking it for) what he believes in. Remarkably, Dr. Hern has the fortitude, the focus, and the capacity to write about abortion politics with special insight, clarity, and style.

Rickie Solinger, *author of* Pregnancy and Power:
A History of Reproductive Politics in the U.S. *(2019, rev. ed.)*
and Reproductive Justice: An Introduction *(2017)*

Reasons to publish Warren Hern's book – or anything he writes: Dr. Hern wears a bullet-proof vest to work because he is one of the last medical practitioners of the last line of skilled help and healing for women whose lives and pregnancies are in danger. You will also find him testifying in the U.S. Congress, the United Nations, the World Health Organization and many other influential places about women's health and the scary politics of reproduction. Now, more than ever, we need his voice, his compassionate stories, and his political analyses from the front of the great debate over reproductive health for women.

Martha Ward, *author of* Poor Women, Powerful Men:
America's Great Experiment in Family Planning;
Professor of Anthropology, University of New Orleans

For sixty years, Dr. Warren Hern has stood in the front lines of the battle for women's reproductive health care, one abortion patient at a time. His passionate commitment and medical skill make him a beacon of hope for women with nowhere else to turn, and he has never shied away from confronting the hypocrisy and cruelty of those who would deny women and their doctors the right that the Supreme Court once recognized. This book is his story, a testament to his courage and to the knowledge acquired through a lifetime of activism.

Linda Greenhouse, *Pulitzer Prize in Journalism, 1998;*
Author, New York Times reporter and columnist;
Co-author of Before Roe v. Wade: Voices that Shaped the
Abortion Debate Before the Supreme Court's Ruling

This lively and well-written book has much to offer those who are interested in the history and evolution of abortion care in the United States and elsewhere. Dr. Hern takes the reader into the early struggles within the medical community over how to incorporate this essential – *albeit* controversial – service. Also, the author was among the first in abortion providing circles to recognize the threat to reproductive freedom posed by the emerging religious right and he shares his astute observations of the damage that continues to be done to this day by that movement.

Carole Joffe, *Professor of Obstetrics, Gynecology and Reproductive Sciences, University of California, San Francisco, co-author,* Obstacle Course: The Everyday Struggle to Get an Abortion in America

No single American has more totally lived through this country's unending struggle for the availability of safe, legal abortions than Dr. Warren M. Hern. While several of his close professional colleagues have been shot dead by political assassins, Warren Hern has both survived and continued operating what is without question America's most important reproductive health facility for late term abortions. What's more, Warren has also quietly led an absolutely fascinating 'second life' as an anthropologist and photographer who has studied and published professionally on some of South America's most remarkable indigenous peoples. In a life that has allowed me to meet countless memorable people, ranging from Hubert Humphrey and George McGovern through Nelson Mandela and Barack Obama, no human being has ever impressed me more than Warren Hern.

David J. Garrow, *author of* Liberty and Sexuality: The Right to Privacy and the Making of Roe v. Wade (1998) *and* Bearing the Cross: Martin Luther King, Jr. and the Southern Christian Leadership Conference (1986), *Pulitzer Prize for Biography, 1987*

Abortion in the Age of Unreason

This vivid account by a nationally prominent doctor reports the daily challenges of offering and receiving abortion services in a volatile political and social atmosphere. In stories from the front lines – from protecting patients and staff from protesters' attacks to the dangers to women of restricted access to abortion services, and the pertinent findings of his remote research in Latin America, Hern's book is strikingly detailed just as it exposes the needs of women and the U.S. national interest. Dr. Hern – an abortion specialist, researcher, scholar, and highly visible public advocate – shows how abortion saves women's lives given the many risks that arise during pregnancy – remarkably more than most people realize. He points to political and national solutions to reverse a reawakened crisis that now threatens democracy. Throughout the book, Dr. Hern shows how the current emergency was largely created by political actors who have exploited and distorted the abortion issue to increase and consolidate their power.

A vital component of women's health care, the crisis over abortion is not new. Yet the reversal of *Roe v. Wade* and the steady accumulation of power by America's right wing has put the issue at a level of urgency and national prominence not seen since the days before legalization. Women's need for safe abortion services will continue as the struggle to secure their rights intensifies. This book is about that struggle during what has evolved, over the last 50 years, to an Age of Unreason.

Warren M. Hern, M.D., is known to the public through his many appearances on CNN, Rachel Maddow/MSNBC, Sixty Minutes, and in the pages of *The Atlantic Magazine*, *New York Times*, *Washington Post*, and dozens more media. A scientist, Hern wrote about the need for safe abortion services before the 1973 *Roe v. Wade* decision and was present at the first Supreme Court arguments. In his research and medical work, he pioneered since 1973 the modern safe practice of early and late abortion in his highly influential books and scholarship. A tireless national activist for women's reproductive rights, he is an adjunct professor of anthropology at the University of Colorado, Boulder, and holds a clinical appointment in obstetrics and gynecology at the University of Colorado medical center. He holds doctorates in medicine and epidemiology. Dr. Hern received the Christopher Tietze Humanitarian Award and awards from the American Public Health Association for his scientific contributions and defense of reproductive freedom. He lives in Boulder with his wife and son.

Abortion in the Age of Unreason

A Doctor's Account of Caring for Women Before and After *Roe v. Wade*

Warren M. Hern

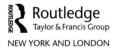
Routledge
Taylor & Francis Group

NEW YORK AND LONDON

Designed cover image: Warren M. Hern

First published 2025
by Routledge
605 Third Avenue, New York, NY 10158

and by Routledge
4 Park Square, Milton Park, Abingdon, Oxon, OX14 4RN

Routledge is an imprint of the Taylor & Francis Group, an informa business

ISBN: 978-1-032-84785-6 (hbk)
ISBN: 978-1-032-84782-5 (pbk)
ISBN: 978-1-003-51496-1 (ebk)

DOI: 10.4324/9781003514961

Typeset in Sabon
by Deanta Global Publishing Services, Chennai, India

Books by Warren Martin Hern

Abortion Services Handbook
Abortion in the Seventies (Warren M. Hern, Bonnie Andrikopoulos, Eds)
Abortion Practice
Risus Sardonicus
Homo Ecophagus: A Deep Diagonosis to Save the Earth

Contents

Figures

"Trust Women"
Dr. George Tiller (1941–2009)

This book is dedicated to all the women whom I have helped to have safe abortions during my medical career.

Acknowledgments

There are certain people in my life who have helped me the most and made the most important contribution to the result you see in this book. Among the most important, of course, are members of my immediate family – my parents, my sisters, and my wife and son. There are many others who gave me critical help and support, such as my mentors in medical school, school of public health graduate work; professional colleagues; inspired teachers, such as John Cassel, Steve Polgar, and Bert Kaplan, Lula Lubchenco, Lyle Saunders, and Ned Hall; medical school classmates. such as Bonnie Camp; people who gave me priceless opportunities and encouragement, such as Dr, Teodor Binder, Dr. Michael Diana, and Dr. Ralph Eichenberger in the Peruvian Amazon and Dr. George Contis in Washington, D.C., along with my cherished workmates in that place; Nan McEvoy, who gave a critical invitation to Preterm Clinic; doctors Mike Burnhill, Ben Branch, Earl Herr, and Jane Hodgson at Preterm; Dr. Louise Tyrer; Dr. Sherburne Macfarlan in Boulder; nurse AnnaGail Oakes, whose help in starting the first clinic in Colorado was indispensable; Dr. Phil Stubblefield, a brother in spirit who is always there for me; Lisa Biello and Darlene Pedersen, Lippincott editors who gave me their total support in creating, writing, and preparing my textbook, *Abortion Practice*, without which that book would not have happened; Dr. John Sciarra, who included me among his contributors to his multi-volume textbook *Gynecology and Obstetrics*; Ralph Wynn, who offered to publish one of my first papers; my friends and colleagues in Colorado Dell Bernstein, Ted Engel, Arlen Ambrose, Don Aptekar, Bill Droegemueller, David Thayer, Ruth Wright, Dorothy Rupert, Vicki Cowart, Savita Ginde, Steve Hindes, Ron Kuseski, Harvey Cohen, and Frank Susman, who argued six abortion cases before the Supreme Court and reviewed the Court chapter in this book for me; Karen Mulhauser and Fran Kissling, who were there at the beginning; Bill Baird, who began inspiring me in 1968 when I got on the stage with him; Ellie Smeal, who, as president of the National Organization for Women, recognized my work and gave me unique opportunities to participate in this struggle; the editors of major journals who published my material; my dear friend, psychotherapist, ski partner, and gruff cheerleader Dr. Bill Rashbaum in New York; Dr. Christopher Tietze and his wife, Sarah Lewit; my book designer friend Polly Christensen, who took an idea of mine and some loose scraps of paper and turned them into a beautiful book of poetry and anecdotes, giving me a sense of artistic creation that I had not experienced and what it really means to assemble a book; the incredible, amazing, dedicated, brilliant women, starting with Sunya, Lolly, AnnaGail, Marcy, Martha, both Vickies, and PJ, who have helped me to take care of our patients for most of the past 50 years; Ann Rose, our far-sighted Internet expert, who dragged me kicking and screaming into the twentieth century cyberworld and her genius associate, Yvonne Morris, without whom we would probably be closed; my current fantastic staff; my friend and colleague Dennis Christensen; my friend and colleague Bernie Smith; my friend and colleague Fred Hopkins, who has been like a brother; Frank Arrieta, my office administrator, whose dedication and hard work to help me take care of my patients while trying to do ten other things is just beyond belief; anthropologist colleagues Robert Carneiro, Payson Sheets, Donna Goldstein, Paul Shankman, and Darna Dufour; and, finally, Dean Birkenkamp, my editor and publisher's representative at Routledge Press, without whose encouragement, critical support, and guidance this book would not have happened – nor the book that preceded it.

My thanks for their invaluable book endorsements as well as friendship and writer's crisis psychotherapy go to Rickie Solinger, a brilliant historian, friend, and author who inspires me, Martha Ward, anthropologist, great spirit, author, and dear friend for decades, Faye Wattleton, who has inspired me for decades and whose warm support for my work (and this book) is irreplaceable, David Garrow, whose scholarship and brilliant writing is an inspiration for my efforts, Linda Greenhouse, one of the great journalists of our time who I am privileged to know, and whose kind words I treasure, Carole Joffe, a dear friend who understands this subject and writes about it with unparalleled depth, and Malcolm Potts, who has inspired and encouraged me for decades. I cannot possibly thank all the dozens of other friends and colleagues who mean as much to me as those mentioned here, and there are literally hundreds of wonderful people who have helped and inspired me from several dozen countries going back 60 years. Many of the most important of these cherished colleagues and close friends, such as Irv Cushner, Bill Rashbaum ("Peace and quiet is for when you're dead"), Judith Rooks, Judy Widdicombe, Mildred Hanson, George Tiller, Henry Morgentaler, Jane Hodson, Louise Tyrer, Jim Armstrong, Priscilla Reining, and Henry David are no longer with us. These are among my best friends in my life. I can only try to pass along what I have learned from them. I learned much and enjoyed their company. I wish I could give them a copy of this book and share some memories of the old days. I miss them all.

I am deeply grateful to and for the young doctors, nurses, counselors, laboratory and records workers, patient coordinators, my superb executive assistant, and all they are doing every day to continue this work for the patients who come to us for help. That's what it's all about.

I am grateful for the wise, courageous and thoughtful volunteer patient escorts who help protect the patients from our antagonists, and who, under the circumstances, are really at risk of anti-abortion violence out there by the entrance to my office, but they come to help in spite of that. Their thoughts and observations are in this book.

The people of Boulder have been supportive from the beginning and continue to be there for us in the city actions and law enforcement, which is more necessary than it should be for my unique medical practice. This work, our safety, and this book would not be possible without the positive support from the people of Boulder, Colorado.

Finally, but not last, I thank my wonderful wife, Odalys, love of my life and life partner, who brought her adorable son, Fernando, into my life along with her love for me and dedication to our life together and to our work in this important field, in which she was already expert when we met in Spain. Her deep humanity and irrepressible Cuban *joi de vivre* complete with irresistible Cuban dance rhythms have enriched my life as has her deep understanding of my commitment to this important life work. She and Fernando sustain me. Fernando, our son, gives me the hope of youth for the future. And he digs epidemiology.

On January 22, 2025, we will observe the 50th anniversary of the opening of Boulder Abortion Clinic, P.C. Here's to another 50 years!

Acknowledgment of Permission Granted

The following publications have granted permission to include excerpts previously published:

The Denver Post
The Daily Camera
The Colorado Statesman
The New York Times
The New Republic
The Progressive
Slate
Springfield News Leader
USA Today

Introduction

The eighteenth century is known as the "Age of Reason" because, following centuries or millennia of blind religious belief in supernatural powers and mystical notions, the way opened for people to understand the world around them, starting with natural phenomena, with observation, and the discovery of facts, reason, and a rational approach to their experiences. The idea of "science" developed as a way of understanding facts about the world.

By contrast, there have been many "Ages of Unreason," such as the Crusades, the Inquisition, the Salem witch hunts, the pogroms against Jews, the rise of fascism in Europe, slavery, the genocide and ethnocide of Native American peoples, the destructiveness of McCarthyism in the United States, and innumerable other examples.

We are now living in a new Age of Unreason in which fundamentalist religious groups and people opposed to scientific facts of all kinds have captured control of parts of the most powerful government on the planet. The terrifying and inexorable process of climate change caused by human activity is denied, and even the historic benefits of public health are being denied by those opposed to vaccination against terrible and fatal diseases. Those opposed to basic facts about the world have become increasingly powerful, culminating with the presidency of Donald J. Trump, who led the most dishonest, corrupt, ignorant, and destructive administration in the history of the United States. Not the least of these denials of and opposition to the benefits of modern science and medicine are shown by those who oppose reproductive health care for women, uncounted millions of whom have died from unsafe abortion and the lack of modern contraceptive care.

Whereas the twentieth century brought historic improvements in these benefits for women and made death from unsafe abortion a rare event in the United States, fundamentalist religious groups joined forces with the radical political right to roll back these advances in many parts of America and to deny these benefits to other women around the world.

The causes and currents of these destructive efforts are complex, and this book is an attempt to portray the broad picture of this conflict and its results. An especially disturbing consequence of the use of the abortion issue by one political party to gain this destructive power was the election of Donald Trump in 2016, whose administration inflicted profound damage on the United States in countless ways.

But this is the culmination of decades of constant fanatic attacks on abortion and abortion services, women, physicians, and the right to basic reproductive health care by the Republican Party, the Roman Catholic Church, a variety of fundamentalist, evangelical Christians, Christian nationalists, the Tea Party and other extreme right-wing groups. Abortion has been an absolutely key and dominant issue in innumerable American

DOI: 10.4324/9781003514961-1

elections at all levels from 1973, starting with the activities of abortion opponents such as Jesse Helms, Bob Dole, Ronald Reagan, and both George H.W. Bush and George W. Bush, and characterized by efforts to secure control of the U.S. Congress, state governments, and legislatures as the result of an essentially symbiotic relationship with religious fanatics and the political right. Some have called this "Christofascism" and others refer to it as a "civic religion" and a "personality cult" of Donald Trump. This book includes fine-grain descriptions of how some of this has happened and how it constitutes an existential threat to democracy in America. It is becoming an example of how a democracy destroys itself.

It is not possible to understand the past 75 years of American political history without a focus on the role of abortion as an issue in electoral and legislative politics. It is worthy of many doctoral dissertations in political science. It is worth paying attention to when going to the polls to vote.

One of the most damaging results of the Republican Party hegemony symbolized by Donald Trump is the assault on reproductive freedom at all levels of American society. It is the culmination of 50 years of constant political attacks on reproductive freedom and the health of women launched immediately after the U.S. Supreme Court decision of *Roe v. Wade*, which struck down anti-abortion laws across the United States in 1973, although this movement started well before that year. Trump's election installed a racist, misogynist American government hostile to reason, facts, constitutional democracy, and science itself. The *Dobbs* decision of 2022 unleashed laws and policies at the state level that pose continuing threats to the health, freedom, and lives of women throughout the United States. Abortion is now illegal in one-third of the United States and highly restricted in many states.

How did this happen? I will try to give some answers in this book.

Last, this book is a way for me to help my fellow American citizens understand the importance of safe abortion services for women and the freedom this means for women to make fundamental decisions about their own lives and families.

If women are not free, none of us are free.

Two of the questions that I am often asked are: why do I perform abortions? and why have I specialized in this work in my professional career? This book is principally an account of how I became involved in abortion services for women and why I have done that. But it is also an attempt to describe some of the formative experiences that I had early in my life that help show the reader what kind of a person I am, how I got that way, and why this matters for the challenges I have experienced as a physician involved in one of the most controversial issues in our society. How I grew up and what I learned in that process may help the reader understand how I have responded to these challenges.

These things matter because there may be no work in medicine that demands more of a person in many ways than specializing in abortion services. It not only requires excellent surgical skills, experience, and judgment, but it also requires a broad understanding of how society works. It requires an understanding of how pregnancy, childbirth, and abortion affect women and how these experiences occur in a biocultural context. It requires an understanding of individual psychology and family dynamics. It may require knowledge of psychopathology. Increasingly over the past 50 years, it has required survival in an intensely political and sometimes violent environment.

Too many times I have felt that medical colleagues and members of the public view physicians who perform abortions as one-dimensional actors in a stark and simple drama that demands no understanding.

Some have asked the reasonable question: how do you protect yourself emotionally and not be destroyed by the torrent of personal attacks, slander, death threats, general bad news, and profound stress of doing this important work? Sometimes, it's pretty tough.

Most important, the patients sustain me and express their profound appreciation in many ways, sometimes for years. They tell me how much it means to them that I (and my staff) helped them at that critical moment in their lives.

Also, check out some of the photos that show me in my natural habitat – the mountains of Colorado – skiing, hiking, and being a natural history/wildlife photographer. You will also see me with the Shipibo people of the Peruvian Amazon, among who I have conducted scientific research and given basic medical care for over 60 years (and counting). They are now, from both their point of view and mine, family – *nokon caibo*! (my family). I have known these people most of my adult life: *euariqui sʳipibão panobaque*! (I am an adopted son of the Shipibo).

Living among these extraordinary people in their remote villages off and on for years in the upper Amazon region has helped to keep me connected to very basic human values and realities. I owe them much.

And I have my wonderful American family and friends all the time, every day. And my wonderful clinic staff is like a second family. And I have many lifelong intellectual and artistic interests, including fine art photography that long preceded my medical career, and music, for which there is not enough time. I have a large repertoire of enjoyable activities and interests in addition to vital friendships and loved ones. This helps a lot.

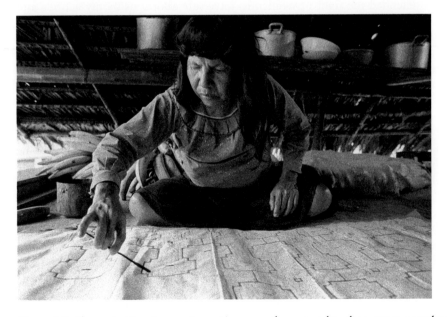

Figure 0.1 Florencia Urquia, master artisan, mother, grandmother, great grandmother, great-great grandmother, hand painting, with dyes she made herself, a hand-woven cloth that she wove with cotton that she spun herself to make a *cushma*, a Shipibo shawl. A dear beloved family friend whose family I have known for five generations and whose children and their families have sustained me and my work for 60 years and as we speak. Photo taken in 1984. Photo © Warren Martin Hern

To the question, "What kind of a person would do this work?" this book is part of my answer. Answering that important question is a serious issue for me requiring self-examination and reflection. This is not an autobiography, but it includes important details about my life that, in my opinion, bear on a responsive answer to that question. Why did I choose to do this rather than any number of other medical, surgical, academic, or public health specialties that I could have chosen? What were the consequences for the lives of those around me and the women I served? What have been the consequences for my life?

In this book, I attempt to explain what all this means for me as a person and what I think it means for our society. I especially want to show what I think it means for women whose lives are at stake.

Why does it matter that I do this work and that I have done it, especially as a total commitment of my energy and resources?

People ask me: How do I feel about doing this work? What has doing this work done to your life?

People ask me: was it worth it? My response: for whom?

For more than 60 years, since my days as a medical student at the University of Colorado, I have seen the despair and tragedy in women's lives as they struggled to control their fertility and, in the early years of my experience, sought unsafe abortions.

Since the early 1970s, I have been part of the work to make safe abortions available to women, first, in support of legal action and public health programs; second, as the founding medical director of Colorado's first nonprofit outpatient abortion clinic in 1973, where I performed all the abortions; and, third, as a private medical practitioner offering this service to women in the safest and most supportive setting I could construct; fourth, I have publicly defended the right of women to have safe abortions by my actions and participation in the public discussion of this issue; fifth, I have used my knowledge as a physician and epidemiologist to determine the safest ways to perform abortions.

My work as both a public health physician and a surgeon in the operating room has given me a special privilege and opportunity to witness historic changes over the past 60 years in abortion services and this deep controversy in American society. It is a privilege to do this work.

During these 60 years I have met and known leaders and architects of safe abortion availability in the United States and other parts of the world, such as Bill Baird, Karl Fossum, Tom Kerenyi, Alan Guttmacher, Christopher Tietze, Henry David, Jane Hodgson, Jeannie Rosoff, Sarah Weddington, Margie Pitts Hames, Harold Schulman, Louis Hellman, Carl Schulz, Roy Lucas, Katherine Kolbert, Janet Benshoof, Terry Beresford, Milan Vuitch, Fran Kissling, Judy Widdicombe, Harriet Pilpel, Malcolm Potts, Lydia Andolsek, Gloria Steinem, Ellie Smeal, Frank Susman, Faye Wattleton, Curtis Boyd, Bob Crist, George Tiller, Henry Morgentaler, Carol Downer, Bill Rashbaum, Mary Steichen Calderone, David Garrow, Mike Burnhill, Phil Stubblefield, Carole Joffe, Louise Tyrer, Karen Mulhauser, Rickie Solinger, Dirk Van Lith, Jack Sciarra, Mark Evans and many others too numerous to mention. I have had the opportunity to publish my medical reports, research, editorials, and observations in a wide variety of important publications, such as *The Progressive*, *The New Republic*, the *New York Times*, the *Washington Post*, the *San Francisco Chronicle*, *Obstetrics and Gynecology*, the *American Journal of Obstetrics and Gynecology*, *Advances in Planned Parenthood*, *Population Studies*, *Natural History*, *Social Science and Medicine*, *Family Planning Perspectives*, the *International Journal of Gynecology and Obstetrics*, and various Colorado newspapers.

In the medical journals I began publishing my research results in the 1970s, showing new procedures, techniques, instruments, and protocols for performing later abortions, and these publications have found an international audience, as has my textbook, *Abortion Practice*, the only single-author medical textbook on the subject. My opinions, thoughts, and observations have been sought by many local and major news media in the United States and other countries, including *60 Minutes*, the *New York Times*, the *Washington Post*, the *Los Angeles Times*, *The Today Show*, CNN, PBS, BBC, *Rachel Maddow*, *Anderson Cooper*, and other MSNBC programs. My work as a physician has been honored by the National Organization for Women, the Colorado Women's Political Caucus, NARAL Pro-Choice Colorado, the National Abortion Federation, the American Public Health Association, and the Colorado Religious Coalition for Reproductive Choice.

My candle has not been under a basket, and I am grateful for my right of free speech in America.

In this book, I hope to give the reader a brief glimpse of this unique experience and my observations about it. But all this has happened in a setting of intense conflict of various kinds. The result is that this book is not a straight linear story. It's bumpy. It's sort of a journal and scrapbook of what I have seen and experienced at the moment and over the years, what I have tried to do, and what has happened on the way. It includes many events and observations outside of the operating room and in the public forum where I have written and spoken about this issue and the stakes for both women and society. It includes unpublished papers that were not submitted to a professional journal but which give the reader a vivid glimpse of the current issues at that moment. It includes a few of the many editorials that I fired off to newspapers after the latest anti-abortion or political outrage. It includes some thoughts I have concerning the politics of the abortion issue and how it has affected our society.

It includes the transcripts of one U.S. Supreme Court oral argument (*Vuitch*) with a fascinating (and confusing) exchange between the justices and one of the defendant's attorneys. It includes a description of a contentious 1995 hearing of a U.S Senate Judiciary Committee on the "Partial Birth Abortion" bill to which I was first an invited, then a disinvited participant, and then a silent witness as my name was invoked.

It includes the excerpted transcript of a 1997 debate on the floor of the U.S. Senate concerning the so-called Partial Birth Abortion bill. My work was discussed in the debate, and I was condemned to jail by Senator Tom Daschle (D-SD). "*Dr. Hern ... will go to jail, will go to jail.*" Thus Spake the Senator from South Dakota. Pretty interesting. So far, no jail time for me.

Some instances are mentioned more than once in different contexts. The contexts matter. Be patient. None of this happened in an orderly way. There are a lot of things happening all at once because that's how it was – and is.

I include my observations and thoughts about the current (2024) political situation in the United States, which is tumultuous and catastrophic for both women and the country because of the fanatic opposition to safe abortion by a highly totalitarian and effective fascist minority. It is impossible to know how this intractable conflict and terrifying possibilities will turn out.

I say what I think, and I mean what I say. There have been horrible moments, such as the assassination of a friend and other medical colleagues, hideous attacks on women who are my patients, terrifying threats to my family and my staff, and terrifying threats to my life from the very beginning of this. At the same time, it has been an intense privilege to do this work and meet the many amazing people I have met while doing it.

This is my account.

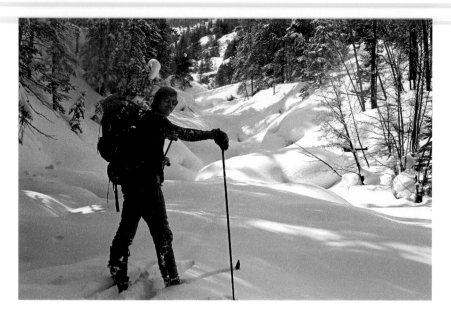

Figure 0.2 Photo by Linda Hodge, 1985. Photo © Warren Martin Hern

Survival is my revenge
Illegitimi non carborundum

1   Terror on the labor deck

Her name was Sharon. I remember her vividly, and I feared for her life. Sharon was in a labor room on the labor deck about to have a baby that she planned to "give up for adoption." I was a junior medical student just starting my third year of medical school with "clinical rotations" – when you actually begin to care for patients. My first clinical rotation was on obstetrics, and Sharon was one of the first patients I was assigned to observe and help. At least, I was participating in her care. But that only lasted until she started bleeding to death.

Sharon was a young woman in her late teens. She was not married. In those days, in the early 1960s, being an unmarried ("unwed") mother was a disgrace. The choice was to get married, possibly to someone you hardly knew or who abused you, or to "give the baby up for adoption." I didn't know anything about Sharon, but that was her choice.

Sharon was in labor, and suddenly she began to spurt blood from her vagina. Within minutes, there was blood on the walls, and Sharon was fading fast. She became white and agitated but quiet.

Sharon had gone from a healthy young woman expecting a healthy baby to dangerously close to losing her life within a few minutes because of a placenta previa. This is when the placenta covers the opening at the lower end of the uterus and a vaginal delivery is not possible. In the days before modern obstetrics, this was a death sentence.

The operating room was not on the same floor as the delivery room. We had to get her to the elevator, down a floor, and to the OR as quickly as possible. An IV had been started earlier, and now a second IV was added to give Sharon fluids so her heart would have something to pump.

Within minutes, Sharon was on the operating table, put to sleep by the anesthesiologist, and one of the obstetrical residents was opening her abdomen. The surgeon made an incision across the lower part of her abdomen, then across the bottom of her uterus, and brought the baby out of Sharon's body. The baby was blue. A pediatrician began clearing its airway and giving it oxygen. The APGAR score was 2 or 3 of a possible 10. The baby was almost dead and was likely to have brain damage.

Sharon was close to death. She was in shock from blood loss. She had a long recovery. I don't know what happened to her baby, but it didn't have a good start in life.

Another patient to whom I was assigned as a junior medical student on my obstetrics rotation was a young woman who had been brought by ambulance from the tiny southern Colorado town of La Jara. She was covered with large bruises head to toe.

Late in her pregnancy, the placenta separated from the wall of the uterus and the fetus died. The large blood clot behind the placenta absorbed all of the patient's fibrinogen and other blood-clotting elements. As a result, she developed a "D.I.C." (disseminated

DOI: 10.4324/9781003514961-2

intravascular coagulation) syndrome, which caused her to start bleeding everywhere within her body and from all orifices. Without rapid evacuation of the uterus by cutting it open, removal of the baby, placenta, and blood clot, and massive blood transfusions, she would die. She survived, but just barely.

On the obstetrics rotation, my favorite resident was a thin cheerful man with a prominent Adam's apple and wonderful smile on his face at all times. He always wore a bow tie. He was cheerful even when he was running up the stairs at 3 AM to see a patient. Dr. Watson Bowes – "Wattie" or "Wat" to all of us – was my idea of a dedicated doctor, a wonderful person and superb teacher. He was kind to the patients and kind to those of us on the lower rungs of the medical hierarchy. With Wat teaching me, I learned how to deliver babies. I thought birth was a miracle and a joyous moment. At least it was for some women. For others, not so much.

Decades later, Wat Bowes and I found ourselves on opposite sides of the abortion issue.

For the women whose husbands were there with them to share in the birth of a new child, it was a moment of pure joy and love. I felt privileged to be a part of their moment and to watch them together with their baby.

The contrast could not have been greater for the young women like Sharon who were alone facing this pain and the danger of childbirth, who had feelings of love and yearning for their new child, anguish for the social isolation, and terrible sadness as they knew they would never know their child. I watched them sob as they stood before the nursery windows looking at their babies for the last time.

There was something very wrong with this picture. It seemed to wrench painfully and ruthlessly with our very biological nature as human beings and especially for women who had carried a pregnancy for nine months expecting to be a mother.

Another patient to whom I was assigned, Maria, was a charming woman from the migrant worker camp in her forties who spoke only Spanish and who was pregnant with her tenth baby. She was suffering from pre-eclampsia, a disease of pregnancy that has been a major cause of death for pregnant women for as long as we have been able to understand the disease and make the diagnosis.

In the early twentieth century in the United States, and throughout Latin America, pre-eclampsia, eclampsia, and other causes of high blood pressure killed up to one-fourth of the women who died from pregnancy. My patient, to whom I was assigned because I spoke Spanish, was cheerful, but she had all the signs of severe pre-eclampsia. She was in great danger of dying before, during, or right after the delivery of her baby. My job was to keep track of all her signs of illness and report them to the intern and resident physicians. When I helped deliver her baby, it was very small, and a lot of the placenta was dead or scarred. This baby also had a difficult start in life.

My next clinical rotation was gynecology. The patient to whom I was assigned, an older Spanish-speaking woman named Anna, was suffering from the terrible effects of radiation treatment for uterine cancer. The radiation had caused the death of tissue deep into her body, and it was my job to clean the wound once a day. The open wound into her groin was several inches deep. The first task was "debridement," which meant carefully removing the specks of dead tissue from Anna's deep wound without hurting her and then placing gauze soaked in "Peruvian balsam" into the wound to stimulate scar tissue growth that would fill the space. It was 1963 in a modern university teaching hospital, but Peruvian balsam, an herb from a tree in South America, was the treatment of choice for this difficult problem. Anna was very patient with me as I picked through her wound trying to get it to heal. Peruvian balsam was a folk remedy, but it worked.

The idea of "debridement" – removal of dead tissue from a wound – was introduced by Ambroise Paré, a battlefield surgeon in the French army in the seventeenth century. The usual treatment of battlefield wounds was to pour boiling oil into the wound to cauterize the flesh, a procedure which produced indescribable agony, more dead tissue, overwhelming infection, and dead soldiers. Paré decided to use a milder treatment combined with removal of the dead tissue, and his soldiers survived.

During every night I was on duty on the gynecology rotation, I was up most of the night with my classmates taking care of women who were sick from having an abortion. I was not really quite sure what was going on because I had never learned anything about abortion. It was a mysterious subject. I had never seen a small fetus, and I had never seen someone who was so desperately sick. We were busy with these patients starting IVs, drawing blood for blood cultures and other tests, and giving them antibiotics. Some of them died.

Abortion was illegal, and no one talked about it. It was considered a hideous crime performed by incompetent and unscrupulous butchers.

During this time, a woman who was several months pregnant went to Denver General Hospital and asked for an abortion. She was refused. In an act of desperation, she went home, shot herself in the uterus with a pistol, and then drove herself to the hospital.

After gynecology, I was on pediatrics with my first stop in the newborn nursery. I loved taking care of the babies, some of whom, in my opinion, showed signs of different personalities from their first days. The saddest thing was watching the mothers of some who had decided on adoption.

At the University of Colorado School of Medicine in the early 1960s, we had a brilliant and compassionate chairman of the pediatrics department, Dr. Henry Kempe. In 1962, the year before I began my rotation on pediatrics, Dr. Kempe and his colleagues published a paper describing the "Battered Child Syndrome."[1] Dr. Kempe had been observing unusual and unexplained injuries in young children for years. His careful study showed that these children were being abused at home by parents who had deep conflicts about having children, how to raise them with care and compassion, or both. Sometimes the parents were psychiatrically disturbed, but not always. Sometimes they were unrealistic in their demands on the child. At other times, they just didn't want the child and hadn't wanted it in the first place. The child was not welcome in the family and was seen as a burden. Crying too long was met with a violent blow.

In my pediatric rotation, I took care of a number of these children. We had a lot of contact and conversations with Dr. Kempe, who helped us understand the complexity of this problem. I saw children who had permanent severe brain damage from head injuries and children who were crippled for life by the abuse they had suffered. The children were very young. Some were infants only a few months old; others were three or four years old. They couldn't defend themselves. They had been horribly beaten and psychologically abused. Their lives, if they survived, were already severely damaged.

One of our field trips as junior medical students was to a place west of Denver called Ridge Home. It was the size of my high school fieldhouse that had a ¼ mile track for running. The floor of the fieldhouse was covered with hundreds of beds full of children waiting to die. Each one was in some kind of vegetative state from brain damage – or no brain. Some of the children were visited by their families once in a while. The families had to pay for this long-term care, for which there was no hope and, seemingly, no end. Many families had no money to pay for this.

Off to Peru

During the summer before medical school, I traveled to West Africa with the Experiment in International Living as a "Community Ambassador" from my hometown of Englewood, Colorado. We lived with African families, and it was an extraordinary experience in many ways. I was an admirer of Albert Schweitzer and his work in Africa, I was interested in African cultures, and I was particularly interested in learning about tropical medicine. My visits to the university teaching hospital in Ibadan helped me learn about childhood diseases such as neonatal tetanus, sickle-cell disease, and *kwashiorkor,* a protein deficiency malnutrition disease related to early weaning when a nursing baby's mother has a new baby. The name of the disease means "red-haired weanling" in Ga, the principal language spoken in Ghana.

Polygyny (multiple wives) has been an African custom throughout the continent, and this was discouraged by Christian missionaries as being immoral. The result of the Christian teachings and abandonment of polygyny meant that African women in monogamous marriages could no longer observe the post-partum sexual abstinence that was part of the custom of polygyny. Women now had babies closer together, and instead of being able to nurse a child for more than a year until it could eat solid food, the new baby was nursed, and the older baby got malnutrition. In African children, the malnutrition caused dyspigmentation, or loss of color, of the dark skin, and this resulted in red hair. But the main effect of the malnutrition was to cause liver failure, brain damage, and other problems. It was a fatal disease.

By the time I came back from Africa in the fall of 1961 to start medical school, I knew that I needed to travel and learn more about the human condition in other places such as developing countries. The next summer, I worked in a mining camp in the back country of Nicaragua and helped with surgery at a hospital in Puerto Cabezas maintained by the Moravian Church. The doctor, Ned Wallace, was an inspiration to me. He also saved my life when I was dying of dysentery.

In 1964, I found a way to work at the *"Hospital Amazonico Albert Schweitzer"* in the Peruvian Amazon. The hospital had been founded and built by Dr. Teodor Binder, a German physician who had been a protégé of Albert Schweitzer, my hero in medicine. Soon after arriving, having just finished my third year of medical school, I was put in charge of the hospital's clinics, where I saw 40–50 patients each afternoon. The patients, most of whom were young children or their mothers, were suffering from a wide variety of serious illnesses, including parasitism and malnutrition among the children. Many of the women had given birth to 8 or 10 children. They begged me for help to keep from getting pregnant. Their bodies were falling apart from repeated childbearing with no obstetrical care. They were desperate to avoid pregnancy. Some women came in suffering from attempts to cause abortion on themselves or who had been treated by an untrained person attempting an abortion. These women were desperately ill, and some died.

A couple of weeks after Dr. Binder left for Europe for a conference and fund-raising for his hospital, Dr. Michael Diana arrived. Dr. Diana was an Italian-American surgeon from New York City who taught surgical anatomy there and had been the chief surgeon at Madison Square Garden. He was *very* Italian and entertained me with hilarious tales of his encounters with *mafiosi* who wouldn't pay his bills and whose hides he promised (in my primitive understanding of Italian) to nail on the wall. He was rough and ready, had worked in many such places as Binder's hospital, and took me under his wing as a surgical assistant. But the operating room was a mess. It was being used for storage. He took one look at it and said, "I'm going home. I'm a surgeon. I have standards." I said, "Give me a couple of weeks to get this ready."

I did, and I trained several members of the hospital staff how to be operating room circulating nurses and scrub nurses. I found some ampules of dried spinal anesthetic in the warehouse that I could mix up with spinal fluid and re-inject to give spinal anesthesia (Yikes!), cleaned up the operating room, and we started.

We did 20 major cases, sometimes with Dr. Diana coaching me as the surgeon. One of the patients was Rosa, a Shipibo Indian woman from the village of Paococha, on whom Dr. Diana performed a hysterectomy because of a history of vaginal bleeding. Rosa's uterus had been largely replaced by cancer, and it was clear she didn't have long to live. Soon after, I went to her village to do research, and she was our neighbor.

After working at the hospital for three months, I went to Paococha, Rosa's Shipibo Indian village about 150 kilometers down the Ucayali River from the hospital so I could conduct research about health practices and beliefs among the Shipibo. A Peace Corps volunteer, Frank Billman, had been living in the village and helping the people with community projects. Part of his job was to provide first aid to people, and that became my responsibility as part of our partnership. He let me share his pole-and-thatch house in the deal.

Our next-door neighbor was my patient, Rosa, and her husband, Pablo. They became dear friends. Frank and I were living in their daughter's pole-and-thatch house with cane poles for walls and a tree-bark floor raised up from the ground in case the nearby river rose to flood stage.

My main purpose in going to the village was to conduct research in what was later called "medical anthropology" – the study of how people in different cultures think

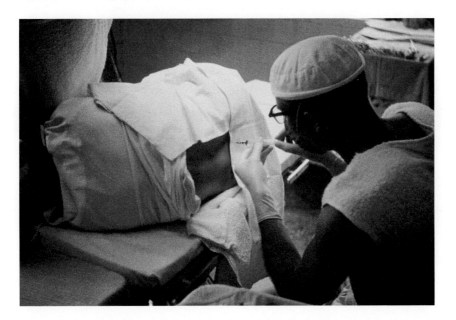

Figure 1.1 Author giving spinal anesthesia to a patient in the *Hospital Amzaonico Albert Schweitzer* in 1964. Photo © Warren Martin Hern

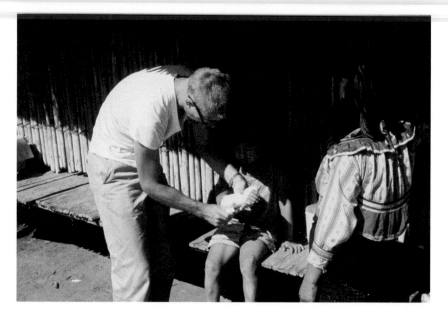

Figure 1.2 Author placing a cast on the arm of an eight-year-old kid known in the 'hood as "tiger."
Photo ©Warren Martin Hern

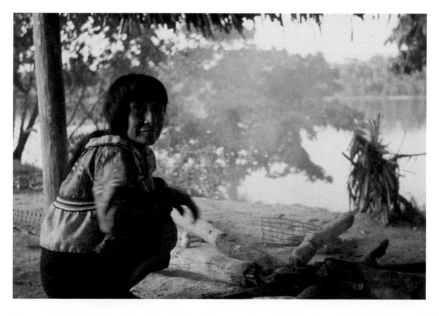

Figure 1.3 My patient (and neighbor) Rosa in her kitchen by the lake. Photo ©Warren Martin
Hern

about health, disease, illness, and the treatment and control of disease. But during my time at the hospital, I had come to know Dr. Ralph Eichenberger, who was the physician for the missionary group called the "Summer Institute of Linguistics," who were dedicated to translating the Bible into the local native Amazonian languages. Ralph and his family lived at the SIL base about five kilometers down the coast of Lake Yarinacocha from the *Hospital Amazonico*. Yarinacocha was an oxbow lake left by an ancient loop of the Ucayali River, the main source of the Amazon River in Peru.

Ralph had studied public health prior to his missionary work, and he encouraged me to spend part of my time conducting a public health survey of the village; so that became one of my objectives in the village.

In doing my health survey of the village, I found myself learning about and treating a wide variety of illnesses. The women had many remedies for avoiding pregnancy, and they had a clear set of beliefs about how they worked. Some of the remedies involved drinking tea made from different herbs, but other remedies required a woman to put caustic substances in her vagina.

On one occasion, a man who was my anthropological "informant," meaning that he taught me about the beliefs and customs concerning health and illness, came to me to tell me that his wife had just had a baby and was bleeding to death. When I examined her under her mosquito net, she was suffering from uterine atony (the uterus was relaxed and not contracted, so it kept bleeding), and she had some retained tissue after the birth. I removed the tissue and gave her medicine to make her uterus contract. She survived, but it was her ninth pregnancy, and her uterus wasn't contracting well. Her baby was brain damaged.

Her husband, Ambrosio, who was helping me understand Shipibo customs, came to me and said, "You saved my wife's life. What can I do for you?" I told him I would like to learn about women's knowledge and beliefs about pregnancy and whether there were medicines that women took to affect pregnancy.

Ambrosio took me to see his aunt, Julia, who was an expert on these things, and she showed me several herbs and preparations designed to prevent pregnancy, to postpone pregnancy, or to stop fertility completely. The Shipibo women had clear ideas about pregnancy and the mechanism of effectiveness of the herbal contraceptives. The uterus was called the *baquenanuti* (nest/ incubator/place for the baby). The different kinds of herbal contraceptives caused the lining of the uterus to dry out so the man's seed couldn't grow. Other herbs were used to make it wet and receptive so the woman could get pregnant.

Learning that any Shipibo person who was sick or taking a folk remedy was required to follow a certain diet regimen and avoid certain foods or actions, I asked Julia and her cousin what regimens women would follow if they were taking herbal contraceptives (*tootimarau!*) (*tooti* – "pregnancy"; *ma* – "negative"; *rau* – "medicine"). The answer was: the woman who was taking *tootimarau* of any kind could not eat *boca chico* (a certain kind of fish), eat salt, eat anything sweet such as honey from bees in the forest, and *she could not have sex*. Well. If she could not have sex while taking *tootimarau*, the epidemiologic term for not getting pregnant would be a "secondary non-causal association." This fact became very important in my later research on the causes of high fertility among the Shipibo.[2]

One of the Shipibo women I was called to see by her husband, Guillermina, was suffering from a constant vaginal discharge. She was one of those who had placed caustic or acidic substances in her vagina to stop having babies. When I did a pelvic exam on Guillermina under her mosquito net with her husband standing by, it was obvious that she had advanced cervical cancer. I arranged for her to go to the cancer hospital in Lima, where I visited her later when I was on my way back home that year. Five years later, she was back in the village but terminally ill from cancer.

As I went through the village conducting my health survey, I found other cases in the small community of a few hundred people of women who had or had recently died from cervical cancer. It became clear to me then and in later studies that cervical cancer was an epidemic among the Shipibo women.

The people of Paococha were very friendly to both Frank and I, and I found myself besieged with requests for both diagnosis and treatment of many ailments ranging from intestinal parasites to broken arms to tuberculosis to cancer. In the process, I began learning about the Shipibo culture, learning the language, and understanding what it was like to live in this fascinating, beautiful, complex and sometimes dangerous environment.

People risked their lives every day to get food, water, and shelter. But it also had important advantages. There was no crime, air pollution, noise from machines or loud-speakers, or danger from getting run over by cars or trucks. There were no orphans, and there was no unemployment. Everyone took care of old people and the children. It was quiet. The sounds of nature were all around. At dawn, the red howler monkeys started singing their songs in a rich baritone, and it sounded ever so much like a Gregorian chant. The night was full of bird calls and animal sounds from the jungle and the river.

When it came time to leave the village and return to Colorado to finish medical school, I didn't want to leave. I felt I was doing exactly what I wanted to do.

Returning to the *Hospital Amazonico* with three young men from the village who were sent with me to learn how to be *sanitarios* (medical corpsmen) to help with first aid in the village, I discovered that there was a smallpox epidemic sweeping through the Peruvian Amazon. Whole villages of native Amazonians were being wiped out. I con-sulted Ralph, who had seen this recently in many villages, and learned that the SIL had smallpox vaccine available. I taught my crew how to help me perform vaccinations, and we returned to Paococha, hitting many logs in the dugout canoe because the water was low in the dry season.

We stopped at a Shipibo village named Sharamashu just upriver from Pao before dawn so that we could tell the people there about the vaccination program and when to come to Pao for their vaccinations. Two men ran back into the jungle to tell their neighbors about this. While we were waiting, as I sat on the riverbank with my companions, one of them said, "*Doctor, mire, una satelita!*" (Doctor, look, there's a satellite!). There we were, hundreds of miles from any major city in a still clear night in the Peruvian Amazon, traveling by dugout canoe in one of the most isolated parts of the planet, and we were watching a satellite in outer space silently pass over in the night sky.

As we approached the landing place for Pao in the pre-dawn dim light, we heard wail-ing coming from the first house right by the riverbank where we would pull in the canoe. "*Lucho baque moa mahuata.*" *El hijo del viejo Lucho ha fallecido*, one of the men said in Shipibo, then in Spanish. "The son of old Luis just died." As we passed by the house, the old man and his two wives sat by the body of the young child, who had been placed in a small battered canoe. The women were wailing, and Lucho was sobbing.

That day, I sent the *sanitario* crew down to Roaboya, the mestizo settlement down the river, and Colonia Roaboya, the Shipibo village next to it, to tell them that we would arrive with the vaccine in two days.

The next day, a missionary pilot, Bob Hettema, expertly set his float plane down on the Ucayali and delivered the vaccine. Bob had been a fighter pilot in the Korean War and was now an expert at navigating across the untracked Peruvian Amazon.

The residents of Sharamashu from up the river arrived that day, and we vaccinated everyone in that village and the residents of Pao. Then we got in the canoe and went down to the two Roaboyas, mestizo and Shipibo.

The Peruvian mestizos regard the Shipibo as subhumans and treat them that way, and the Shipibo regard the mestizos with great fear and suspicion.

As we finished the vaccination program in the larger mestizo village of Roaboya, the village authorities invited us to come to the local *tienda* for dinner. I accepted, and we walked over to the small house up on stilts that featured a general store and a one-table restaurant. There were four places set, and there were three village officials as well as me. They invited me to take a place at the table. "Where are my Shipibo companions?" I asked. "Oh, they're out in back eating with the help." "No," I said, "they eat here with me." The village authorities were mortified, but they called my Shipibo crew, and the four of us sat down to a nice dinner of chicken, rice, beans, and plantains. The village authorities watched us eat. The Shipibo have never forgotten this incident.

We returned to Paococha that evening, navigating up the river through the floating logs to the riverbank entrance to the village.

The next day, I became very sick with a fever, severe headache and stiff neck, and I thought I had all the signs and symptoms of encephalitis. I thought I was going to die, but I recovered, and I returned to the hospital a few days later.

A man who I had admitted to the hospital a month before suffering from a poisonous snake bite was now critically ill with a rotten leg and bleeding. The bones of his lower leg, the tibia and fibula, were exposed and completely bare of flesh for their entire length. We all gave a unit of blood to help him, but Dr. Binder, who had just returned from Europe, would not let me amputate the man's leg. He died in spite of everything else we did.

My three-day hitchhiking trip back over the Andes as the only passenger in a soft drink truck was eventful. Maximo, the driver, forgot his papers at Huanaco and had to go back to get them. I lay down to sleep in the cab of the truck. We were at Cerro de Pasco, site of one of the world's largest open-pit copper mines. I slept because I had not rested well the night before as I was trying to sleep in my hammock slung under the truck. It was cold in the high Andes, and I had no warm clothes.

After a while, I woke up in the truck with a severe headache, gasping for breath, and my fingernails were blue. I was about to die from *soroche*, the high-altitude sickness, while waiting for Maximo to get back from Huanaco. Even though I was from Colorado, I had lived at a very low elevation for six months, I had just given a unit of blood, and I had hookworm from walking through the meadow in my sandals with Dr. Diana to paddle a canoe and swim in Yarinacocha. Also, Cerro de Pasco was at 14,000 feet.

Some soldiers at the guard station heard me honking the horn, carried me into the guard station, and got a 5 liter bag of oxygen from the local hospital. They saved my life. They put me on the Arrellano bus that was coming through on its way to Lima. I got the last seat by the front door, and we went hurtling across the *altiplano* and down the canyons to Lima, where I got myself to the missionary headquarters. They took me in, and the next day, my Peruvian friends gave me a place to stay. I then went to see the Peace Corps physician, Tom Hakala, who had done surgery earlier at the *Hospital Amazonico*. I told Tom that I wanted to stay, but I was sick and out of money. "Go back home and finish medical school," he said. "Otherwise you will get drafted and you're just a well-meaning biologist." So I went home, getting there just in time to start my last year of medical school. My classmates thought I was crazy to go to Peru for six months much less wanting to stay there. They had a point, but it was an incredible experience, one of the most important in my life.

From the experiences in Africa, Nicaragua, and the Peruvian Amazon, I began to develop a public health perspective in medicine.

Notes

1 Kempe, C.H., Silverman, F.N., Steele, B.F., Droegemueller, W., and Silver, H.K. The battered child syndrome. *Journal of the American Medical Association* 181(1):17–24, 1962. doi:10.1001/jama.1962.03050270019004
2 Hern, W.M. Knowledge and use of herbal contraceptives in a Peruvian Amazon village. *Human Organization* 35(1): 9–19, 1976 https://doi.org/10.17730/humo.35.1.b7h6706718u56412

2 Abortion and public health in the Americas

Back in medical school, I was relieved to be home, and I enjoyed my last year. Everything was interesting. I excelled in surgery, but I felt that the field of surgery was full of bullies.

One hulking surgery resident at the VA hospital ("Eric, The Rat"), where they did venocaval shunts on alcoholic veterans with terminal liver cirrhosis, was reputed to eat junior medical students alive for breakfast. Another resident, Bob Malowney, who was a Navy veteran, was a superb surgeon who liked me and wanted me as his first assistant. He let me do a hernia repair as the principal surgeon. I was good at it, but Malowney was a little rough. "Hern, you work like old people make love: slowly and ineffectually." I replied with some smart-ass comment as I sewed up the patient. I had worked with a lot of people like Bob on construction jobs, and we got along fine. He liked that I gave as good as I got.

I did have the extraordinary opportunity to scrub with Dr. Tom Starzl, who had started the kidney transplant program at Colorado. One of my days was spent looking at the back of Starzl's neck as I held up the liver while he did a baboon kidney transplant on one of my patients from internal medicine. Starzl leaned on my arm, which cut off the circulation in my arm and made it difficult to hold up the patient's liver as well as Starzl's body, and he then complained that I wasn't holding up the liver well enough. At the end of the eight-hour operation, I went home and put my feet up to let all the clots run out of my legs. I got an appointment with the orthopedic surgeons to release all the flexion contractures in my forearms that resulted from muscle necrosis and spasms over eight hours. Tough work.

Dr. Bill Droegemueller, one of my residents in gynecology when I was in my senior year, told me in the middle of an operation that I was "the pushiest medical student" at the operating table that he had ever seen. He did not mean it as a criticism because he liked my enthusiasm for learning good surgical technique.

"Droeges" and I became close friends later, and he invited me to lecture his residents and students on abortion wherever he was chair of an ob/gyn department. He valued my work in and out of the operating room. In the midst of thundering and raging controversy about my work in performing late abortions years later, he was one of the few medical colleagues I could call and have a calm discussion about technical issues in patient care. His support and advice was the best.

Because I had now worked in Latin America and spoke Spanish, and I was interested in tropical medicine, I applied for a rotating internship at Gorgas Hospital in the Canal Zone. It was one of the few places I could go where I could continue learning Spanish and also learn as much as possible about tropical medicine. I had stopped in Panama on my way south to Peru in 1964 to learn about the riots that had occurred there as students

DOI: 10.4324/9781003514961-3

protested the continued colonial domination of Panama by the United States. That was an interesting adventure.

At the Miami airport, waiting for my prop-jet plane to Panama, I met a young Black man named Gene Kelly. He was from a Jamaican family that lived in Colón, a port city on the northern (Caribbean) coast of Panama where the country bends in the middle. Gene invited me to visit his family, so after we got me a hotel room in Panama City, he and I went out to walk around and see the effects and scars of the riots that had occurred the previous year. There were bullet holes in most of the buildings, and there was a wooden vendor's cart sitting in the middle of one of the plazas near the border of the American-controlled Canal Zone. On the side of the cart that would have been an open window for selling fruit, there were bullet holes, all encircled with red paint. The caption by one of the bullet holes, written in red paint, was the message, "*Esta bala mató un humilde anciano*" ("This bullet killed a humble old man.").

As we walked around the city, we found ourselves accompanied by a squad of heavily armed soldiers. Accompanied by Gene, I was the only white person in sight. There were no other tourists of any kind to be seen. There was tension because the riots had only ended a few weeks before my arrival. I knew that there had been riots, and I wanted to learn about the issues, but I did not realize that many Panamanian people had been killed in their protests over American colonialism.

Gene and I took the train over to Colón, which was home to many people from Jamaica whose ancestors had been brought to the Caribbean islands as slaves. Gene's family and friends were eager to meet me, and they told me how much they had grieved when President Kennedy was assassinated. They had faith in him and his "*Alianza para el Progreso*" ("Alliance for Progress"), Kennedy's program for helping Latin America. "On the night that Kennedy died, there was a candle in every window here," Gene's mother told me.

My train ride back to Panama City was uneventful, but I became acutely conscious of a potentially dangerous situation as I was followed by soldiers from the train station to my hotel. For dinner, I decided to go to a bar next door to the hotel. As I walked through the swinging doors and went to take a seat at the bar, silence fell in what had been a noisy place. As I sat down at the bar, I smiled and greeted those around me in my primitive Spanish. Everyone was looking at me intensely with great wariness. They were Panamanian students, and they suspected that I was an American spy. I was afraid.

After I explained that I was a medical student on my way to Peru and wanted to know what the Panamanians thought about the Canal Zone and why they had rioted, I was taken to a large table and surrounded by university students eager to tell me what they thought.

It seemed like a close call, but I learned a lot, and it helped me the next year when I came back to Panama to do my internship at Gorgas Hospital in the Canal Zone.

By the summer of 1965, when I was about to start my internship, Gorgas had only one-half the number of interns that it needed. Few had applied for intern positions because of the violent riots in 1964. As a result, all of us who were there were working double shifts all year. Even then, two of our eight interns dropped out of the program. This meant, aside from a lot of sleepless nights, that we got to do many things as interns that were normally reserved solely for residents.

Once more, on the gynecology service, I saw patients who were suffering from the terrible and sometimes fatal consequences of unsafe abortion, and I saw children who were battered and abused in the pediatric service.

Since Gorgas was responsible for the medical care of all U.S. diplomatic and military personnel in Latin America, we took care of young soldiers who were about to be shipped off as cannon fodder for the U.S. war in Vietnam. We also were responsible for taking care of American Peace Corps volunteers from Latin America, and I knew some of their Peace Corps doctors. Volunteers who came to Gorgas from Brazil pleaded with me to come there as a Peace Corps physician, especially Bahia, where they did not have a Peace Corps doctor. As a result, I applied for a commission in the U.S. Public Health Service, which assigned its commissioned officers to the Peace Corps. I applied for Peru as my first choice since I had been there and wanted to go back, and I applied for Brazil as my second choice.Since I spoke Spanish, the Peace Corps assigned me to Brazil, where they speak Portuguese. From there, I received intensive training in Brazilian Portuguese, so I spoke it fluently by the time I got to Brazil.

My principal duty post was Salvador, Bahia, the first capitol of Brazil, and it was a fascinating place. Salvador has an underlying African culture, with various African languages spoken in the marketplace because it had been the main arrival point for slaves being brought from Africa from the seventeenth to the nineteenth centuries. Forte São Marcelo, the prison for slaves arriving from Africa, sits in the middle of the bay facing the city of Salvador.

The principal part of the old city is located on a high bluff overlooking the bay, and the center of the old city of Salvador is Pelorinho, a plaza where the slave auctions were held. It is a popular place for tourists whose charm and color conceals a sordid and painful past. Children play there, and young men practice *capoeira*, a highly athletic and coordinated fight/dance that developed as a martial art defense by the Brazilian slaves. Capoeira is the principal origin of what is known as "break-dancing" in the United States. The slaves practiced the moves as artful self-defense but told the slave masters that they were just "dancing" when their owners showed up.

The roots of African culture are very deep in Bahia, and this is reflected in the food, language, expressions, music, religion, and social structure.

As a Peace Corps physician speaking Portuguese with a local accent, I was welcomed with open arms by my Brazilian colleagues. One was Dr. Elsimar Coutinho, who was doing original research on injectable contraceptives known later as "Depo-Provera." Elsimar asked one of his colleagues to take me through the maternity hospital that was part of the University of Bahia medical school. One ward was full of women recovering from childbirth. There were two wards full of women recovering from unsafe abortion, and half of these women died. They were too sick to save by the time they reached the hospital.

At that time, unsafe abortion was the leading cause of death among women in the child-bearing age range in Latin America.

In medical school, I had been encouraged by Dr. Lula Lubchenco, a pediatrician with international experience, to read an article about this in the *Revista Medica de Chile*, the principal medical journal in Chile. In this article, written by Drs. Rolando Armijo and Tegualda Monreal, the authors gave details about the large number of women who were seen each year in hospitals in Santiago, Chile.[1] They showed that the women had major and fatal complications from unsafe abortion, that most of them already had children and were married, and that they were seeking abortions because of severe economic difficulties in caring for the children they already had.

In time, I came to know the physicians who were starting an organization they called *Sociedade Brasileira Bem-Estar Familiar* ("*BEM-FAM*") – The Brazilian Society for

Family Well-Being. Their patriarch, the most distinguished obstetrician/gynecologist in Brazil, was Dr. Octavio Rodriguez-Lima. His son, Dr. Walter Rodriguez, became a great friend, and Walter was the head of BEM-FAM. We met several times in Rio de Janeiro when I was there on Peace Corps business. Their main purpose was to launch national family planning programs to help women avoid unplanned pregnancies and therefore avoid having to have abortions.

At one point in 1966, my Brazilian friends told me about a major conference that they wanted to attend in 1967 in Santiago, Chile. The meeting was the Eighth International Congress of the International Planned Parenthood Federation, and physicians as well as other program officers would be coming from all over the world.[2] They wanted to attend this meeting, but they had no money. Could I help?

I then went to the U.S. Embassy and spoke to people running the Agency for International Development (AID) local program. With this, I was able to obtain funding for ten of my Brazilian colleagues to attend the meeting. In fact, I decided to take one of my two weeks' vacation time as a USPHS officer and attend the meeting as a "busman's holiday."

On my way to Santiago, we had a stopover and change of planes in Montevideo, Uruguay, and one of my new seatmates was a young Pakistani obstetrician/gynecologist, Nafis Sadik. She was head of the Pakistani maternal-child health programs in her country. This was remarkable because here was a highly educated woman from a Muslim country with super professional credentials and a national responsibility for this critical problem. We became friends and worked together many years later when she had become the president of the UN Population Fund. This included the 1994 International Conference on Population and Development sponsored by the UN Population Fund, which was held in Cairo. At that meeting, I was the American representative of the American Public Health Association since I was chairman at that time of the APHA Population, Family Planning and Reproductive Health section.

The Santiago meeting was extraordinary. I found myself sitting by physicians from Cuba (one of whom, Dr. Laonchera, I saw later on a 1978 trip to Cuba), Africa, Asia, Europe, and all of Latin America. I met many American leaders, including Dr. Alan Guttmacher and Dr. Christopher Tietze. Chris and I later had a close working relationship on various matters.

A turning point for me occurred at the Santiago meeting when I met Dr. Chuck Arnold, a professor of public health at the University of North Carolina School of Public Health, the *alma mater* of my missionary doctor friend from Peru, Dr. Ralph Eichenberger. Chuck encouraged me to apply to UNC since I was especially interested in epidemiology. I learned from Chuck that one of my heroes in public health, Dr. John Cassel, was now chairman of the Department of Epidemiology at UNC. As an undergraduate studying applied cultural anthropology, I had read Dr. Cassel's studies and publications on the health effects of cultural change among the Zulu of South Africa. I was planning to do research on this subject among the Shipibo of the Peruvian Amazon. This encounter led to my application at UNC and help from Dr. Cassel in getting a U.S. Public Health Service grant for studying epidemiology at UNC.

In reviewing the Santiago program, I was astounded to see that another one of my public health heroes, Dr. Rolando Armijo, was giving a presentation in a symposium on the epidemiology of unsafe abortion in Chile. I attended, and I then went up to Dr. Armijo to introduce myself after his talk. He was most gracious, and he invited me to join him for coffee at a shop on the Via España by the conference center. We had a great visit for over an hour.

The conference had arranged for each participant to have a Chilean sponsor, and mine was Dr. Mariano Requena.[3] Both he and his wife, Beatriz, were physicians, and they were gracious hosts at a dinner for me at their home. Our friendship continued for decades. Mariano came to speak at a class of mine at the University of North Carolina School of Public Health about a year later, and I visited him and Beatriz in Santiago in 2011. A difficult time for Mariano had occurred in 1973 when he was serving as the deputy minister of health under the Chilean president, Dr. Salvador Allende, who was thought to be assassinated in a *coup d'état* organized by the American Central Intelligence Agency in support of General Augusto Pinochet. Some reports are that Allende committed suicide rather than being taken prisoner.

Pinochet became a ruthless military dictator. Mariano was imprisoned by Pinochet for a long time, and his cellmate happened to be Angel Parra, a renowned Chilean folksinger, who I also met during my visit to Santiago. Angel and his sister, Isabel, specialized in songs of protest against unfair labor practices and social conditions. They had continued the great tradition of their mother, Violeta, and they were unpopular with the authoritarian political leaders.

One of my favorite experiences ever, and especially during the Santiago meeting, was visiting their club, *La Peña de Los Parra*, attended principally by students, social protest movement leaders, and young Peace Corps physicians. It was an enormous treat to listen to their live performances of fantastic music while enjoying a modest traditional snack of *anticuchos* (chunks of marinated beef heart), *choclos* (Andean white corn on the cob), a little bread, and a cup of excellent Chilean red wine. *Peña* means "sorrow" or "grief" in Spanish, and many of the songs spoke of the longing for justice and suffering of the *Chilenos* who were deprived of it.

On returning to the United States in 1968, I started my public health studies at the University of North Carolina School of Public Health. The best thing about the whole experience was having Dr. John Cassel as my mentor and advisor. His leadership in the school and in the Department of Epidemiology was nothing short of brilliant and inspiring. The department faculty had great depth in scholarship and teaching, with numerous social scientists – anthropologists, sociologists, and psychologists – who fulfilled the department's ethos of studying the epidemiology of health and illness in a social and cultural context.[4]

John Cassel's definition of epidemiology was "the study of the distribution and determinants of health and illness." Having been grounded in a classical medical education and having been fascinated by the history of medicine going back to the Greeks, I marveled at how physicians over the centuries had figured out basic physiology and the origins of many diseases without modern technology. They did it by careful observation and logic.

Some of the best and most life-saving examples included Ignaz Semmelweis's discovery of the causes of "childbed fever" in the early nineteenth century. At the Vienna maternity hospital where he worked and studied, the best medical teaching facility in Europe at the time, a large proportion of the women having babies died a few days after giving birth from terrible raging infection. The infections seemingly sprang from nowhere to kill healthy young women, who left orphans. Then Semmelweis discovered that most of these deaths were among women who were being cared for by medical students and other physicians learning to be obstetricians. Among women who were having their babies delivered by nurse midwives in a separate maternity ward, far fewer of the women died. One of the main differences in the activities of the midwives and physicians was that the physicians always did autopsies on the women who had just died. From the autopsy room, the physicians went right back to the delivery rooms to deliver babies.

At the time, of course, there were no sterile rubber gloves used in surgical operating rooms. Handwashing was not practiced. Semmelweis wondered if the physicians were carrying something from the women who had died from infection to the women whose babies they were delivering. He urged the doctors to wash their hands with a mild acid solution after performing the autopsies. The microbial causes of infection were unknown at the time. Those discoveries would come much later in the nineteenth century, but Semmelweis suspected that handwashing might prevent the terrible infections.

One of Semmelweis's mentors in obstetrics cut himself while performing an autopsy. When Semmelweis came back from a brief vacation, his mentor was dead. He had died of an overwhelming infection that was identical to those killing the recently delivered women. Semmelweis saw the connection even though there was no knowledge of bacteria or bacterial infection at this time in history.

Semmelweis went on a campaign to persuade his colleagues to wash their hands as he had recommended, but he was regarded as a fool and a troublemaker. The women continued to die. Eventually, he was taken to an insane asylum where he was beaten to death. We know now that Semmelweis was right, and his discovery saved the lives of countless hundreds of millions of women.[5]

Another pioneer in epidemiology was John Snow. Snow was a family doctor in England when a cholera epidemic broke out in London in 1835. London secured its water from the Thames River through private companies that brought the water to different parts of the city. One company sourced its water intake above London, and the other one acquired the water from downstream from the city. Cholera was killing many people in some parts of London, but other parts of the city had very little of the disease.

Snow was puzzled by the fact that none of the men in the brewery in his neighborhood got sick, but many other people were dying from cholera. Everyone in the neighborhood got their water from the Broad Street pump, which was supplied by the water company that took its water downstream from London. The men from the brewery, however, got their water from the well within the brewery.

After seeing that more people were getting sick when their water came from the downstream Thames, with lower rates of illness when the water came from both sources, and even lower rates when the water came from above London, Snow decided that there was something wrong with the water after it flowed through London. Again, no one knew anything about bacteria as a source of disease, but Snow decided that the Broad Street pump was a source of illness. He took the handle off the pump, and the epidemic stopped in his neighborhood.[6]

Is pregnancy really normal?

As I was interested in population issues, the Carolina Population Center offered extraordinary depth and instruction in those disciplines. A member of that faculty was Steven Polgar, a Hungarian anthropologist who came from the University of Chicago Ph.D. program – one of the best – and the Harvard School of Public Health. Steve had worked with family planning programs in New York and had a perspective that ranged from cultural adaptation and cultural ecology to the details of specific health programs designed to help people with problems of fertility control. Steve taught two graduate seminars, one of which was Culture and Fertility. He took us through the history of human population growth and some of the theories about it, including the "Demographic Transition Theory" that states that modernization of traditional societies will result in declines in both death rates and birth rates. In this analysis, death rates decline more rapidly than birth rates, and the result is a "population explosion" that levels off after birth rates also decline. Whether that is really true is another discussion for another book.

Steve's second seminar the next fall was Cultural Ecology, in which we studied how human cultures adapt to and exploit different environments. A fascinating part of Steve's seminar was the study of how various societies deal with health and illness. I was especially interested in how this applied to pregnancy. My reading included Margaret Mead's book, *Cultural Patterns and Technological Change* in which she raised the question of the definition of health.[7] Is a state of "health" one defined by the existing average or by an ideal to be attained? Mead noted that among Native Americans, one-sided hip dislocation was extremely common in older men, especially in the Apache tribe, and this was accepted as the "normal" condition for old men. She also described other situations in which diseases like iodine-deficient goiter were so common in some communities it was considered "normal" to have a goiter.

In other societies, Mead said, "health" is more likely to be considered an ideal to be obtained rather than the existing average. This is obviously influenced by the availability of medical care that is specific to and part of the local culture.

These questions made me reflect on my experiences as a medical student when I read in my obstetrics textbook of "normal" pregnancy and the idea that a woman is most "normal" when she's pregnant. If that's what she is when she's pregnant, what is she when she *isn't* pregnant? Does it mean that her existence is not meaningful unless she's pregnant and having babies? Is having babies what she's *for*? How many pregnancies during a woman's lifetime are "normal?"

I had just spent time in a Shipibo village in the Amazon where most women were pregnant most of the time, and where the women had a relatively sophisticated set of beliefs about pregnancy as well as a system of herbal medications to prevent pregnancy. These things indicated that they didn't think it was "normal" to be pregnant *all the time*. In fact, I later calculated that the average Shipibo woman was pregnant 45% of the time during her "child-bearing years," as they are called, from 15 to 45 years of age. I also compared this to the fact that the average American woman with two or three children was pregnant for only about 5% of her reproductive years.

In addition to this analysis, I had spent a lot of my time as a medical student and intern helping women to keep from dying as a result of being pregnant. And my textbook on obstetrics was full of information about the ways that pregnancy can kill women. Not only that, there was a death rate due to pregnancy called the "maternal mortality ratio" – the number of women who die as the result of pregnancy per 100,000 live births. I thought of our patient Sharon from my third year of medical school. Pregnancy is not a benign condition. It can kill you.

The result of this exercise was a paper I wrote for Steve's 1969 fall seminar for which my title was "Cultural definitions of normality in pregnancy." In 1970, Steve helped me present this paper at a seminar he organized at a meeting of the American Anthropological Association. The information and concepts that I worked with and developed in this paper became an important part of the events described in this book.

Another mentor with whom I studied and worked closely at Chapel Hill was Dr. Abdel Omran, an Egyptian population epidemiologist who had devised the Epidemiologic Transition Theory, which states that the major causes of morbidity and mortality change, along with economic development and cultural change from acute infectious illnesses, for example, to chronic illnesses that result from more sedentary lifestyles.[8]

With Abdel, I studied issues of epidemiologic methodology, and I taught his course in population epidemiology in the fall of 1969, one of the best experiences of my life. I decided that teaching and doing research in epidemiology was what I wanted to do in my medical career. I enjoyed it very much.

During a visit to my family in Colorado over Christmas in 1968, I learned that Colorado had passed an abortion reform law – the first in the country – in 1967. I thought this was a very important development. I wrote to freshman Democratic state Representative Richard Lamm, who had sponsored the successful state legislation, to congratulate him and ask him whether he thought I should study law instead of public health. His legislation had broken through an important barrier and promised to help millions of women. His friendly but laconic reply was that lawyers spend most of their time moving money from one pocket to another and that I should stick to public health. His own career as an innovative legislator and subsequent three terms as governor of Colorado refuted that admonition, but I followed his advice and stuck to public health.

Another important moment came in the fall of 1968 when I learned that Bill Baird would be giving a presentation on his challenges to the laws against birth control at Duke University, right around the corner from my pad in Durham. I went to the meeting out of curiosity. Bill talked eloquently about his challenges to the laws in Massachusetts that prevented unmarried women from getting oral contraceptives or other contraceptive devices and how this kept them from making choices about their own lives. He then said that he had been speaking all over the country about this issue, and that he had yet to be joined on the platform by a single physician who supported his efforts. I got up and walked on to the stage with Bill. We are still friends.

Although he is neither a lawyer nor physician, Bill had two successful challenges to laws against dispensing contraception and permitting minors to have abortions without parental consent in the U.S. Supreme Court: *Baird v. Bellotti* and *Eisenstadt v. Baird*. He made history and a difference in people's lives by his dedication and persistence.

Since I had repeatedly seen terrible problems and suffering from unsafe abortion throughout Latin America and in Colorado as a medical student, I focused on the epidemiology of abortion mortality in my public health studies. In the midst of this, I was recruited to help run the Office of Economic Opportunity's (OEO) Family Planning Division in Washington, D.C., in the spring of 1970. One of my classmates from UNC had recommended me to Dr. George Contis, director of the OEO Family Planning Division, and he offered me the job when he came to speak at the Carolina Population Center about the OEO program.

In March 1970 I moved to Washington to start my new job working for the federal government. Richard Nixon was president, the Vietnam War was raging, the civil rights movement was making progress, the women's liberation movement was driving changes that were long overdue, and the OEO family planning program, which had been launched in 1964 as a part of President Johnson's War on Poverty initiative, looked like a way to make an important contribution to some basic issues in women's health care.

A short time before I left North Carolina, I drove by a Ku Klux Klan cross that had burned overnight on a hill right by the highway near my apartment. I was on my way from Durham, where I had my apartment, to Chapel Hill. The burnt cross and the rantings of Jesse Helms on the local television station reminded me that belligerent ignorance and violent racism were alive and well in North Carolina.

Notes

1 Armijo, R., and Monreal, T. Epidemología del aborto provocado en Santiago, Chile. *Revista Medica de Chile*, 7:548–86, 1964. PMID: 14223384
2 Hankinson, R.K.B., Kleinman, R.L., Eckstein, P., and Romero, H (Spanish edition). *Proceedings of the Eighth International Conference of the International Planned Parenthood Federation, Santiago, Chile 9–15 April 1967*. Hartford, UK: International Planned Parenthood Federation 1967.
3 Requena, M.B. Social and economic correlates of induced abortion in Santiago, Chile. *Demography* 2:33–49, 1965.
4 Cassel, J. Social science theory as a source of hypothesis in epidemiological research. *American Journal of Public Health* 54:1482, 1964.
5 Carter, K.C., and Carter, B.R. *Childbed Fever: A Scientific Biography of Ignaz Semmelweis*. Westport, CT: Greenwood Press, 1994; Semmelweis, I. *The Etiology, Concept, and Prophylaxis of Childbed Fever*. Translated by K.C. Carter. Madison: University of Wisconsin Press, 1983.
6 Snow. J. *Snow on Cholera: Being A Reprint of Two Papers by John Snow, M.D. Together with A Biographical Memoir by P.W. Richardson and an Introduction by Wade Hampton Frost, M.D.* New York and London: Harper, 1965 (Facsimile of 1936 edition).
7 Mead, M. *Cultural Patterns and Technological Change*. Paris: UNESCO, 1953
8 Omran, A.R. The Epidemiologic Transition: A Theory of the Epidemiology of Population Change. *Milbank Memorial Fund Quarterly* 49:509–38, 1971.

3   Focus on family planning

Arriving in Washington, D.C., to begin my new job as a medical officer in a big federal program, I found myself in the company of agreeable young people who shared my values and who had important previous experience. Three of the young women had been Peace Corps volunteers in India, one had been one of my classmates at the school of public health in North Carolina, and our boss, Dr. George Contis, was a highly experienced pediatrician with public health training. Although George and I were at the opposite ends of the political spectrum and from very different life experiences, we got along famously. We not only enjoyed each other's company, we agreed on the basic public health issues of the day, especially in our agency's focus, namely the need for family planning services for poor women and their families.

To help about 350,000 women across the country who were receiving health care at the OEO Community Health Centers get the contraceptive care they were requesting, we had an operating budget of $24 million, which is about the amount spent by the Pentagon on erasers in its public relations department in a single afternoon. But George was a highly skilled negotiator, and he managed to get a contract with Syntex, one of the manufacturers of oral contraceptives, for OEO to get birth control pills at the rate of 26 cents per cycle, a tiny fraction of the going retail cost. George dealt directly with Carl Djerassi, the brilliant Hungarian biochemist who was a chief architect of oral contraceptives. George also got condom manufacturers to provide these items to our programs at a heavily reduced cost. In addition to being a skilled physician, George was a Republican, a good businessman, and an effective negotiator for our goals.

During the two tumultuous years that I worked at OEO from the spring of 1970 until June 1972, I had the opportunity to help start various new programs and to meet extraordinary people who were national leaders in our field. My work also brought me into contact with some national political leaders.

Washington was an exciting place to be, and many public officials were quite accessible. One would encounter them, especially members of Congress, walking around the streets by the Capitol and in the halls of the Senate and House of Representatives. It was inspiring to get to know personally people who were running our country. But we were constantly reminded of the carnage and suffering going on in Vietnam and the rest of Southeast Asia and the struggles for racial justice and equality going on in our own country. As a member of the Medical Committee for Human Rights, I participated in numerous anti-war demonstrations and gave medical care to some overzealous and overheated participants. One had a cardiac arrest, but I gave him CPR, got him started, and turned him over to an emergency crew.

DOI: 10.4324/9781003514961-4

The women's movement was becoming more energetic and visible, and I found myself marching in the streets with women's groups and meeting with representatives of groups such as the Women's National Abortion Action Coalition (WONAAC), the newly formed National Association for the Repeal of Abortion Laws (NARAL), and the National Organization for Women (NOW). Many of these groups had common members. The legalization of abortion in New York State in the spring of 1970 energized the pro-choice movement and made it seem inevitable that abortion would soon be legalized throughout the country.

Since I walked several miles to and from work each day through the Dupont Circle area to Kalorama Road, I found myself one day walking by the offices of *The New Republic* that had famously been founded by Walter Lippman and his associates. Being an admirer of the magazine, I decided to stop in to meet the staff. They were interested in my work, so I wrote an article, "Family planning and the poor," about what we were doing at OEO, and it was published in November 1970.[1]

Earlier that fall, I had an opportunity to present my paper on the cultural and epidemiologic aspects of pregnancy at the annual meeting of the American Anthropological Association in San Diego along with my mentor, Steve Polgar. A few weeks later, I attended a Planned Parenthood luncheon in New York in my capacity as an OEO official and found myself talking with Dick Lincoln, the editor of the new publication, *Family Planning Perspectives*. Dick found my perspective interesting and asked me to submit my paper to him for publication in *Perspectives*, so I did. The paper, published under the title, "Is pregnancy really normal?" in January 1971, caused a bit of a sensation.[2] The New York–based Association for the Study of Abortion (ASA), led by Dr. Mary Steichen Calderone, decided to include it in their standard reprint literature and circulated it widely. It elicited a mixed reaction from the feminists.

One of the consequences stemming from both these publications was a series of invitations to meet with people who were working to make abortion legal in the United States. They included Joe Nellis, a Washington, D.C., attorney who had deep roots in the Democratic Party and who was the attorney for Dr. Milan Vuitch, a Yugoslav surgeon who was performing abortions in Washington. Joe invited me to join him and Dr. Vuitch for lunch, where I learned that Dr. Vuitch was challenging the Washington, D.C., statute restricting abortion. Then I was invited to be present when Joe and Norman Dorsen from the American Civil Liberties Union argued Dr. Vuitch's case before the U.S. Supreme Court on January 12, 1971. Something very interesting happened.

The issue of whether a pregnancy is "normal" became the focus of a bizarre and fascinating exchange between several U.S. Supreme Court justices, including Justices White, Blackmun, Marshall, and Chief Justice Burger, and Norman Dorsen, one of the attorneys for Dr. Vuitch.

At the January 1971 hearing before the Court, Dr. Vuitch was challenging the Washington, D.C., statute prohibiting abortion.[3]

The premise of the government's case against Dr. Vuitch was that he had violated the D.C. statute by performing abortions on women without a "health" justification. Dorsen asserted that it was the woman's right to make the decision to have an abortion. The justices and Dorsen were discussing the "justification" for abortion. The overall premise of the argument – which prevailed in virtually all public discussions of this issue at the time – was that pregnancy is "normal," and therefore some reason had to be found to "justify" the abortion.

Justice Blackmun opened the line of questioning by asking Dorsen (since Dorsen asserted that the woman had the right to do what she wished with her body) if she had the right to commit suicide. Dorsen wasn't sure, but he said that he thought so. Justice Blackmun then pressed Dorsen to admit that the logical conclusion of his argument was that since she could do with this a fetus, she could prevail upon the doctor to saw off her arm. Dorsen said the doctor could exercise medical judgment and do so if there was a "disease situation." Burger then asked Dorsen whether he hadn't already said "there need be no diseased condition, no other factor except the direction of the woman to authorize the abortion?" "Well, that is correct," said Dorsen. Chief Justice Burger then asked, "Why should it be different on amputating the arm? She just doesn't, she just…" Justice Marshall: "just doesn't want the arm?" Chief Justice Burger: "She just wants to mutilate herself and she wants to do it in a safe sort of way?" Dorsen: "Well, I do have problems with that, I do have problems with that." Justice White: "Why do you have problems with that, Mr. Dorsen, if you're not [taking] that position?" Dorsen: "Well, I take the position because abortion is a well-recognized medical operation without any indication at all perhaps traces out the question. I would…" Justice White: "Then I am talking…if you have trouble with the arm, I think you would have trouble with the abortion, especially and *a fortiori* if you recall….and you even thought that the unborn child had some rights?" Dorsen: "I don't think that this court…" Justice White: "Certainly an arm doesn't?" "Dorsen: "That's right."

The rest of the exchange did not improve in clarity, facts, or logic, but it continued until Dorsen finally escaped this blind alley and said, "Our contention is that this language is unconstitutionally vague, that it cannot be cured, and that this Court should therefore affirm the judgement of the court below."

The Supreme Court reversed Judge Gerhard Gesell's U.S. District Court for the District of Columbia decision that the D.C. statute was unconstitutional. But in the process, Justice Black asserted that the burden of proof for violating the abortion statute was not on the doctor to prove that there was a "health" reason for performing the abortion but on the prosecution to show that there was no "health" issue at stake. This critical assertion has been generally lost in the mists of time throughout the abortion controversy.

The question of whether a woman's health was affected by being pregnant was left hanging in the air.

Dorsen was stuck with the idea of cutting off a normal arm because he accepted the same premise as the justices – that pregnancy is "normal" and therefore you can't perform an abortion without finding some other justification. His answers were not clear, but he said it was not a normal practice to remove the arm if it was healthy. It was surreal. If he said no, it can't be removed because it is normal, Justice White and others would have him impaled on the conventional wisdom that pregnancy is "normal," and therefore you can't justify interrupting it unless you have some compelling, overriding reason. Then - which reason, on what basis, and who decides? Dorsen's discomfort reflected the unreality of the entire controversy. No one distinguished themselves in that discussion. The intellectual mousetrap of pregnancy being "normal" remained undisturbed.

As I settled into my responsibilities at the OEO office, I was given a title: Chief, Program Development and Evaluation Branch. I was the branch or, you might say, the twig. I had no staff under my direction, and I shared an excellent secretary, a young woman high school graduate named Vickie from a hardscrabble place in West Virginia, with the rest of our Family Planning Division staff. I was placed in charge of starting new programs and figuring out whether what we were doing was getting any results. I was also the staff liaison with many private organizations, such as Planned Parenthood's Center for Family Planning Research and Development, Columbia University's Center for Family Planning Research, and the American Public Health Association's Subcommittee on Family Planning Methods. These responsibilities took me to many places across the country, especially New York City, to investigate programs.

One month after I began working at the OEO Family Planning Division, the state of New York legalized abortion up to 24 menstrual weeks. Even though OEO had no funding for abortion services, this was obviously a major development from a public health and public policy perspective, not to mention what it meant to women everywhere who needed abortions.

Soon after this, I was invited to attend a board meeting of the New York City Department of Health at which the board would take up rules and policies governing the performance of abortions within the city. One of the main questions was whether abortions would be permitted on an outpatient basis or if they would have to be performed in hospitals, which were already overworked. The solution was to require abortions after about 12 weeks of pregnancy to be performed in hospital settings.

One of the city's outstanding medical officials with whom I met was Dr. Jean Pakter, who was director of the maternal health division in the city's health department. We worked together years later on other projects.

One day George opened our staff meeting with a challenge: he wanted to see if we could start statewide family planning programs anywhere and asked if anyone knew of a good place to start. I volunteered to call Sheri Tepper, the director of the Planned Parenthood program in Denver, Colorado, who I had known since my time as a medical student in Denver. I called Sheri, and I asked her, "How would you like to start a statewide family planning program in Colorado?" "Of course," she replied, so we agreed to have a meeting with the critical people at her home in Denver on a fall morning that year.

The meeting at Sheri's home in Denver was attended by, among others, my former mentor from medical school, Dr. Bill Droegemueller, who was now the medical director of Planned Parenthood in addition to his duties on the faculty of the medical school in the Department of Obstetrics and Gynecology. Also in attendance was Sylvia Clark, a nurse who was Sheri's deputy, and State Representative Dick Lamm. Lamm's presence was significant because he had been the initial sponsor of Colorado's first abortion reform bill, which was signed into law in April 1967 and which was the first abortion reform law in the United States. We had corresponded when I was studying public health in North Carolina, but this was the first time that I met him. I congratulated him on the success of his abortion reform law, which made U.S. history, and then we talked politics. "Are you going to run for the Senate?" I asked. "No, I think it would be a lot more fun to be governor." He was elected governor of Colorado in 1974 and served for three terms. Contrary to warnings he had been given as the sponsor of the abortion reform bill, his leadership on this issue did not constitute his political death warrant.

My job back in Washington was to get Sheri's grant proposal through the government bureaucracy to the point of approval and disbursement of funds. The grant to Rocky Mountain Planned Parenthood in 1971 was for $270,000. This was its first federal grant, and the agency's budget is now $40 million a year and serves thousands of women throughout Colorado and several states. It took about a year, and it was a good example of how government works to create new programs that are helpful to people.

The sterilization guidelines controversy

In the part of my job that required me to evaluate our family planning programs, I visited clinics and hospitals across the country as well as analyzing stacks of reports and statistics. It became clear that 80 percent of all the OEO family planning programs wanted to offer voluntary sterilization services to both men and women in addition to the standard temporary contraceptives, such as condoms, foam, diaphragms, and birth control pills. There were several problems with doing this.

Under the first director of OEO, Sargent Shriver, a staunch Catholic, it had been difficult to get even "family planning" included in the OEO health clinic programs. Inclusion of abortion was out because it was illegal, and voluntary sterilization services were even more unacceptable to Shriver. Second, "Black Power" leaders in the African American community were opposed to family planning programs for Black women for their own political reasons, and white supremacists were opposed to them for white women. Both groups wanted women to have more babies of their preferred color. It constituted a classic example of men using women's bodies to achieve political goals, not a new thing in human history.

A third problem was that white doctors throughout the South (and some other places) had been performing involuntary sterilizations on Black women when the women were under anesthesia for other reasons. The same circumstances occurred for Hispanic and Native American women according to reports we received. Since people coming in for help in OEO health services were, by definition, poor, this included many women in minority groups who were anxious about these issues.

One day I received a call from Jeanette Smith, a nurse running the OEO family planning clinic in Anderson County, Tennessee. She said that many of their patients, who were from poor white families living in the hills around Oak Ridge, were requesting voluntary sterilization services that were not available anywhere. She wanted to know if there was a way that she and her colleagues could start offering these services.

A few weeks later, I traveled to Oak Ridge and met with Jeanette, and she introduced me to Bob Brooks, a man native to the Appalachian hills who understood and was sympathetic to the problems of the poor coal miners' families the program was serving. Bob's day job was running the maintenance programs for the Oak Ridge nuclear plant.

Bob and I hit it off, and we went up into the hills to visit some of the families that he knew wanted this help. Here is an excerpt from my article I wrote for *The New Republic* after I got back to Washington:

> The site that Eleanor Roosevelt visited in West Virginia during the Depression and described as the poorest place in America is still, according to local inhabitants, as miserable as ever, if not worse. The mountains, long denuded of their finest timber, are heavily eroded and gouged by strip mines. They look like partly plucked and badly butchered chickens. Their topsoil is buried beneath the eviscerated hillsides or silted into black streams choked with coal dust and sulfuric acid. An ugly industrial slum winds through the valleys from Huntington to Charleston and is overlain with a yellowish grey pall which impartially dissolves lung tissue and automobile finish. The rivers are a stinking cauldron of industrial poisons.
>
> Into this mutilated landscape the newly born miner's child is thrust. The mother, battered by repeated childbearing, struggles against sheer physical exhaustion. Years in the mines have left the father with a chronic cough, frequent chest pain, shortness

of breath, and other symptoms of severe lung disease and early heart failure. If he is lucky enough to have a job at all in the mines, he may earn as little as $2.75 a car loaded with 1 to 1 ½ tons of coal; and he loads seven cars a day in a 12-to-14-hour day. The work is dangerous and sporadic. In the smaller mines, he buys his own equipment. There are no fringe benefits. The coal is sold for up to $12 a ton to others, or perhaps slightly less if he buys it to heat his own tumbledown shack. The shack has no running water, sanitation or privacy. When it is available, electricity powers a few naked light bulbs and, if work has been steady recently, perhaps a new refrigerator. Except for a TV and a telephone, which works only occasionally, the refrigerator is the only appliance. For this, the miner pays "so much a month" – perhaps up to four times the real retail price.

To the south of West Virginia, the strip mines are invading the beautiful Smoky Mountains of eastern Tennessee, and the inhabitants are becoming impoverished in an environment unfit for humans.

On a crisp, sunny November morning, I stood in the littered front yard of a Tennessee mountain family's household talking with Robert Brooks of Oak Ridge. Brooks is a 45-year-old chemical plant worker who became so enthusiastic about his wife's activities as an OEO family-planning outreach worker that he decided to help in his spare time. Brooks is a poor coal miner's son from one of the remote "hollers" of Tennessee.

We had come to visit one of the poorest families near the unemployment-stricken village of Fratersville, and we stood well out in the yard waiting to be invited in. We looked across the valley at the fading but still splendid autumn foliage and watched as a strip mining operation ripped a brown, ragged wound across the hillside. A few days before, water accumulating from heavy rains had broken through some of these abandoned shelves, unleashing a destructive flash flood on the hollow near Fratersville.

A woman finally asked us to come in. She invited us to sit on a tattered sofa in a room otherwise barren except for a potbelly iron stove and a broken wooden chair. She pulled the chair near the glowing stove and sat down. As we talked, she slumped forward and watched her children listlessly, her arms crossed. She spoke in a monotone. She was 38 years old. She and her husband had nine living children. She was six months pregnant. "I tuck them pills for awhile, but my stumick got to botherin' me like it did afor I tuck 'em so I quit for three months. Couldn't afford 'em, no how." Brooks told her that she could get free medical exams and birth control help at the OEO clinic, and she said, "Well, I'll be down after the baby's got borned, but ain't there some way asides a pill?"

Similar requests from families with all the children they want are commonly heard by Brooks and his fellow OEO outreach workers in Tennessee. Mrs. Jeanette Smith, the nurse directing the OEO-funded Anderson County family planning project through the local Planned Parenthood organization, estimates that her office receives four to five sterilization requests a week from poor families. A recent program-management survey of OEO family planning projects, which are currently serving more than 300,000 patients, indicates that this is far from unusual. Eighty percent of the projects reported that they wanted to provide sterilization as part of their regular services, which already include pelvic exams, cancer detection, VD screening, counseling, and education as well as contraceptives and referral for other medical problems. Project directors such as Mrs. Smith, however, feel that many of the patients want sterilization and that a complete program should include this service.

Perhaps the most surprising aspect of this experience in Tennessee is the frequency of requests by men for vasectomy, the male sterilizing operation. In his contacts with the mountain men of Tennessee, Robert Brooks makes no secret of the fact that he had a vasectomy done after he and his wife had their child 15 years ago. Since vasectomy cannot now be offered by OEO programs, he does not bring up the subject deliberately.

One man, a seasonally employed garage mechanic, wanted a vasectomy done on himself as soon as it could be arranged. He and his 26-year-old wife have three children. She has also had two miscarriages. She cannot take birth control pills because of chronic kidney disease, high blood pressure, chronic urinary tract infections, and rheumatic heart disease. Other forms of contraception have been ineffective or unsuitable for her. Yet she will be risking pregnancy for the next 20 years. Her last unplanned child was delivered by Caesarean section. Any future pregnancy would probably require a similar operation. Some of their medical bills are paid by public sources, but one more child would plunge them even deeper into debt.

Another woman in her early twenties, an outreach worker for one of the Tennessee family planning projects, is plagued by extreme obesity, made worse with each pregnancy. She weighs close to 300 pounds. The obesity is also aggravated by taking birth control pills, but she is so fearful of pregnancy she doesn't want to stop taking them. Her anxiety about pregnancy causes her to eat more and the problem gets worse. She and her husband have three children "...all we can handle. We don't want any more children." Her last pregnancy was unwanted. All three children have been ill and have had recent hospital stays. Her husband was seriously injured nearly a year ago and is unable to work. They want sterilization for either one but can't afford it.

A young woman in her late twenties told me that neither she nor her middle-aged unemployed husband, who has had two heart attacks, wants any more children. None of her three children was intended. Her first child was born out of wedlock; the others have been born since she married in 1968. She was using foam and the rhythm method, respectively, when she became pregnant with the last two. They came 13 months apart. Her first thought, she says, when she discovered her last pregnancy, was "...how can I get rid of it?" They live in a cramped trailer house, and she says, "Each one makes it harder on the ones we already got. We couldn't really afford them, but here they are so what can you do?" She wants to be sterilized and "...would go this afternoon if I thought I could get it done," but they don't have the money to pay. Her youngest child is six months old.

A dejected, tobacco-chewing young man shifted nervously in front of a squat iron stove which provided the only heat for his one-room tarpaper shelter. He looked past his 31-year-old wife at one of their seven children, who was screaming and pummeling a younger brother, and said, "I git another I reckon I'll shoot myself." Their house burned down two years ago Christmas and he has been unemployed "for a long time." He takes odd jobs and they get food surplus, but there seems to be no way to get ahead. Their "house" has no running water, toilet, adequate cooking facilities; they have no refrigerator. His wife looks nearly 20 years older than her age. The youngest child is three months old. All the children are anemic and dirty. Two appear to be mentally retarded. The others go to school only when the weather is warm. They have no shoes or warm clothes. The man wants his hernia fixed and a vasectomy done at the same time. "We got all we kin handle." His wife became pregnant with their youngest child when she ran out of birth control pills and couldn't afford to buy more at the time. She was recently contacted by the local OEO family-planning outreach worker and has begun attending the clinic, but both she and her husband feel that temporary measures such as the "pill" are not enough to suit their need. However, they cannot afford an operation, which would cost around $100 for the man's vasectomy or as much as $400 for the woman.

Families like these need jobs, decent housing, a healthy environment, adequate food, clean water, sanitation, and education. OEO health programs, including the 450 projects primarily concerned with family planning, provide a network of services which are meeting some of these individual needs. *But one of the most important needs is freedom from the tyranny of their own biology* [Italics supplied].[4]

It was obvious from this glimpse into the lives of some of the poorest people in America that their struggle for survival in a devastated landscape destroyed by coal mining was desperate, and that a major part of their suffering was related to their inability or lack of resources to control their own fertility. Pregnancy was not a blessing for these people.

At the OEO office, I began reviewing guidelines for voluntary sterilization services I had helped prepare for the American Public Health Association Subcommittee on Family Planning Methods, and I made connections with doctors and agencies that were attempting to provide these services. At about this time, an interesting thing happened when the leaders of OEO went to Congress and asked for money for the OEO programs.

The director of OEO at this time was Frank Carlucci, a Nixon appointee who followed his college roommate, Don Rumsfeld, as transitory OEO directors on their way to higher political appointments. During routine budget hearings for the Office of Economic Opportunity, Carlucci appeared before Congresswoman Edith Green (D-OR) to explain and justify OEO's budget requests. At his side was Dr. Tom Bryant, director of the Office of Health Affairs at OEO, who was our direct supervisor in the Family Planning Division. Tom was a very congenial person, and we got along with him well. He was extraordinarily well prepared for his job as both a physician and an attorney.

At the hearing with Congresswoman Green, Carlucci presented the program details of the various OEO programs, but she interrupted him with a sharp question: why weren't the OEO Family Planning programs providing vasectomies for men as well as oral contraceptives for women?

Taken aback by this question for which he was not prepared, Carlucci turned to Tom Bryant for guidance. Tom whispered to Carlucci that we were "working on it" at the OEO family planning office, and Carlucci repeated this to the congresswoman.

It turns out that Congresswoman Green had seen my article in *The New Republic* and wanted to know why sterilization services were not being offered even though they were needed by those we were serving.

Within a few days, I had the green light to go ahead with plans for offering voluntary sterilization services in OEO family planning programs. I got in touch with Jeanette Smith in Tennessee and asked her to prepare a grant request for this. I also began working on developing a set of guidelines for voluntary sterilization services since I was aware of the constant stories and rumors of abuse of this operation in the South and elsewhere in the country. I used the framework that we had developed with the American Public

Health Association standards that I had helped write and began circulating drafts among my medical colleagues across the country.

There were many levels of approval for the sterilization guidelines I was preparing, which I regarded as essential prior to a formal change in the OEO policy permitting these services. There was a long history of sterilization procedures being used in punitive ways toward minority women, especially in the South against Black women. I wanted to make sure these actions couldn't occur in our programs.

It was a serious lesson on how the government really works in the middle levels where I was the technical mover of the project just under the higher level directors who reported to the president and Congress. One of the men I worked with was a fellow named Dan Zwick, a balding, unassuming middle-aged man who really knew the nuts and bolts of government and how you put together a program that actually accomplishes something. Dan seemed to me to be the best example of an expert, dedicated public servant who was using the power of the government to help large groups of people who would not otherwise secure help. That was the essence of the OEO Community Action Programs (CAPs) and all their various branches. We would get the ideas and the permissions from those at higher levels, and he would make it happen. We had to get our documents approved, for example, through the Office of Management and Budget and various other agencies before the program could be listed in the Federal Register, and since we were officially in the Executive Office of the President, this couldn't happen until it was approved by someone in the Nixon White House.

One of my vivid memories from various occasions was watching Dan Zwick sitting at the conference table, sweating, hard at work in his white shirt and tie (no jacket) with the sleeves rolled up, going through budget documents line by line, doing calculations, and figuring out which numbers were going to get past the budget people at OMB (Office of Management and Budget).

Much later, I learned that Dan had an incredibly distinguished background, a Ph.D. in economics and a career that included teaching economics at Harvard with one of the great public intellectuals of our time, John Kenneth Galbraith. Dan came to OEO because of his idealism for public service. He is one of the persons I think about when some ignorant person condemns the "deep state" and "faceless bureaucrats in Washington."

In this process, I met with Howard Phillips, who, according to the rumors at OEO, was a hatchet man sent by Nixon to kill OEO. OEO, an outgrowth of the "War on Poverty," was the creation of Lyndon Johnson, it symbolized liberal "do good" programs that the Republicans hated, and it represented a vestige of the Johnson programs that Nixon wanted to end. Phillips was Nixon's man. Phillips was large, intense, with black curly hair, seemed to be aggressively pursuing some goal and barely tolerant of me. Contempt would be more accurate.

It was only years later that I learned that Phillips was part of the "New Right" in the Republican Party that was vigorously opposed to social welfare programs like OEO and many other such programs loved by the liberals in the Democratic Party. I didn't realize right away that I was caught in the crossfire of this ideological conflict. Phillips was not seriously unpleasant to me, but he was officious, abrupt, curt, and, shall we say, highly restrained in his elemental courtesy. He tolerated my presence. I sensed that he really didn't want my project to succeed, but I couldn't identify the reasons or specific actions – until later.

In Michelle Goldberg's indispensable book, *Kingdom Coming: The Rise of Christian Nationalism*, she describes Howard Phillip's rise to power in OEO and the radical New

Right and descent from Judaism and a Harvard education to a radical proponent of Christian reconstructionism and a fascist theocracy.[5]

Along with Tom Coburn, Phillips advocated the execution of doctors who perform abortions. He was on the cusp of this transformation when I knew him in my capacity as a low-level OEO federal medical officer in 1972. He would have me marked for execution if he had attained the power that he sought. Since he didn't, my life has been spared. I think.

Another character in the drama at OEO was a man named Wes Hjornevik, who was the deputy director just under Don Rumsfeld, our OEO director at that time. Wes was another man who had held various high government jobs, including running the Houston space agency, and he was quite powerful at OEO. He was always pleasant and professional toward me in spite of my youth, inexperience, and lack of familiarity with government procedures.

On May 18, 1971, Wes Hjornevik approved my initiative to include voluntary sterilization services in OEO family planning programs by issuing a directive that only abortion services would be banned. This directive overruled the previous policy set by Sargent Shriver in 1964 banning abortion and sterilization services from OEO programs. Following this, I was able to get the guidelines approved all the way through the maze of federal agencies and get them published in the Federal Register. I then authorized 25,000 copies to be printed by the Government Printing Office for distribution to all OEO programs throughout the country.

Then the shit hit the fan.

The first notice that I had was when the man who ran the administration department of OEO came to my office and demanded all the copies I had of the sterilization guidelines. I was so flabbergasted by this demand that I gave him the few copies that I had. My boss, George Contis, went ballistic. He went to the office of Leon Cooper, MD, who had just been appointed head of the Office of Health Affairs. Cooper was now the new person to whom George reported. There had already been personal conflict. George was a very conservative Republican of Greek descent with a Harvard education and strong East Coast ethos who was very much a part of the institutional medical establishment, and Leon was an aggressively liberal Black physician from Atlanta who had operated community health programs at the local level and who harbored serious resentment against the White Medical Establishment. George had been running his successful program for over two years, and Leon was the new kid on the block. Even though George was highly qualified, with many years of experience as a pediatric public health physician and in the agency, he was passed over for promotion to the office that Cooper now held.

The two had already begun to disagree on all kinds of policy issues, and their operating styles were starkly different. George believed in following organizational principles and procedures, and Leon operated in a more informal manner. George dressed elegantly in perfectly tailored three-piece suits and Leon didn't. We learned that the directive to confiscate the guidelines in my office came from Leon.

Realizing that I had made a major error in not keeping any copy of the guidelines I had prepared and which I regarded as critical to the safety of the women we were trying to help, I went to Shami Lubin, who worked in the public relations section of OEO and with whom I had a warm friendship as a professional colleague. I had given a copy to Shami, and she gave it back to me. This was the original copy I would hand over to Senator Ted Kennedy (D-MA) in 1973 at a congressional hearing on this episode.

In January 1972 I began sending memos to Cooper insisting that the sterilization guidelines should be issued as planned. We had changed the sterilization policy, money had been disbursed for the programs, there was now a pilot sterilization operating in Tennessee, and lives were at risk. The program was getting national attention.[6] It was essential that OEO provide guidance for the sterilization programs and official protection against sterilization abuse. Cooper was unmoved. After a half dozen such memos, one of which told me that the guidelines could not be released until after the 1972 election (what???), I decided that I could not in good conscience continue to participate in the program, so I resigned in protest on June 2, 1972. My resignation was effective on June 17, 1972, which happened also to be the day of the Watergate break-in that ended the presidency of Richard Nixon.

One year later, on July 10, 1973, I was back in Washington testifying before Senator Ted Kennedy's Senate subcommittee concerning the OEO sterilization guidelines that had been suppressed. What follows is an excerpt of my testimony before Senator Kennedy:

Introduction by Senator Kennedy:	When [Dr. Hern] was with the Office of Economic Opportunity, he Opportunity, he was primarily responsible for the guidelines, and will have some important testimony on what happened to those guidelines. Now tell us your story.
Dr. Hern:	I have come voluntarily from Colorado to appear before this subcommittee in order to describe for Congress and the public a series of events that occurred last year in the Office of Economic Opportunity. *[description of development of the guidelines and efforts to get them through the approval process]* On numerous occasions, I made attempts to find out when the guidelines would be issued and why they were being held up. I was told that they were being reviewed by the White House and they would not be issued until after the 1972 elections.
Senator Kennedy:	That is a rather extraordinary statement. Who told you this?
Dr. Hern:	Several people told me that....I was not given any explanation of what the 1972 elections had to do with it. I felt that many people's lives were at stake, and we knew that many programs were going ahead without the guidelines even though we had requested them not to do so. And we felt this was a very dangerous situation. I tried on many occasions to get Mr. Howard Phillips to tell me what he knew about this, because everyone recognized him as the policy hatchet man at OEO. He refused my calls. *[Details of intra-office communications within OEO]*
Senator Kennedy:	What sort of dangers did you foresee if they did not issue the guidelines?
Dr. Hern:	I felt in the first place that sound medical and surgical procedures be taken, and also for patients requesting to, but only for patients requesting services could do so with informed consent, that they could not be coerced, and that patients be adequately counseled. This was a major aspect of the guidelines.
Senator Kennedy:	Why did you think you needed guidelines in those areas?

Dr. Hern:	We felt that this is a highly sensitive and irreversible procedure... we felt there were possibilities of abuse.

Dr. Hern: We felt that this is a highly sensitive and irreversible procedure... we felt there were possibilities of abuse.

We felt that there were possibilities that people who were not adequately informed, or able to consent for themselves, who would perhaps be vulnerable to a procedure that would render them sterile, in which they were really unable to really protect themselves against this sort of thing. Now, we really had in mind the kind of situation that we have down in Alabama.

Senator Kennedy: Do you think that if the guidelines had been in effect and adequately enforced, this situation could have been prevented?

Dr. Hern: That is the objective, and I think so. I do not think there is any absolute guarantee.

[*continued testimony by Dr. Hern*]

On March 30, 1972, I sent a memorandum to Dr. Leon Cooper asking him to look into the immediate release of the guidelines. On that afternoon, I had a conversation with Dr. Cooper about another matter, and I raised the question of the guidelines at that time. He told me then that there would not be any chance that the guidelines would come out before the 1972 elections, and that they were being held up by the White House.

On April 5, I made an attempt to find out whether...the guidelines were at the bottom of somebody's in-box over at the White House.

The closest thing I knew about how to find out about this was to call the White House General Counsel, and I had some personal contacts, and I found out that this must mean John Dean's office. I was told that Fred Fielding was the person who would handle that, if anyone did.

So I left a message for Mr. Fielding in his office and asked him about their status. He called me at home and told me they had never received the guidelines in that office, and he had no record of it in his logs, in the file, or anything like that.

[*after trying to call the OMB*]

I got a call from Dr. Cooper telling me that I must refrain from any contact with the Executive Office, White House, or OMB. I said I was doing my job and trying to find out where the guidelines were. He said if I wanted to talk to people over there, I would have to quit.

I told him I was not planning to quit.

My attempts to find out about the status of the guidelines were met with hostility, harassment, attempts at intimidation, and pointed invitations to resign.

On May 28, 1972, the *New York Times* published an article in which Dr. Cooper identified himself as the person responsible for stopping the issuance of the guidelines. He said this was not an "administration decision" contrary to what he had told me previously. [*end of excerpt of testimony to Senator Kennedy*]

* * *

At the end of the hearing, I handed my only copy of the OEO sterilization guidelines that I had prepared to Senator Kennedy, and he published them in the Congressional Record along with all the testimony.[7]

(*Note: Coincidentally, the day of my testimony was the same day that White House Counsel John Dean gave his "cancer on the presidency" testimony before the Watergate Committee*).

From my testimony, Bill Kovach of the *New York Times* called me, pursued the story and found the 25,000 copies of the guidelines still locked in the federal warehouse. OEO officials denied this and said that they had been distributed. But there they were.[8] Mark Bloom, a reporter from *Medical World News*, caught up with me at a medical meeting, went to see the stored documents, and his magazine published a front-page cover story about it in November 1973.[9]

In his book, *The Politics of Population Control*, Tom Littlewood gives a detailed description of this controversy, including my role in it and its resolution.[10]

The guidelines that I wrote and pushed through to completion had an important purpose: to protect women, especially minority women, from sterilization abuse.

Prior to their suppression at OEO and within the government, we submitted a copy of the OEO sterilization guidelines with commentary to the *American Journal of Public Health*. The paper was accepted, and publication of our paper was scheduled to be published in the journal in Volume 63:150, 1973 (January). It was in press with page proofs when the editors of the journal agreed to delete and suppress it at the demand of the Nixon White House. Somewhere I have these page proofs.

In early 1973 two young Black girls, Minnie Lee Relf and Mary Alice Relf, who were 12 and 14 years old, respectively, were involuntarily sterilized in Montgomery, Alabama, by a surgeon employed by an OEO health program. The two girls were regarded as mentally disabled by the OEO outreach workers and were taken to the hospital for these operations by the OEO agents. Their unemployed parents were illiterate, but they discovered the surgical scars after the girls were brought home from the hospital.

It was exactly this kind of involuntary sterilization that I had sought to prevent by preparing the OEO guidelines that were suppressed. This became a *cause célèbre*, and I was called to testify before Senator Kennedy, who was investigating this incident. As noted before, after I completed my testimony, I handed my only copy of the guidelines to Senator Kennedy, and he published them in the Congressional Record.[11]

The incident with the Relf sisters came to symbolize the misuse of sterilization procedures, particularly in an atmosphere of racial discrimination, and of abuse of power by government officials. Dr. Cooper was held responsible for the immediate action of preventing distribution of the guidelines, but the order to do so came from the Nixon White House on the recommendation of Paul O'Neill, who was serving at the time in the Office of Management and Budget.

Nixon was running for reelection in 1972, and his advisors were terrified that any health actions between the neck and the knees – particularly a controversial operation like voluntary sterilization – would sink Nixon's chances for reelection. As it turned out, Nixon successfully portrayed a highly decorated World War II hero, B-24 bomber pilot George McGovern, as a weak-kneed anti-war peacenik wimp who wouldn't stand up to dictators (as McGovern had done by risking his life on 35 combat bombing missions over

Germany). Nixon won the election by 520 electoral votes to 17 for Senator McGovern. The Vietnam War continued at the cost of thousands of more lives.

Notes

1 Hern, W.M. Family planning and the poor. *The New Republic.* November 14, 1970.
2 Hern, W.M. Is pregnancy really normal? *Family Planning Perspectives* 3(1): 1–6, January 1971. https://www.drhern.com/wp-content/uploads/2019/10/Is-Pregnancy-Really-Normal.pdf
3 *United States v. Vuitch*, 402 U.S. 62 (1971). https://www.oyez.org/cases/1970/84 at 1:26:12 to 1:31:04.
4 Hern, W.M. Biological Tyranny. *The New Republic,* February 27, 1971. https://www.drhern.com/wp-content/uploads/2019/10/biological-tyranny.pdf
5 Goldberg, M. *Kingdom Coming: The Rise of Christian Nationalism.* New York: W.W. Norton, 2006. Pp. 165–67.
6 Vecsey, G. U.S. agency financing sterilizations. *New York Times,* October 11, 1971. https://www.nytimes.com/1971/10/11/archives/u-s-agency-financing-sterilizations-u-s-antipoverty-agency-is.html?searchResultPosition=1; Vecsey, G. Federal sterilization program in doubt. *New York Times,* May 26, 1972. https://www.nytimes.com/1972/05/28/archives/federal-sterilization-program-in-doubt.html?searchResultPosition=2; CBS Reports, June, 1972. Voluntary sterilization program in Anderson County, Tennessee.
7 U.S. Senate hearings, Subcommittee on Health, U.S. Senate Committee on Labor and Public Welfare on "Quality of Health Care – Human Experimentation, 1973," Part 4, July 10, 1973, pp 1446 ff. Chaired by Senator Ted Kennedy; my testimony pp. 1503–13. https://books.google.com/books?id=lBc2AAAAIAAJ&pg=PA1443&lpg=PA1443&dq=RELF+HEARINGS+US+SENATE+JULY+10+1973&source=bl&ots=Zky0SP9Beq&sig=ACfU3U2K0VgxYC6RoAXdCLKtija3XEsGeQ&hl=en&sa=X&ved=2ahUKEwiE3b35m6qEAxVS8MkDHTRYCiYQ6AF6BAgkEAM#v=onepage&q=RELF%20HEARINGS%20US%20SENATE%20JULY%2010%201973&f=false
8 Kovach, B. Guidelines found on sterilization: Discovered in a warehouse: physician disputes OEO. *New York Times,* July 7, 1973. https://www.nytimes.com/1973/07/07/archives/guidelines-found-on-sterilization-discovered-in-a-warehouse.html?searchResultPo
9 Bloom, M. Sterilization guidelines: 22 months on the shelf. *Medical World News,* November 9, 1973, p. 53.
10 Littlewood, T. Richard Nixon's Catholic strategy – and the murky business of sterilization (Chapter 7). In Littlewood, T. *The Politics of Population Control.* Notre Dame, IN: University of Notre Dame Press, 1977, pp. 107–32.
11 U.S. Senate hearings, Subcommittee on Health, "Quality of Health Care – Human Experimentation, 1973."

4   Abortion becomes an issue in America

Although I had studied abortion as a public health issue and had taken care of desperate women who were dying from an unsafe abortion, and I had seen wards full of women dying from this cause in Brazil, I did not see myself as being directly involved with abortion services. After all, abortion was illegal almost everywhere in the United States, and it wasn't even a question in my mind. I increasingly saw myself having an academic career in public health, in general, and in epidemiology, in particular. Still, I was keenly interested in the efforts across the country to make abortion legal. Through my work at OEO, I quickly came into contact with people who were either performing abortions under the new law in New York or who were actively trying to expand the number of states where abortion was legal.

My article on the epidemiologic aspects of pregnancy and my assertion that abortion was the treatment of choice for pregnancy unless a woman wanted to be pregnant and have a baby caught the attention of various people involved in this issue. One of the calls came from Nan McEvoy, a wealthy philanthropist who had joined businessman Harry Levin in setting up an excellent private non-profit abortion clinic in Washington, D.C. I knew nothing about Ms. McEvoy at the time except that she was one of the owners or founders of Preterm Clinic. She invited me to come to work for them performing abortions. I replied that I was quite occupied with a very important job at OEO, but I would visit the clinic and spend the day to learn more about it. It was clear from my conversation with McEvoy that she and Harry Levin were trying to make a difference by offering safe abortions for women in Washington. She had learned about me from my January 1971 paper in *Family Planning Perspectives*, "Is pregnancy really normal?" (not my title).

My guide and mentor for the day was Dr. Ben Branch, an obstetrician/ gynecologist who was the medical director of the clinic. Ben showed me around and instructed me on the basic procedures that were being used to perform early surgical abortions by vacuum aspiration and sharp curettage (checking the empty uterus to make sure no tissue was left behind after the vacuum had been applied). Then he turned me over to Dr. Earl Herr, who had me watch him perform several early abortions. Then Earl invited me to perform one. I was terrified.

In medical school, I had learned how to perform a "D & C" (dilation and curettage) with the patient under general anesthesia with the old (nineteenth century) Hegar cervical dilators that were exclusively used by the medical school and curettes but with none of the modern vacuum aspiration technology. I had a lot of surgical experience in medical school, internship, and in South America, I was quite confident of my surgical skills, but I had never done exactly this before.

DOI: 10.4324/9781003514961-5

My patient was a young woman who was 17 years old, a senior in high school from a neighboring state, who wanted to go to medical school and become an anesthesiologist. She was terrified, also. I reassured her as much as I could and told her that Dr. Herr, who was quite experienced, would be helping me.

The procedure went well and exactly as planned, and I was tremendously relieved that we had got through it safely without my causing her any injury. I went to the head of the table and told her that we were finished and that she did well, and she cried with relief. So did I. Tears came to my eyes.

It was a very intense moment. I had discovered a new meaning in practicing medicine, a new form of helping another human being in distress and whose life was threatened in various ways by a medical condition that I could change as a physician and surgeon. It gave me a new understanding of the Oath of Maimonides:

May I never see in the patient anything but a fellow creature in pain.

At the end of the day, I thanked Ben and Earl, the nurses, counselors, and other staff members for an important and memorable experience. It was a revelation for me.

About a year later, when I resigned my job at OEO, Ben Branch learned of my departure and invited me to come back to Preterm for a few weeks and conduct a management study of the whole operation.

In the intervening time, I had not only attended the U.S. Supreme Court hearing for Dr. Vuitch's case in January 1971, I had joined him in his office in downtown Washington where he was performing surgical abortions for $300 per patient. He had been a surgeon in World War II and had performed tens of thousands of abortions in Yugoslavia, his native country, before coming to the United States. He had been operating illegally in Washington for years.

In Dr. Vuitch's office, there was no counseling, no lab work, no physical exam, a few forms to fill out, payment was made, and the patient went into the operating room. Dr. Vuitch spoke to me about his work while he was operating, bloody instruments clattering into a basin. He was a burly, vigorous man who operated with supreme confidence. He had performed tens of thousands. if not hundreds of thousands, of abortions.

Dr. Vuitch spoke about going to the U.S. Supreme Court, which was still considering his case. "*I go zer and plant zee flag!*" he exclaimed. His was the first abortion case heard by the Court. He had been arrested for performing an abortion without showing, as required by the Washington, D.C., statute, that the abortion was being performed "for the health of the woman." Dr. Vuitch claimed that he was doing exactly that.

Ultimately, the *Vuitch* decision was muddled and did not come down with a clear prohibition against abortion or nullification of the law. The lower court's dismissal of Dr. Vuitch's prosecution on the grounds that the D.C. statute was unconstitutional was overturned, but the Supreme Court did not press for his prosecution.

Later that year, on December 13, 1971, Sarah Weddington argued the *Roe v. Wade* case before the U.S. Supreme Court for the first time. She was 26 years old at the time, had practiced little law beyond a divorce case and family will settlement, and had bypassed the appeals process to come directly to the Supreme Court. In spite of an inappropriate attempted humor by the attorney arguing for Texas, Sarah retained her poise and presented her case. She was articulate, clear in her arguments, and extremely well prepared for the justices' questions. She appeared to carry the day, but the Court had only seven justices at the time, and she was invited to argue the case once more in 1972.

The companion case for the case was *Doe v. Bolton*, which was argued by Atlanta civil rights attorney Margie Pitts Hames, whose argument attacked the hospital's requirement for a committee to decide whether a woman could have an abortion.

After the arguments, Sarah and Margie invited me to join them for coffee in the cafeteria downstairs, which I did. Soon after we sat down, Chief Justice Warren Burger and Justice Harry Blackmun sat down at the next table. Justice Blackmun gave us a friendly wave and a smile, and Burger also gave us a friendly smile. I was stunned to be in their presence.

Abortion in New York; APHA standards

The first year at OEO for me was marked by the new experience of working in a government agency with multimillion dollar programs to understand, evaluate, and guide on the basis of my own clinical experience and training in public health. I was impressed by the idealism of the people at OEO in all the departments, especially our own, which was staffed primarily by young people, some younger than me, several of whom had worked as Peace Corps volunteers in India. They wanted to Do Good. The chief of our office, George Contis, was a little older and had experience as a distinguished public health pediatrician. Even though he came from a deeply traditional and culturally conservative Greek family and was a strong Republican, he treated all of us with affable good humor in spite of the fact that we were clearly of a new generation that was informal, liberal to progressive, and ready to implement new ideas about how society should operate, especially for women. I, for one, had long hair, sideburns, declined to wear a tie, and wore a Shipibo bead necklace from the Amazon instead of standard business dress. We were ready to make things happen, and we did. We saw our program as an enormous lifetime opportunity to get help to poor families and especially women who desperately needed to control their own fertility for reasons of their own health and the health of their families. My experience with the Appalachian coal miner families in the hills of Tennessee exemplified the problems that we were tackling.

Almost immediately after I arrived at OEO, we learned of the decision of the New York legislature to legalize abortion in that state by passing a bill – with a one-vote margin cast famously by legislator Constance Cook – that was signed into law by New York governor Nelson Rockefeller.

At the same time, we were approached by Dr. Don Harting, a retired pediatrician, who came to us from the American Public Health Association with a request for OEO to provide money for the newly created APHA Task Force on Family Planning Methods. Dr. Harting had assembled a group of nationally recognized experts on various aspects of fertility control to form this group. Their purpose was to set out standards of care for, among other things, abortion services and voluntary sterilization. The group would be chaired by Dr. Carl Tyler, head of the Abortion Surveillance Unit at the Centers for Disease Control in Atlanta, and he would be accompanied by several of his CDC staff members, including Dr. John Asher and nurse Judith Bourne. Among the other distinguished members of this group were Dr. Bill Rashbaum, a practicing obstetrician/gynecologist in New York who had been performing abortions and was a recognized expert on the subject; Dr. Jean Pakter, head of the maternal health section of the New York City Department of Health; and Dr. Sadja Goldsmith, an idealistic young obstetrician/gynecologist who had set up teen clinics in the San Francisco Bay area to help young people secure access to birth control methods. The Haight-Ashbury / hippie / drugs-and-sex / youth culture in San Francisco, especially, had resulted in a large number of unplanned pregnancies and sexually transmitted diseases among young people, which needed attention. A San Francisco psychologist, Harvey Karman, had devised a small flexible plastic cannula with a notch at the tip that could be used for an early vacuum aspiration abortion. This instrument was rapidly gaining popularity throughout the nation. Sadja was a key person who was at the center of these developments.

The most distinguished member of the APHA group was Dr. Christopher Tietze, who was head of research at the Population Council. Dr. Tietze, who left Vienna just ahead of the Nazis takeover of Austria in 1938, had been a key consultant in the formulation of the 1970 New York abortion law, and he was currently conducting the Joint Program for the Study of Abortion (JPSA) for the Population Council to document the clinical facts of different abortion procedures, such as complication rates by week of pregnancy. He was working closely with the CDC Abortion Surveillance Unit. These studies served as the essential public health guide to the safety and risks of abortion services when they were first published in 1972.

As the person in our office in charge of program development, my task was to respond to the grant request from Dr. Harting and to be the liaison person from OEO to the APHA committee. Our first meeting was in New York City in the summer of 1970, and I was astounded by the depth of experience and expertise in that small group. All members were dedicated without reservation to making safe abortion services as available as possible to women throughout the country. They were also dedicated to gathering as much scientific information about abortion as possible, and they were supremely prepared to do it. It was an amazing collection of brilliant, dedicated people.

During this first visit, I was invited to go with Dr. Jean Pakter to the first meeting of the New York City Board of Health, chaired by Dr. Ed Daily, where the board members would discuss the new abortion law and decide what restrictions would apply to the services. Would abortions be allowed on an outpatient basis or would they have to be performed in hospitals? If allowed in outpatient clinics, up to what point in pregnancy could they be performed and under what conditions? What would be the licensure requirements for those who were performing or assisting with abortions? What were the techniques and operative procedures that would be allowed or required? These questions were being discussed even though various abortion clinics had already been opened in New York City.

One clinic was opened in early 1970 by Dr. Karl Fossum, a New York psychiatrist originally from Sweden, who felt the urgent need to make abortion services available as soon as possible now that it was legal in that state. He soon found himself overwhelmed with the demand and hired Dr. Thomas Kerenyi, a Hungarian obstetrician/gynecologist who was at Mount Sinai Hospital, to organize the abortion services. Dr. Kerenyi had already developed techniques for performing second trimester abortions using the saline method, which required injecting hypertonic saline solution into the amniotic cavity. Following the lead of his mentor at Mount Sinai, Dr. Alan Guttmacher, Dr. Kerenyi had become a strong advocate for the availability of safe abortion services.

One of Dr. Kerenyi's vivid experiences that reinforced this commitment was caring for a young woman who presented in his emergency room with catastrophic vaginal bleeding one evening. She reported that she had experienced a miscarriage. On examination, Dr. Kerenyi discovered a white Lysol tablet high in her vagina. The patient had placed this poisonous substance into her vagina in her attempt to abort a pregnancy. The corrosive

Lysol had eroded through the wall of her vagina into an artery, and she was bleeding to death.

Dr. Kerenyi and his colleagues repaired this grievous injury and offered to perform the abortion for her, but she refused. She came back a few weeks later following another attempted abortion with a high fever and her lower abdomen full of pus from an incompletely performed abortion procedure. It was necessary to remove her uterus and ovaries to save her life. She was 17 years old. From this experience, Dr. Kerenyi became more committed to the availability of safe abortions for women, and he spent much of his life and career doing that. This led to his role in establishing one of the first abortion clinics in New York City and in the nation.

On this same trip, I was invited to go with Sadja Goldsmith to a new high-volume abortion clinic that was operating in the basement of an office building in Greenwich Village. The clinic doctors were using Harvey Karman's plastic cannula for the early abortions, and they were performing upwards of one hundred abortions or more per week. Women were coming from all over the United States and many foreign countries to have abortions in New York City. Harvey was present at the clinic with his associate Merle Goldberg when we visited.

Meanwhile, George and I were being asked to prepare a paper for the *American Journal of Public Health* concerning the availability of abortions for military personnel and the official policies of the federal government concerning abortion services. After reviewing all the information with George, I wrote the paper, George reviewed it and added his information, and George presented the paper at the annual meeting of the American Public Health Association in Houston that year (1970).

Many of the national leaders of the family planning field were present, including Harriet Pilpel, the attorney who had successfully argued the landmark *Griswold v. Connecticut* case before the U.S. Supreme Court. The *Griswold* decision established the constitutional right of privacy for married couples to use contraception, a use that had been prohibited under Connecticut law. Carl Tyler and his Abortion Surveillance Unit staff from the CDC was present also and presented a paper. Our paper from OEO, "US Government policy on abortion," was published early the next year in the *American Journal of Public Health*.[1]

In the context of the current national political hysteria concerning abortion in the United States, it is worth quoting from this article: "*The first [consideration (in policy choices)] is the role of abortion in the total context of health services. Our unofficial position is that abortion should be an essential part of complete family planning and comprehensive health services.*" (italics supplied)

Also at this time, various techniques and procedures for performing second trimester abortions, which were much more complicated and carried greater risks for women, were emerging. Among these was the "saline" abortion, which required injecting a hypertonic saline solution into the woman's uterus after the pregnancy was advanced enough for there to be amniotic fluid surrounding the fetus. Although it was generally effective, there were many hazards associated with saline abortions that included fatal derangement of the woman's electrolyte balance – too much or too little salt in her circulating blood, for example – that caused physicians to look for safer ways of performing second trimester abortions.[2]

One was the use of synthetic prostaglandins injected into the uterus. Prostaglandins occur naturally in the body, but concentrated synthetic prostaglandins will cause the uterus to contract, and medical scientists began using them with great effectiveness to induce abortions in the second trimester. One of the problems was that many of the fetuses were born alive or with agonal movements, which was highly disconcerting to the medical and nursing staffs of hospitals where this was occurring, and especially disconcerting to the patients.

In 1971 the APHA, Planned Parenthood, and various other organizations organized an international conference on abortion techniques and services. This conference, which was held at the Barbizon Plaza Hotel in New York City, brought together experts on abortion from all parts of the world, including Doctors Mark Bygdeman from Sweden and Sultan Karim from Malaysia. Also among those attending was Dr. Rea Ravenholt, head of the U.S. AID population program, who I had met at the 1967 IPPF Congress in Santiago, Chile. It was a remarkable world review of the global status of abortion services.[3] Dr. Thomas Kerenyi from New York was the leading expert on the saline abortion technique, which was being eclipsed by widespread use of prostaglandins. The latter were being advocated by Dr. Bygdeman and Dr. Karim. There was considerable controversy over which methods were best and safest.

One of the persons speaking was Dr. Zigmond Lebenson, who had written about the psychiatric aspects of unwanted pregnancy and abortion. When he mentioned something about how some pregnant women felt that they were stricken with a serious illness, I decided to approach him and tell him about my new paper on the epidemiology of pregnancy that had just been published in *Family Planning Perspectives*. He had seen my paper and told me about a textbook by François Mauriceau published in 1668 in which Mauriceau had called pregnancy a *"malade de neuf mois"* (a disease of nine months).[4] He told me I could find Hugh Chamberlen's 1680 translation of Mauriceau's book in the National Library of Medicine, and I did.[5] I found the indispensable quote and used in later publications.

At the end of this incredibly interesting and important conference with the world leaders of my field, I went down to the Village Gate to hear my hero in jazz music, Ahmad Jamal, play his gig there. As usual, his group started by playing his classic arrangement of "Poinciana." It was addictive. As I was preparing to leave, I saw Jamal sitting by himself having dinner. I spoke to him, he invited me to sit down, and I asked if I could study jazz piano with him. He said he would be happy to be my jazz piano teacher. Unfortunately, I did not find time to do that, and I have regretted it ever since, although we got acquainted on several other occasions. I did get to study classical and Brazilian jazz guitar with Frank Mullen, who was Charlie Byrd's partner, and who taught just down the street from where I worked in Washington.

Leaving OEO: clinical experience with abortion

The beginning of 1971 was marked by the U.S. Supreme Court hearing of the *Vuitch* case, which I attended, and punctuated in December by the U.S. Supreme Court arguments on the *Roe v. Wade* case.

At OEO it was increasingly evident in early 1972 that there was permanent conflict between Dr. George Contis in our office and his nominal superior, Dr. Leon Cooper, head of the Office of Health Affairs. It was also increasingly obvious that Nixon, who was running for reelection, was determined to close down OEO as a symbol of previous

Democratic administrations, whose legislative efforts were anathema to conservative Republicans. They hated the efforts within OEO to provide legal assistance to poor communities and citizens and to support health and nutrition and community organization programs. Republicans saw the OEO Community Action Programs as daggers at the heart of Republican power since most if not all of the CAP centers were in communities heavily populated by members of minority groups who voted Democratic. Hence, Howard Phillips, the Nixon White House hatchet man, and, hence, the rapid turnover of OEO directors, who were political appointees moving on to higher level positions (Don Rumsfeld, Frank Carlucci, Philip Sanchez), and whose transitory leadership signaled a lack of commitment if not hostility to OEO's principal goals.

OEO was, of course, a main engine of Lyndon Johnson's War on Poverty, which not only attempted to lift people from poverty but also worked to enable them to shape their own destinies. These goals and programs stood in direct conflict with Republican political objectives, which were focused on the maintenance of white authoritarian political power throughout the country. It was no coincidence that this paralleled the Nixon White House "Southern strategy," which set out to get the white supremacists in the Democratic Party in the southern United States to switch their support to the Republican Party. As history shows, this strategy was completely successful and shifted the balance of power in U.S. politics and government over the next 50 years.

Somehow, the news that I was leaving OEO reached various people, and I received important invitations, some of which I accepted. One of them was to be interviewed for the position of medical director of the Planned Parenthood Federation of America, whose offices were in New York City. This position also carried the title of vice president for medical affairs. I considered it one of the most important public health jobs in the world, if not *the* most important. But I didn't want to live in New York City. I wanted to go back to Colorado. The idea of working in a Manhattan skyscraper office building did not appeal to me even though I found New York City an interesting place.

A second invitation was from Ben Branch at Preterm Clinic. Ben wanted me to evaluate their operation. "Tell us what we're doing wrong," he said. "I couldn't see anything you were doing wrong when I was there last year," I said. "Come back and take a look," he said. So I stayed in Washington another three weeks.

By this time, Dr. Jane Hodgson was the medical director of Preterm. Ben had gone to part-time status. Dr. Hodgson was already legendary for her challenge of the Minnesota abortion law, which landed her in jail. No firebrand, Jane was a pleasant, calm, self-confident middle-aged professional woman who was clearly an expert in her field and who was totally dedicated to the purpose of helping women have safe abortions. She welcomed me and the project for which I had been invited.

It was also my first contact with Dr. Mike Burnhill, who, with his father, had been one of the inventors of one of the first intrauterine devices, the Birnberg Bow, which I had learned about in my third year of medical school. Mike was a delightful, energetic person with a great sense of humor and a passion for his work. He spoke to the patient as he was performing the abortion and made everyone in the operating room at ease. There were several other physicians from Tennessee and other states who were helping at the clinic.

At Preterm, there was a professional counseling staff, and each patient was assigned to a counselor, who spent individual private time with the patient and explained all the procedures she would experience. I was impressed with the level of total individual support for each patient and the highly modern, well-kept facility.

My experience as a participant-observer (as an anthropologist visiting an exotic tribe) included performing about a half-dozen abortions under the supervision of Mike Burnhill and Jane Hodgson. The procedure was not complicated, but it had to be done carefully to assure complete emptying of the uterus to prevent complications.

In my management report, I raised questions only about the advisability and necessity of a sex education project aimed at both the staff and the patients that included all patients. The sex education was a good thing for those who requested it, but it appeared that the time and energy spent on it was a distraction from the main purpose of performing safe abortions for women who needed and wanted them. One staff member commented, "Teaching people how to screw is fine, but we have other more important things to do."

What Preterm really offered was a new model of medical care that gave the patient maximum emotional and social support as well as excellence in surgical care. It was a model I would follow later when the need arose.

Several years later, I combined my observations at Preterm with the observations of two of my colleagues in my private medical practice in a report for anthropologists about abortion clinics as organizations, "Administrative incongruity and authority conflict in four abortion clinics," which was published in *Human Organization*, the journal of the Society for Applied Anthropology.[6]

The third invitation I received was from Leveo Sanchez, a New Mexico businessman who had founded Development Associates, a consulting business that helped government programs with evaluation and improvements in organization. Leveo invited me to lunch, and, by the end of the lunch, I was the medical director of a family planning training program for the Rocky Mountain region of the U.S. Department of Health, Education and Welfare (HEW). Region VIII consisted of Colorado, Wyoming, Utah, Montana, and the Dakotas. I was to travel to visit federally financed family planning programs in these states and conduct training programs for their personnel in Denver. It was officially a part-time job, but I would be on the road a lot visiting these programs. I was to begin as soon as I returned to Colorado at the end of the summer.

Leveo also made me the medical director of his Latin American family planning training program, and I soon left for South America with Eric Hoffman, who had been the Peace Corps director in Ecuador. We visited programs in Colombia, Venezuela, Peru, Ecuador, and Panama. At our last stop in Panama, I noticed with alarm that I had almost complete atrophy of all my right arm and shoulder muscles, which I concluded was the result of my having been mugged one evening in Washington. I went to see one of my medical school classmates who was doing his residency in surgery at Gorgas Hospital, where I had done my internship, and he confirmed my suspicions. His diagnosis was that I had a brachial plexus stretch injury from getting mugged in Washington and that I would be lucky to get back any function much less full function in my right arm and shoulder.

After returning to Washington from this trip, I headed back to Colorado.

Notes

1 Contis, G., and Hern, W.M. U.S. government policy on abortion. *American Journal of Public Health* 61:1038–41, May 1971. https://www.drhern.com/wp-content/uploads/2018/06/usgovtabpolicy.pdf
2 Kerenyi, T.D. Outpatient intra-amniotic injection of hypertonic saline. *Clinical Obstetrics and Gynecology* 14:124–40, March 1971. PMID: 5568237 DOI: 10.1097/00003081-197103000-00012
3 Lewit, S (ed.). *Abortion Techniques and Services: Proceedings of the Conference*, New York, June 3–6, 1971. Amsterdam: Excerpta Medica, 1972.
4 Mauriçeau, F. *Des maladies des femmes grosses et accouchées*. Paris, 1668
5 Chamberlen, H. *The Diseases of Women with Child, and in Child-Bed*. Translation of *Des maladies des femmes grosses et accouchées* by François Mauriceau. London: 1673.
6 Hern, W.M., Gold, M., and Oakes, A. Administrative incongruence and authority conflict in four abortion clinics. *Human Organization* 36:376–83, 1977. https://www.drhern.com/wp-content/uploads/2018/05/aiac-four-ab-clinics.pdf

5   Making safe abortion real for women

Rolling across the eastern high plains of Colorado in the summer of 1972, watching Pike's Peak and other high mountains come into view, I began to feel at home again. Except for occasional brief family visits and skiing, I had been gone for over seven years in Latin America and on the East Coast. I missed Colorado. An offer of the best public health job in the world in New York City could not keep me away.

It was the first time in my life I had felt free from any serious immediate obligation.

My only job at the moment, which I had not yet begun, was as the medical director of a family planning advisory program with a private consulting firm, Development Associates. The program was set up to help family planning programs, now funded by the Title X Act, get started and provide these services for low-income families in the Rocky Mountain region (region VIII: Colorado, Wyoming, Montana, the Dakotas, and Utah). I was to conduct training seminars in Denver and travel to community clinics in all those states. But it was only part-time work. To make up the difference, I signed up as an attending physician in the emergency room of Denver General Hospital (affectionately known among health-care workers as "The Saturday Night Knife and Gun Club"). I was paid $9/hour.

One evening, I helped unload a victim of a neighborhood fight from the arriving ambulance. There was a knife sticking out of his chest. As we wheeled him down the hall to the operating room, the knife wavered back and forth with each heartbeat. He survived.

Brain-dead motorcycle crash and gun-shot victims were brought in, still alive but with massive head injuries. My former mentor in the kidney transplant program from CU medical school, Dr. Tom Starzl, showed up with his retinue, black ravens on their shoulders, to salvage the kidneys. Never a dull moment.

My consulting job took me to dozens of small towns in the northern midwestern states to work with the idealistic and dedicated people who were setting up and running the family planning clinics. I had met some of them at the training seminars in Denver and others for the first time in their natural habitats. There were, of course, rainbow trout needing and yearning to be caught in the Yellowstone River. But they played hard to get. It was a battle of wits, and sometimes I won and had a delicious trout dinner.

I was astonished to learn that in some small towns in Montana, Wyoming, and Utah, especially, doctors who began helping in the family planning programs were forced to leave town by religious conservatives. The same was true in other states.

Dr. Jim Armstrong, a family doctor in Kalispell, became one of my best friends, and we made long backpacking trips into the Montana wilderness. We had different approaches to the experience. I would be carrying 50 or 60 pounds in my pack, which included a 4"x 5" classical view camera with all its paraphernalia as well as survival gear, stopping to

DOI: 10.4324/9781003514961-6

take a picture of each animal, flower, rock, bug, and breathtaking view, and a Canon F-1 35mm camera with a heavy 400mm lens for wildlife plus other lenses. On the other hand, Jim's idea was to run through the forest with a 20-pound pack while scaring all the animals out of the way. My footprints were visible in the otherwise smooth glacier-polished rocks after we passed by. But Jim was the one who ran out of gas on Boulder Pass, so we had to camp illegally with his .357 Magnum bear repellent under his pillow. At dawn, I got one of the best landscape photos in my life with my view camera.

Jim Armstrong was one of those quintessential ideal Americans who was the pillar of his community and his society. He was a graduate of Princeton University. He and his wife were leaders in their church and had two wonderful children. Jim was on the town school board, he led a Boy Scout troop, and his family medical practice helped thousands of people in and around Kalispell. His favorite activity was going into the remotest parts of the Glacier National Park wilderness by himself and enjoying the beauty and solitude of that place.

With my help, Jim began performing early surgical abortions in his Kalispell office. He led the legal fight to protect the right to safe abortion in Montana. Anti-abortion firebombs twice destroyed his office. The complete losses included Jim's treasured copy of that dawn landscape photo that I had made on our first trip into Glacier National Park in 1978.

Anti-abortion fanatics destroyed his medical practice. They later destroyed the abortion practice of Susan Cahill, the physician's assistant who Jim taught to do early abortions.

During the fall of 1972, I started getting ready to build a house for myself on some property in the mountains west of Denver that I had bought along with my parents while I was working in Washington. I had always wanted to live in the Colorado mountains. I

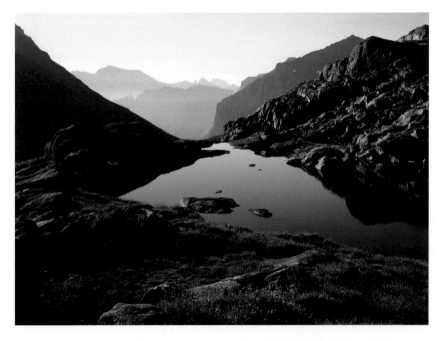

Figure 5.1 Tarn on Boulder Pass, Glacier National Park, 1978. Photo © Warren Martin Hern

designed the house with the help of an architect, got a construction loan, and my father agreed to build it for me. He was a highly experienced carpenter/contractor who was skilled at many trades. We hired one of my sister's friends to be the laborer to help my dad. I would help with chores in between my other two jobs.

We bulldozed a small site near the top of a hill at 9,600 ft. elevation with a spectacular view of the Continental Divide, and I helped my father pour the cement footings for the house in mild autumn weather. A curious deer rambled onto the building site while my father was building the footing forms. We were headed for one of the coldest winters in Colorado history with heavy snowfall at that altitude. We worked in freezing weather, sometimes in sub-zero temperatures, most of the time.

Because of national news about my work in Washington, D.C., I began receiving calls from political people asking for my help. The main request was from the McGovern campaign, and I joined with some other physicians to start the Colorado Physicians for McGovern organization. Some people wanted me to run for Congress, but I had no desire for that even though I was strongly against the war in Vietnam.

After working in Washington, I decided that I would rather inform and influence people in power than to try to seek to have power myself. In the process, though, I found myself meeting some really incredible and important people, such as Archibald Cox, who had been fired by Nixon during the "Saturday Night Massacre," and Pat Schroeder, a brilliant and charismatic young lawyer who was elected to the first of her 12 terms in Congress representing Denver. We became fast friends.

In preparation for my family planning seminars, I got back in touch with my former and new colleagues at the University of Colorado Medical School, including Dr. Bill Droegemueller, who taught me about the use of *Laminaria japonicum*, a sterilized seaweed stalk from Japan. It had clear advantages in safety over the standard method of dilating the cervix for an abortion by forcing steel metal dilators through the cervix to stretch it open.

That November, just after the reelection of Nixon, my article, "The Politics of Abortion," was published in *The Progressive* magazine alongside an article by George McGovern criticizing U.S. policy in Vietnam.[1] In the article, I described the national efforts to legalize abortion on a state-by-state basis and offered my advice that male politicians had better start listening to women. Two months later, on January 22, 1973, the *Roe v. Wade* decision was handed down by the U.S. Supreme Court legalizing abortion throughout the nation.

Soon after this decision came down, letters to the editor criticizing it began appearing in the *Denver Post*. I responded to some and defended *Roe v. Wade* on the grounds of women's health and public health. I stated that women need to be able to make these decisions.

A few weeks later, I got a call from Mort Stern, editor of the *Denver Post*, asking me to have lunch with him at the Platte River Yacht Club (the Platte River is historically known to be "an inch deep and a mile wide"). I agreed, and, when we met, Mort asked me to explain the *Roe vs. Wade* decision to him. I attempted to do so, then he asked me to write an editorial for him for the paper explaining this in detail, which I did. The editorial, "Abortion: The need for rational policy and safe standards," was published in the *Denver Post* on May 27.[2] But before that happened, I got a call from a doctor in Boulder, Robert McFarland, asking me if I would be interested in helping a group in Boulder start a private, non-profit abortion clinic there.

Although I was surprised by the call, I said I would be interested in doing that. I felt that the Supreme Court decision wouldn't mean anything if physicians weren't ready to perform abortions. Since I had some experience and knew how to perform early abortions, I thought I would help the clinic get started, work there for a year or so, save some money, then go back to school in North Carolina to get my Ph.D. in epidemiology. I wanted to have a career in teaching and research. I thought epidemiology was the most interesting and stimulating subject in medicine and public health.

"How did you get my name, and why are you calling me?" I asked McFarland. "Ben Greer gave me your name." Months before, as I was preparing for my family planning seminars, I had visited Ben and other colleagues at the CU medical school inquiring about the latest technologies in contraception, abortion, and sterilization. Ben had told me about some new aspects of vacuum aspiration abortion (which I had learned about and practiced at Preterm in Washington, D.C.), and he told me of a new book, *Abortion Techniques*, by two New York physicians, Neubart and Schulman.[3] It didn't occur to me that I would find an immediate need for these publications for my own medical practice. I just wanted some background information to share with my trainees.

Soon after my call from Bob McFarland, I attended a meeting with the group that he had mentioned. Our meeting was in a large room with cushions to sit on but without much furniture in the private medical office of Dr. Ran Sclar, a Boulder psychiatrist. The ten or so members of the group were diverse: one was a publisher of a right-wing magazine for mercenary soldiers of fortune, one was an accomplished laboratory scientist, another was a local businesswoman who had seen terrible results from illegal abortion, and another was a graduate student in sociology. And there was Bob, a family practice physician who was deeply involved with issues of social justice and public health care who had helped start a drug rehabilitation program for local hippies and who later helped open a general health clinic for low-income citizens of Boulder.

No one knew anything about abortion except they thought it was a good idea to open the clinic. They wanted me to organize the clinic and set it up. I wrote a program plan and budget with myself as the medical director and the sociology graduate student, Roger W., as the executive director. Roger found a vacant office at 1000 Alpine up the street from Boulder Community Hospital, and the board signed a lease. But the anti-abortion tenants, including a plastic surgeon and an obstetrician/gynecologist, raised hell with the building's owner in Kansas City, and the lease was canceled. We found another place, a remodeled house on Broadway that had been used as a real estate office, and I set about arranging for the equipment, such as an operating room table, operating room light, autoclaves, instruments, and other materials we needed for patient care. I installed the operating room light and other equipment myself.

As we were preparing to open the clinic to see patients in the fall of 1973, I attended, as usual, the annual meeting of the American Public Health Association, which was held that year in Los Angeles. At a session on abortion, I found myself sitting next to Carl Tyler, a friend and colleague from my days at OEO when Carl, a nationally known obstetrician/gynecologist, had created and become chief of the Abortion Surveillance Unit at the Centers for Disease Control in Atlanta. He and his team were in the process of defining the best practices in abortion services nationally by looking at complication and death rates.

When I told Carl that I was planning to use overnight laminaria placement for cervical dilation instead of conventional manual dilation with steel rods, Carl gave me a baleful look of disapproval and told me that he would worry about a high rate of serious and potentially fatal infections with this protocol. I told him I was going to be using a very thorough antiseptic and sterile technique and coated the laminaria in antibiotic ointment before inserting, but his glowering response to this unconventional approach made me nervous, to say the least. I wanted him of all people on my side. We were now under national scrutiny.

In my conversations with my friend, Dr. Bill Rashbaum, from whom I had learned some abortion procedures at the ParkMed clinic where he was working in New York City, I learned that his chief nurse, AnnaGail Oakes, had just moved to Colorado with her husband. "She's the best," he said. I found Gail and asked her to be our head nurse. Since she had helped with many thousands more abortions than I had performed, it was a great good fortune to have her with us.

I organized the operating room and a recovery room, and we soon had a volunteer staff of abortion counselors, one of whom Ran hired as the head counselor who had worked for a time at a busy abortion clinic in New York City.

Rob Pudim, a local lab technician, biologist, and lepidopterist who was also a brilliant artist and political cartoonist, took over the lab work, at which he was highly skilled.

There was no money for the equipment lease, which was for about $10,000, so I signed the lease. I found what we needed at a surgical supply house in Denver. This included a very large hospital-size autoclave for sterilizing instruments. I decided that all instruments, including vaginal speculums, would be individually wrapped and sterilized in the autoclave. This was not always standard practice.

To have adequate medical records for each patient, I prepared forms for each patient to complete and drew up an operative record for each patient's procedure showing the physical exam, vital signs, lab work, procedure times, blood loss, and tissue weight. The back page was for the follow-up exams three weeks after the procedure.

Since I had some nice carved African masks from my visit to West Africa in 1961, I put up several of them around the clinic for decoration.

I then got the names of as many physicians as I could find in the telephone books and medical society records to inform the medical community that we would be performing abortions for patients in the first trimester. I visited several physicians in Boulder who we knew to be sympathetic or at least neutral about our work, the principal one being Dr. Sherburne Macfarlan, who had been practicing obstetrics and gynecology in Boulder for about ten years at that time. Mac was friendly but very professional and asked me about my previous experience in surgery and in performing abortions in particular. I had performed about a half-dozen first-trimester vacuum aspiration abortions at Preterm, and I described my experiences in general surgery as a student, intern, and physician in Brazil and Peru. His help was critical in the next months. He had treated many women suffering from severe complications from illegal abortions and strongly supported our efforts.

One doctor, Jake, who was about to retire, was very supportive and gave me a set of Hegar dilators (designed in the nineteenth century), the kind I had used in medical school, and some good advice on managing patients.

The next challenge was getting hospital privileges at the local hospital.

After completing my application forms and submitting them to the hospital staff office, I was told to come to the regular monthly OB/GYN department staff meeting on Monday, November 5 at 7 AM. It was normally held in a corner of the hospital dining room set off by some sliding plastic curtain walls.

At 7 AM on the appointed morning, I found the hospital dining room, but it took me a few minutes to see the partially closed-off area where a meeting was going on. I cautiously parted two of the sliding walls and looked in. I didn't recognize anyone at first.

The conversation completely stopped. I walked in and was offered a seat. There was what is politely called "an awkward silence." Dr. Ned Brown, my former OB/GYN attending physician from when I was in medical school, who was apparently chairman of the department, was leading the meeting. He asked me to identify myself, which I did. He told me that they were expecting me and that they would come to my business in a few minutes. My entrance had clearly disrupted the proceedings as I had come in a few minutes after 7. There were about a half-dozen men in suits at the table. There were no women members of the ob/gyn staff.

When the meeting focused on my request for staff membership with admitting privileges, I began to get some harsh questions. Although I had a lot of surgical experience and had performed a few early abortions, and I had a Colorado medical license, I had not done any residency training beyond internship. My home was in the mountains, not in Boulder. There were no other physicians on the staff of the new clinic; I was the medical director. Who was going to take night call for the clinic? I said that I would be doing that 24/7/365.

At this point, a burly man with an aggressive attitude and a Scottish last name asked, in a gravelly voice that would have turned a hardened *mafioso* into ice with fear, "Who's gonna take the *shit* calls?" This man, who we shall call RM, became one of my most vigorous adversaries. He was performing abortions in his office for $135 each and doing "sucks fer bucks," as he put it. I didn't know this at that moment, but he saw the clinic that I was helping start up as highly threatening economic competition.

One of the OB/GYN specialists offered his contemptuous opinion that someone without an ob/gyn residency should not be performing abortions, although the general attitude among his colleagues was that performing abortions was below their status and skill level. It was "scut" work beneath the dignity of real doctors.

In response to RM's outburst, a gentlemanly man, who turned out to be Dr. Art Klemme, an associate of Dr. Sherburne Macfarlan, quietly said he would help me with emergency calls. The rest of the group was silent. My former mentor, Dr. Brown, who I was sure did not recognize me from my days as one of his students, was correct but cold. The committee heard me out, then the meeting was over. I was discouraged. It went downhill from there.

Two days later, we saw our first patients at Boulder Valley Clinic. Even though I felt confident of my skills as a physician and surgeon, I felt out on a limb. I had only done a few abortions, and I knew I had a lot to learn. I had read my Neubart and Schulman book through a dozen times and everything else I could read about abortion.

The "Fight the Abortion Clinic Committee" was now getting headlines by going to the Boulder City Council and demanding that we be shut down. Zenon Raskowski, head of the FTAC Committee, accused me of "corrupting the youth" because the clinic was only a block from the Catholic school. I was pleased to be in the company of Socrates, who had been accused of this same crime in Athens 2,400 years ago.

I heard from my close friend, medical school lab partner and classmate Jerry Hickman, who was a family doctor in Boulder, about a resolution offered at the November meeting of the Boulder County Medical Society. The resolution was that the clinic was a "clear and present danger to health and public welfare." The authors of the resolution wanted it to be sent to the Boulder County Department of Health and to the Colorado Department of Health. Jerry had stood up in the meeting to say that he knew me as a conscientious physician and that the medical society should investigate the clinic before passing such a resolution. A committee was formed to do so. It was headed by Gil Kloster, a plastic surgeon who was against abortion and who, along with Ned Brown, had caused the original lease at 1000 Alpine to be canceled, and Ted Appel, one of the anti-abortion OB/GYNs on the hospital staff.

We started seeing patients on Wednesday, November 8. I had set up the patient protocol to begin with medical history forms that I had designed, routine lab work (urine analysis, hematocrit, rH test), and vital signs (heart rate, temperature, blood pressure) with the patient ready sitting on the exam table in a hospital gown. I would perform a physical exam on each patient, including routine breast exam, bimanual pelvic exam, Pap smear, and gonorrhea culture, and then I would place one laminaria stalk into the cervix to allow the cervix to dilate overnight. The patient was given overnight instructions and a phone number to call in an emergency.

I decided to have each speculum and all instruments washed thoroughly, individually wrapped, and sterilized in the autoclave. A separate instrument pack was made and sterilized for each patient. I wanted there to be a zero risk of infection.

The next morning, the patient would come in, replace her clothes with an exam gown, have her blood pressure taken, and I would remove the laminaria placed the day before. Using a sterile speculum, I would then prep the vagina, put in local anesthesia around the cervix (a paracervical block), place a curved plastic cannula into the cervix and uterus, and apply a vacuum with the standard vacuum aspiration machine. After the uterus was empty, I would then use a small forceps to explore the uterine cavity to assure no tissue was left, perform a sharp curettage with different sizes of curettes to further assure myself that the uterus was empty, then apply a final suction toward the same goal. Then I would have the nurse give the patient an injection of a drug called Methergine to make the uterus contract along with oxytocin, another drug that had the same kind of action.

A basic principle of surgery is the "removal of devitalized tissue" from any wound. This idea comes to us from Ambroise Paré, a seventeenth-century French battlefield surgeon who discovered that cleaning a wound instead of pouring boiling oil into it allowed the soldiers to survive and recover from their injuries. The post-abortion uterus is a raw wound in a closed space, and dead tissue can result in fatal infection. That's why this is so important, and I wanted our patients to have a zero risk of fatal infection or hemorrhage from retained dead tissue.

After each procedure, I would empty the cotton sock in the suction bottle of its contents, spread the tissue out on a glass plate, and look at it carefully over a light box so I could identify the chorionic villi (part of the early placenta). This was the way to be sure that the pregnancy was actually in the uterus instead of in the Fallopian tube. It was also a way to make sure that the abortion was complete. If I could identify parts of the embryo, it could help me determine the actual length of the pregnancy, which was important to know.

As I was doing this, the patient would be taken to the recovery room, where she would have her blood pressure taken and be observed for an hour by the nurse. We would have the patient empty her bladder to allow her uterus to contract. At the end of an hour, the nurse would examine her abdomen to be sure the patient had no abdominal pain that might indicate a uterine perforation, press on her uterus to make sure there was no heavy bleeding, have the patient get dressed, and give the patient her follow-up instructions. Most of the patients came from Boulder or nearby towns, and we would give the patients appointments for a follow-up exam three weeks after the abortion. I did the follow-up exams when the patients returned.

We had about ten patients the first week, and soon we were seeing about 20 patients a week.

We started getting anti-abortion demonstrations in front of the clinic every day.

Two weeks after we started seeing patients, I got an obscene death threat at 3 AM at my isolated house in the mountains, which was 30 miles from Boulder. I was terrified. How did they get my phone number? I expected to be assassinated when I arrived at home late at night (usually 6 or 7 PM) or when I left my home (usually about 7 AM).

The calls continued and got worse. I started sleeping with a rifle by my bed in case someone tried to break into my house during the night. Each morning, I looked out around the house to see if anyone was waiting for me outside. When I came home at night, I waited before I got out of my car so I could escape in it if I needed to do so. I changed the phone number and got it unlisted. I installed an alarm system.

Since I lived so far from Boulder, I had a contractor install a shower in the clinic's single bathroom by the recovery room so I could take a shower after my evening run around the park and so I could sleep at the clinic two nights a week (Wednesday and Friday nights). I couldn't afford to get a place in Boulder. I thought I should be immediately available in case there were an overnight emergency with one of the patients in whom I had placed a laminaria. This became especially important in the winter with heavy snow and slow driving in the mountains.

One day I got a call from Tommy Thompson, the chairman of the Department of Obstetrics and Gynecology at Denver General Hospital, who had defended the legalization of abortion in Colorado in 1967 and had continued to do so. "Be careful," Tommy said. "I don't want to read bad things about you and the clinic in the newspaper." "I'm working hard to make it perfect," I told Tommy. "Safety is my main concern. We have some good people to do this." Message: we were being watched. There was a lot on the line.

At about this time, a new public controversy erupted because Dr. Frank Bolles, a family doctor who was head of the local Right to Life Committee, arranged to have about 80,000 pieces of hideously graphic anti-abortion mail with photos of bloody fetuses in different states of dismemberment sent out to every household in Boulder. Alex Hunter, the district attorney, attacked the mailing. I defended it to the newspapers on grounds of free speech even though I criticized the mailing as obscene, sensational, and hateful. Alex was a friend of mine from college, and I agreed with his anger, but I thought he was wrong.

One day, Bob McFarland told me that he had arranged for me to meet the medical community and general hospital staff at a meeting at the Adventist Memorial Hospital up the hill from Boulder Community Hospital. This would be a good opportunity for me to let the medical community know what we were doing and to get some support.

On the morning of this meeting, Bob introduced me to a room full of about 25 physicians, and I explained our medical/surgical protocol. Then I took questions. I was confronted with a barrage of hostile questions, including an accusation (from one of my former residents in orthopedics from medical school) that I was bringing "socialized medicine" to Boulder.

RM was livid with me, probably because the clinic's board of directors had set our fee at $110, well below RM's fee of $135, but his accusation was that I was damaging his reputation. It turns out that he had fit one of his patients with a diaphragm after performing an abortion on her, but she got pregnant anyway and then came to us for another abortion before accusing him of doing a lousy job of fitting the diaphragm.

Ted Appel accused me of not knowing how to treat a pelvic infection because I had called a colleague at Denver General Hospital to ask for his advice and confirm my understanding of the correct antibiotic dosage for a vaginal infection. That's what teaching hospitals are for. But the doctor I called, who I knew on friendly terms when I was on the emergency room staff, was against abortion, and he used my call as an excuse to call Appel and accuse me of not knowing what I was doing.

My effort to give my patient the best treatment through a routine academic consultation resulted in an unwarranted, vengeful public accusation of incompetence. So much for collegial professional relationships to improve medical care for women. I was getting a taste of the ruthless, cynical, dishonest hypocrisy from anti-abortion members of the medical community that I would encounter on numerous occasions in the future.

When I got back to the clinic to begin seeing patients for the day, I was demoralized. "How did it go?" asked Roger. "Terrible. It was horrible. I got raked over the coals," I replied. "I'm having a great time," said Bob Mcfarland. "Well, I'm not," I said.

I felt like the point of the spear for somebody else's war on society.

A couple of weeks later, I got a call from Appel telling me that he and another member of the medical society committee to investigate the clinic wanted to come over and visit on the first Wednesday of December. I agreed, and Appel showed up with Ned Brown, the head of the OB/GYN department at the hospital.

I showed them the equipment I had set up for our work, including a very large autoclave that blew them away. It was the same size as the one they used at the hospital. I went through our whole protocol for preparing patients, including medical history, lab work, counseling, physical exam, and laminaria placement for cervical dilation, and I then described the procedures that I used in the operating room. I showed them my instrument packs and how I used them. I described the post-op care and recovery room care and showed them the medical charts I had designed. We were now getting patients back for their three-week follow-up exams, and there had been no complications. They invited me to come to the medical society meeting that evening, and then they left. I went back to work.

That evening, I went to the medical society meeting expecting the worst. Outside the meeting, I was met by Bolles's equally anti-abortion medical practice partner, a nice man who had the attitude of a mournful, patronizing Baptist preacher trying to save the soul of a misguided lost member of his flock. He unfortunately had no shepherd's hook. I was polite, listened to his sermon, and thanked him for the instruction.

The meeting opened with a lot of boring medical society business and special meeting notices, and then they got down to brass tacks. The head of the committee to investigate Boulder Valley Clinic, our plastic surgeon adversary Gil Kloster, stood up to speak. "Our committee visited the Boulder Valley Clinic and found that the standard of medical care being practiced there is exemplary and commendable. It is equal to or exceeds the best standards of medical care in the community." Then he sat down. There was a stunned silence. I was pretty stunned myself. Our aggressively hostile OB/GYN adversary, RM, was silent.

At that point, Dr. Bill Takahashi, a Boulder pediatrician, stood up and moved that the motion to declare Boulder Valley Clinic a "clear and present danger to public health" be tabled indefinitely. His motion passed. There followed more boring medical society business including date and time of the next meeting, and then the group dissolved and headed for the bar although without the Baptists.

The last quarterly hospital medical staff meeting was held a week later. There were plenty of high-calorie artery-clogging snacks supplied by the cardiologists to browse on. There was good cheer and comradeship that I observed from a respectful distance. The quarterly staff meeting was the occasion on which specialty committees recommended (or offered) the names of prospective new members of the hospital staff for membership and admitting privileges. The acceptance by voice vote normally took between three and five seconds each between snack bites and wine swallows.

In my case, the debate erupted and lasted for 45 minutes. There was concerted and vociferous opposition based on the fact that I was new in town, I had not done a residency, I hadn't delivered any babies at the hospital, I had long hair, and I didn't know how to do crossword puzzles. A principal objection was that I lived out of town and couldn't be available to be the first to see one of my own patients in the emergency room if she showed up as a local practitioner would be expected to do. Then someone pointed out that the staff had just accepted a neurosurgeon who lived in Denver for full privileges.

After 45 minutes, the crowd began to get restless, the snacks were running out, and Dr. Sherburne Macfarlan stood up. He was one of the most respected and admired physicians in the community. "If Warren has a patient come to the ER and can't get there immediately, I'll see her first and take care of his patient." Then he sat down. My staff membership and admitting privileges were passed by a close vote.

For decades after that, I brought Mac a bottle of champagne every New Year's Eve until I learned that he didn't like champagne. True to his heritage, he drank only single-malt Scotch, whatever that is, so I started getting him that stuff.

And then there was more. By this time, in mid-December, the Fight the Abortion Clinic Committee had successfully prevailed upon the Colorado Board of Health to convene a special meeting to consider the FACC's accusation that we were a "clear and present danger to public health" and that we were running a "butcher shop" a block from the Catholic school. The meeting was held in the Colorado Department of Health building, and I was invited to make a presentation. The entire press corps of Denver was present, including staff from all the TV and radio stations and wire services. The FACC leaders made their hysterical accusations accompanied by statements that we were "killing babies" at the clinic and that we were "corrupting the youth" (thank you again, Socrates). Then I was invited to speak.

Using the intellectually demanding ultra-modern current technology of letter-size IBM printed punch cards with marked places to be punched all around the edges of each card, a beautifully finished chrome single-punch ticket puncher, and an elegant, specially designed blunt ice pick with a nice plastic handle, I had made a card for each patient with punched-out holes for her demographic information, length of pregnancy, measured blood loss, and follow-up information The challenging part of this technology was running the ice pick (too delicate for ice) through all the unpunched holes, lifting up the intact cards in a smooth movement to allow the punched cards to fall out, finding a suitably sharpened wood pencil, and counting all the punched-out cards for that variable. Whew! I had mastered this complex mind-bending technology enough to prepare my report, and I presented this information to the Board of Health in a few minutes.

After giving my credentials and qualifications, I stated that during the first six weeks of operation, we had seen about 100 patients up to 12 weeks of pregnancy, none of them had experienced any complication, and our follow-up rate was almost 100 percent for those who were three weeks post-op or more. I answered questions for ten or 15 minutes. The board discussed the matter for about the same length of time, took a vote, and decided to take no action to close the clinic.

It was an eventful first month for the clinic's operation.

Notes

1 Hern, W.M. The politics of abortion. *The Progressive*, November 1972. https://www.research-gate.net/publication/271966828_The politics_of_abortion
2 Hern, W.M. Abortion: The need for rational policy and safe standards. *Denver Post*, May 27, 1973. https://www.academia.edu/45269732/Abortion_The_Need_for_Rational_Policy_and_Safe_Standards; https://www.drhern.com/wp-content/uploads/2018/06/abortion-policy-safe-standards-1972.pdf
3 Neubart, S., and Schulman, H. *Techniques of Abortion*. Boston: Little, Brown and Company, 1972.

6   "Please don't ever stop doing this"

A few weeks after we opened Boulder Valley Clinic, we observed the first anniversary of the *Roe v. Wade* decision that had made possible what we were doing. It was nothing special. We started a new group of patients that morning. Their abortions would be performed the next day.

The demonstrations and political turmoil outside the clinic continued, but now, what we were doing was normal health care for women.

The patients were almost all young, healthy women in their early twenties who had their lives before them and who wanted to shape their own lives. They weren't ready to start a family, and most weren't sure that the man with whom they became pregnant was their choice for a partner in life. Sometimes the partner came with them, but oftentimes not. Sometimes the partner was supportive, but sometimes not.

Many of the patients were students at the university up the hill, but they were also teachers, clerks, lawyers, nurses, waitresses, budding journalists, airline attendants, carpenters, bank tellers, and truck drivers. One was a telephone lineman (lineperson?). Some were mothers with small children who didn't want more or who just did not feel ready to have another child. They were overwhelmed with the responsibilities of the children they already had. Some never wanted to have children – ever. They wanted to make that choice for themselves.

The common theme was that the current pregnancy, if carried to term, would disrupt everything about their lives as they were living them. It would mean giving up plans to get an education, to learn a profession, to have economic independence, and to be free of unwanted repetitive childbearing. It would mean less money, time, and attention for children they already had. And birth control had failed. Most patients had been using some form of contraception that didn't succeed in preventing the pregnancy. Some were using "cosmic energy," a popular but obviously ineffective option.

Sometimes the circumstances of the pregnancy were funny.

One patient told me that she got pregnant during a "streaking" event. "Streaking" meant that all the students removed all their clothes and went running naked together through the campus for fun, to shock everyone else, and as a kind of rebellion against dull conformity. This particular patient told me that she spotted one of her male friends and they got behind a bush for a while. "How was it?" I asked. "Great," she said with a smile. "Great fun. But now I have this, and I have to have an abortion."

The Defenders of Public Virtue will have a field day with this story.

There were other, sadder stories. Several patients told me that they had been raped and were living through the trauma of that experience. They had abusive partners. The partner left the relationship after the patient discovered she was pregnant. She felt abandoned

DOI: 10.4324/9781003514961-7

and had no way of supporting a child alone. Numerous women told me that they had had illegal abortions in the past and were eloquent in describing what it had been like.

One day, I walked into the operating room to do the patient's physical exam and laminaria placement as the first step of her abortion procedure, and she was shaking uncontrollably. I remember her vividly. She was in her surgical gown, she had red hair, and she was in her mid-thirties. Before going ahead, I stopped and asked her, "What's wrong? What's bothering you?" She was terrified. "Tell me how you feel," I said.

"It's so different," she said. "You're a doctor. It's clean. The lights are on. The windows are open." Then she told me about her illegal abortion she had had many years before. It was the most frightening and humiliating experience of her life. She looked up at me and said, "Please don't ever stop doing this." So I didn't.

Aside from being fanatically obsessed with patient safety, I had an underlying fear of something going catastrophically wrong that would mean a major complication or death for a patient. This anxiety was increased when I found myself performing a procedure on a patient whose pregnancy was much further advanced than I had anticipated. There was no ultrasound for preoperative diagnosis of the length of pregnancy. I was at the mercy of the patient's history of the date of her last menstrual period (which was often incorrect or misleading) and my own physical exam of the patient via a bimanual exam (one hand on the abdomen to feel the uterus from outside the body and the other gloved fingers in the vagina to feel it from below so I could get a sense of the uterine size – the only way to make that judgment). It was very easy to be wrong.

One day a procedure that I began on a woman (Mary) who was older than most (about 40 years old) turned into a frightening experience because it quickly became apparent that she was at least a month further along that I thought. She was about 15 weeks pregnant, and I had never done a procedure with the pregnancy that advanced. I feared for the patient's life. I did not have the proper instruments to do this procedure, but I improvised and got through it. Her blood loss was more than usual but not catastrophic. The fetal tissue was much larger and more identifiable than what I had come to expect in a first trimester abortion procedure. After the procedure, I was so shaken that I had to leave the operating area for an hour just to recover my composure. I was alarmed at how easy it was to get into this extremely difficult situation.

In my Neubart and Schulman *Abortion Techniques* book, I had read Dr. Neubart's account of the use by Japanese physicians of a serial multiple laminaria technique for later or more complicated abortions, especially for patients with a hydatidiform mole (an abnormal pregnancy that looks like a bunch of white grapes). In this protocol, the physician would place one or more laminaria in the cervix to begin cervical dilation, leaving it in overnight, then begin changing and enlarging the number of laminaria each day until the uterus expelled the pregnancy.

One day, I encountered a situation similar to Mary's, but this time, I discovered that the pregnancy was about a month further along than I thought *before* I started the abortion procedure. Both her own doctor and I had determined that she was about 12 weeks pregnant, which was consistent with her menstrual dates, and I had placed a single laminaria in her cervix the first day. But when I examined her on the second day prior to starting the abortion, I realized that she might be at least one month further along. Being off one month on the menstrual dates was pretty common, and I then estimated that she was 16 weeks pregnant. At that, I stopped what I was doing and went to the head of the exam table to talk with the patient. I told her what the situation was and presented her with some alternatives. First, I could remove the laminaria and send her on her way with the hope that nothing would happen and she could continue the pregnancy, or she might be able to find someone who would do a saline injection abortion for her (the customary second trimester procedure in 1974). Third, I could try the serial multiple laminaria protocol that I had learned about but not used. In this protocol, I would replace the laminaria from the first day with two or three new laminaria that (second) day and then have her come back the next (third) day for her procedure. She agreed on the last alternative, so that's what we did. The next day, I started an IV, removed the several new laminaria placed on the second visit, ruptured the membranes to reduce the risk of amniotic fluid embolism (which could be fatal), and started the procedure. I used a ring forceps that was larger than my normal early first trimester forceps to empty the uterus, gave her lots of oxytocin to make the uterus contract, and finished the procedure with minimal blood loss in a few minutes. It worked. I was relieved and grateful. So was the patient. This proved to be a very important experience in my future clinical practice.

At the hospital, I began going routinely to the monthly ob/gyn staff meetings that started every first Monday at 7 AM. The only person who would speak to me, when he was there, was Dr. Macfarlan, who had defended me at the quarterly staff meeting. I did not speak. Monday was a day I had off, and I wanted to go skiing, but I felt it was essential that I maintain my presence at the staff meetings. I thought it would make it possible to develop acquaintances with other members of the ob/gyn staff in case I needed their help for a patient and to show that I was serious about the hospital staff membership.

To have continuity of care and good communication with the medical community, I brought my typewriter to the clinic so I could write letters to the physicians, nurses, and family planning clinics that had referred patients. I made it clear that I was referring patients back to them for continuing care so they would realize we weren't stealing their patients, and I also made clear that I was responsible if there was a complication with the abortion procedure. I felt this was an essential step in maintaining good relations with the medical community and that we were following normal standards of medical care and communication. The credibility of what we were doing and of the clinic itself was at stake.

Even though I had left Washington, I kept in touch with my former colleagues there and in public health and family planning across the country. I decided that what we were doing in Colorado was important enough to report it at the coming annual American Public Health Association (APHA) meeting that would take place in New Orleans that fall, so I submitted an abstract about the use of laminaria for cervical dilation in first trimester abortion. There was only one other report in the medical literature that I knew about. It seemed like a normal and reasonable thing to do. I also made plans to continue my research in the Peruvian Amazon among the Shipibo.

In the summer of 1974, Channel 4 in Denver decided to do a special program on the abortion issue, and the news director, Sue O'Brien, asked me to represent the pro-choice side of the debate. My opponent was to be Dr. Frank Bolles, the family doctor who had sent out the lurid anti-abortion pamphlets in the fall of 1973. Dr. Bolles had met Jesus on a park bench in Chicago and had learned that abortion was wrong.

Both Dr. Bolles and I would be flanked by two or three allies of our own point of view. The program was carried on live TV.

Soon after that, the Colorado chapter of the National Organization for Women sponsored a special event and award ceremony at East High School in Denver in order to recognize people who had made important contributions to women's roles in society. One of the persons recognized was Reynelda Muse, a Black TV journalist who had become a trusted and beloved celebrity among the Denver news media. I was also invited to attend and be recognized for my work in abortion services.

After Reynelda spoke, I came forward to receive my award certificate. As I began to speak, the anti-abortion fanatics in the crowd erupted in frenzied shouts of "baby killer" and other epithets and surged forward toward me. Their faces were contorted in anger and hatred. They were only a few yards from me. The intensity of their hatred literally made the hair stand on the back of my neck. I had never seen such ferocity in human beings. I could not understand this anger or why what I was doing was so controversial. We were helping women in a singularly important way. For the first time in human history, women could end a pregnancy safely, and this was an astounding step forward for the health of women and for public health in general.

That summer, I made one of my brief research trips to the Shipibo Indian village in the Peruvian Amazon where I was conducting my long-term study of the health effects of cultural change. My first study was done in 1964 when I was a medical student, my next visit for six weeks was in 1969 when I was doing the research for my Master of Public Health thesis at the University of North Carolina, and we were now at another five-year interval. I arranged for a young doctor who was doing his residency in obstetrics and gynecology in Colorado to see patients for me for a few weeks at Boulder Valley Clinic while I was gone.

When I returned from Peru, points of conflict that had been simmering at the clinic became more difficult to avoid. We were extremely busy, and we didn't have enough instruments. We couldn't sterilize enough instruments quickly enough to keep up. Gail and I decided we needed more vaginal speculums, for example. I went to Roger to ask him to buy some more. "We can't afford it," he said. We were only charging $110 per procedure, which included all administrative costs, building lease, utilities, lab work, two clinic visits, staff pay, follow-up exams, and building maintenance. The board had wanted to charge only $100, but I argued that we had to cover the costs of the routine pathology that was being done on each tissue specimen to confirm that it was from an intrauterine pregnancy instead of an ectopic pregnancy. The counselors, except for the head counselor that Sclar hired, were all volunteers. Two of the nurses were volunteers. Rob Pudim, who did the lab work, was a volunteer. I was being paid $600 per week with no benefits, which amounted to about $9/hour since I was working 60–70 hours a week not counting nights I slept at the clinic to take call. I was paying for my own malpractice insurance, medical society dues, and health insurance. "Well, let's raise the fees so we can afford to get the instruments we need," I told Roger. "We're not gonna do that. You and Gail just need to work out your relationship. You don't need more instruments," he said.

The operating rooms were insufferably hot, and we couldn't afford air conditioning.

The head counselor hired by Ran Sclar made it clear that she considered having an abortion to be "a horrible experience." That was the script. In my view, it certainly had been that way in the past for a lot of people, but we had a different, positive approach that made it a normal component of women's health care. Under these new circumstances, which we were creating and which others such as those at Preterm had created, it wasn't and shouldn't be "a horrible experience." We were past that. It wasn't necessary or healthy to impose that view on patients.

One morning before patients arrived, I walked into the operating room and saw dust balls on the floor. Roger and some others were sitting in the tiny staff area, which was not closed in, having coffee and discussing the doctor's poor attitude. I said, "We can't work in a dirty operating room. This needs to be cleaned up," I said. "Clean it up yourself," Roger said. "Look," I said, "I can do every single job in this place including cleaning the rooms and the lab work as well as washing the instruments and performing the abortions, but we will only see a half-dozen patients a week." I grabbed a broom and headed for the operating room. I made my point, and the cleaning was done. But there was resistance.

There were other issues such as the patients' charts being kept in open cardboard boxes in plain view under the open stairway in the waiting room instead of in locked steel file cabinets. My concern about this was considered abnormal and annoying.

At the next meeting of the clinic's board of directors, we discussed these problems. There was disagreement among the board members about what should be done. No decision could be reached. There were petty personal conflicts. At one point, I remarked, "This sounds more like a psychotherapy group than a board meeting." "Well, it is," one of the members said. This is when I learned that *it really was a psychotherapy group.*

The group that had called me in April 1973, and which I visited in Ran Sclar's office on that occasion, was a psychotherapy group that Ran conducted weekly in his office. The group had decided that it would be therapeutic for everyone to have some common project on which they would work together, and the project they settled on was starting a non-profit abortion clinic. Bob McFarland was a member of the group, and, as a practicing family physician, he was designated to find a doctor who would help the group develop this project idea. That's when he called Ben Greer to see if Ben knew a possible candidate, and that's when Ben recommended that Bob call me.

Suddenly, the dynamics of the board of directors and (overlapping) staff became clear. While the results were good in many ways for patients, and I became increasingly convinced that it was a vital activity for many reasons, it started as a psychotherapy group. Sweet are the uses of adversity.

Roger assigned himself to the activity of visiting with the patients' partners. On one occasion, the partner asked for confirmation that the woman's pregnancy was his since he suspected that she got pregnant before he met her. He wanted to know how far along she was when I did the abortion for her. Roger got the chart and told him that the length of the pregnancy didn't coincide with his information of when his girlfriend got pregnant. She got pregnant with somebody else before he had met her. There was a row when the patient found this out. At this moment, I angrily told Roger that he had violated a basic principle of the patient's confidentiality, and that this was unacceptable and outrageous. He was defiant that he had the right to do it.

There were other issues. It was apparent to me that the economics of the arrangement that had been set up were not compatible with long-term survival of the clinic. Most of the staff were not being paid or were being paid token amounts. A new person came to work for a while and said she only needed to be paid enough "to get by." It was as if this were a Peace Corps project where people would work for a while to feel good about themselves and say they had done it and then go back to a real job after "doing good."

The tensions grew more severe when I flew to New Orleans to present my paper on the experience of laminaria use for cervical dilation in over 1,000 first trimester abortion patients with no major complications. My presentation was well attended, went well, and many of my colleagues from around the country, including Dr. Irv Cushner, were sitting in the front row. It was well received, and I began preparing the paper for publication in the *Rocky Mountain Medical Journal.* Among the APHA audience, what we were doing was considered important.

Roger, the head counselor, and others excoriated me for making the trip (at my own expense) and presenting the paper. They said that they hated the "professionalism" that this presentation represented. What I did was "elitist."

One staff member made it clear that she hated doctors, and she hated male doctors in particular. I was a target of her antagonism. Doctors were a necessary evil. There should be no "hierarchy" in the clinic. "Nobody should be in charge." I pointed out that if one of our patients died, the board of medical examiners would come after me and my medical license. I had to have the authority to set and maintain high medical standards at the clinic. "There has to be accountability and responsibility," I argued. No dice. Nobody agreed with me. My point of view was "elitist."

Things came to a head when we were having a routine staff meeting and dinner at Fred's Café downtown where Fred played the guitar and sang folk songs for his counterculture Boulder dining customers. Roger announced that he would be spending his days in the clinic basement writing a book about his experiences in abortion work. "We can't afford a writer-in-residence," I said. "We can't pay the bills we have and don't have enough money to do the work. We need to raise the fee to $125 to meet the expenses." At that point, Roger furiously stood up and got ready to punch me in the face. I stood up and faced him and got ready to punch back. I was also furious and ready to quit on the spot.

I called my younger sister and asked her and her boyfriend to meet me at my house in the mountains where I had a stiff drink of 151 proof rum that I normally used for cooking Cornish game hen flambé. I was so angry I was worried about having a heart attack and decided that the anti-coagulant drink would be a good way to prevent that.

At the next meeting of the clinic's board of directors, the decision was made to have no executive director and that the clinic should operate as a "commune." Next, the board abolished my job of medical director. I was told to continue performing the abortions as a technician, but I had no authority over anything. I left the building and never went back. It had been a little over a year since we had started the clinic.

My choices were to find another job, save some money, and go back to school for my Ph.D. and pursue an academic career as I had planned or open my own office as a private medical practice specializing in abortion services. I immediately decided to open my own practice. I did not consider the possibility that this would change my life radically, and I didn't examine other alternatives.

In retrospect, I would say it was a "calling," but there were no supernatural voices. I heard the women.

"Please don't ever stop doing this."

Starting over

By this time, I had decided that performing abortions was the most important thing I could do in medicine. I still wanted to pursue an academic career, at least on a part-time basis, I still wanted to do my research in Peru, but my priority became finding a way to continue performing abortions. I had no doubt about that. But how?

I had $600 to my name and a mortgage to pay. I was still working in the emergency room and still doing the consulting work in family planning training. But I no longer had a steady job. I couldn't afford to go back to school for my graduate work. I decided to set up my own private practice specializing in outpatient abortion services as my main activity and see if I could work out the other stuff somehow.

The first step was finding a place to work. A few blocks from the first clinic, and just across the street from Boulder Community Hospital, I found a small vacant space that I could rent for a modest amount, but it needed remodeling so I could work in it. It was on the bottom floor ("garden level") of a combination of what had been a surgeon's small office and a dentist's office. Just beyond the old dentist's office was a dermatologist who was pleasant, and around the corner another way was an aging orthopedic surgeon. Beyond the orthopedic surgeon was an ophthalmologist and his associated optical dispensary. The Associated Internists, with six doctors, worked upstairs. I decided I could remove a bathroom, making a common hallway between my two small offices, knock out part of another wall, and have a place to work. I then went to the bank where I had my checking account and secured a conference with a *very* conservative banker who complained to me about the "troublemakers" up the street who had started the abortion clinic. He didn't realize that he was talking with one of the "troublemakers."

I borrowed $7,000, hired a contractor, and opened my new office on January 22, 1975, the second anniversary of the *Roe v. Wade* decision. The first week, I had three patients. My one employee was Sunya Plattner, a Ph.D. candidate graduate student in psychology with whom I had worked at Boulder Valley Clinic. Within a short time, I persuaded Gail to come join me as the head nurse. I continued my other jobs so I could pay the bills.

A month or two after I opened my office, a charming young woman named Maggie came in to see us. She had wanted me to perform her abortion but couldn't find me so she went to the guy named RM and was intensely unhappy about the result. She wanted to work for me, so I hired her to work as a counselor. "Why don't you call your office 'Boulder Abortion Clinic?'" she asked. "What a good idea," I said. I had been thinking about this, but Maggie's question got me energized. I incorporated my practice as Boulder Abortion Clinic, and we have continued under that name for almost 50 years.

A principal reason for calling my office Boulder Abortion Clinic is that it is a step toward the social legitimization of abortion and abortion services. If there is a Boulder Allergy Clinic and a Boulder Orthopedic Clinic and a Denver Skin Clinic, why can't there be a Boulder Abortion Clinic? It lets people know immediately what we are doing and conveys the message (I hope) that women can walk in the front door, be accepted and respected, and know that we are here to offer excellent abortion services. Some people won't like it, but I can't help that. It's a straightforward message, and that's the point.

One problem that immediately became apparent was that people assumed I was still working at Boulder Valley Clinic and they kept sending patients there instead of to me. I had helped to give that clinic a good reputation. I was now competing with my previous association and good work. I started visiting doctors around the Denver/Boulder metro area to inform them about my new private practice. I was well received, but the first year in my own private practice was a struggle. In December of that year, I had to borrow $1,000 on my 1972 Ford Bronco in order to make my mortgage payment for the month. But I was free to make my own decisions about how to give my patients the best medical care possible.

It was my clear purpose to offer women the safest abortion procedure possible under the best medical conditions possible with total social and emotional support for each individual patient and her family.

My standing in the medical community improved a little when my paper on the use of laminaria for cervical dilation and reduction of risks of uterine perforation was published in 1975 in the *Rocky Mountain Medical Journal*.[1] My ambition to make first trimester abortion safer was supported by the publication of this paper.

Within a few months after I opened my own practice, I decided that I would try to perform early second trimester abortions using the technique that I had learned about by reading Neubart and Schulman's book and by my own experience, but I would approach it in a more systematic way. I would inform the patient of the plan for her and the risks (some of them not so clearly known) as well as the benefits. I would only do this for patients for whom I had a rather precise idea of the length of pregnancy; I would do it over a period of three days to give the maximum opportunity for the *laminaria* to do its work; and I got special instruments, including larger forceps, for performing the procedure.

Eventually, a patient with the right specifications presented herself and requested an abortion. We went through the protocol I had designed. The procedure went smoothly. The patient had no pain. There was minimal blood loss. I was able to empty the uterus completely to my satisfaction within a few minutes. It was a success. I looked at Gail and said, "I think we have something important here." She agreed.

What I had done, in terms of standard abortion practice care at that time, was to violate the Old Testament, the Sharia, the Talmud, the Qu'ran, the Bhagavad-Gita, and any number of other sacred texts. The patient was saved from a more dangerous saline abortion not to mention a term pregnancy, which was even more dangerous. The only acceptable conventional protocol for early second trimester abortion at that time was to wait until the patient was 16 weeks pregnant and had enough amniotic fluid to be able to inject a concentrated saline solution into the uterus. This would kill the fetus and cause the patient to go into labor. In spite of the best efforts, it had a high complication and death rate for the women for whom this method of abortion was used. The information that I had from Chris Tietze's JPSA study appeared to back up my view that what I was doing was much safer for the patients.

At a conference early the next year (1976), I drew aside Dr. Irv Cushner, a friend and colleague who I knew well and who had a distinguished reputation in his general field as well as abortion services, speaking with him in an empty coffee shop near the meeting place and told him about what I had done. I had performed this procedure dozens of times with excellent results. He said, "Warren, if you can show that this is a safe procedure in the early second trimester, that is really revolutionary."

Later that year, in December 1976, I presented my paper on 150 patients whose early second trimester pregnancies I had ended, of whom 110 had received the serial multiple laminaria treatment. It was published in 1977 in *Advances in Planned Parenthood*, and it was the first publication in the American medical literature of the serial multiple laminaria technique.[2] It became the procedure of choice for early second trimester abortion.

From that time on, with some variations, the protocol in my office for second trimester and later abortion procedures has been the placement of one laminaria on the first day, replacement of that laminaria with five or six laminaria on the second day, removal of the laminaria on the third day followed by a paracervical block, rupture of the amniotic sac to allow the amniotic fluid to flow out, reducing the risk of an amniotic fluid embolism, and removal of the fetus and placenta with instruments.

My relationship with the medical community in Boulder remained tenuous. Dr. Sherburne Macfarlan continued to be a friendly and indispensable ally. Other physicians tolerated my presence. My best friend, medical school classmate and lab partner had a family practice in Boulder and remained my friend. He spoke up for me at critical times.

Also in 1975, that first year of my practice, my paper, "The illness parameters of pregnancy" was published in the British journal *Social Science and Medicine*.[3] In that paper,

I continued and expanded my discussion of the idea that pregnancy fits into the cognitive framework of illness. It has an etiology (known cause), pathogenesis, pathophysiology, signs, symptoms, laboratory findings, diagnosis, prognosis (over in nine months or earlier), clinical course, physiologic changes, illness behavior, sick role behavior, incidence, prevalence, distribution, susceptibility (females more than males), duration, recovery period (post-partum period), and case fatality/death rate (maternal mortality ratio).

Pregnancy may not be an illness, but in what way is it *not* an illness? This is independent of whether the pregnancy is desired or not. *The treatment of choice for pregnancy is abortion unless the woman wants to carry the pregnancy to term and have a baby.* In that case, she should have the best medical care possible to assure that she survives and has a healthy baby.

Well. This is not a popular point of view, but it underlies a fundamental and essential component of women's health care. That is a view that is abhorrent to those who believe that the purpose of women, aside from giving men sexual pleasure and doing the housework, is for them to have as many babies as possible. After all, that's what women are *for*.

The latter view was promoted in the Colorado legislature, where, at the beginning of 1975, there were several bills introduced to make abortion illegal in Colorado. One of the bills was sponsored by Representative Gerry Frank (D).

Let's play a little hardball

Ruth Steel, a well-known Colorado champion of women's reproductive rights and access to birth control and abortion, called me to tip me off that Frank's bill would be considered in a legislative committee meeting the next morning. Ruth gave me the time of the meeting and the room number.

To Representative Frank's surprise and dismay, I showed up, listened to the presentation, and then attacked the bill. I listed the reasons why the bill was wrong and not reasonable. The bill was defeated in the committee's vote.

The next thing I did was to arrange a meeting with Sheila Kowal, the current chair of the Colorado Democratic Party. I knew Sheila from my work with the McGovern campaign. We had a friendly relationship. I told Sheila that because of Gerry Frank's sponsorship of this anti-abortion bill, we would d work to defeat his reelection and do everything possible to keep him from being elected even a precinct captain much less reelected to the Colorado General Assembly. Sheila was horrified and pleaded with me to let up on Gerry. We agreed that he was a nice guy, but I said that his introduction of this bill put him on the wrong side of this issue, and that we would deal with anybody else in the Democratic Party who sponsors anti-abortion legislation the same way.

Frank was defeated in his next election, and, although we had nothing to do with it, the message was out that we were playing hardball on this issue.

Ruth, who had included me in her meetings in her home to discuss ways of countering these bills, was horrified. Ruth was a very correct, conservative person in many ways whose approach to these conflicts was to go to the legislature, well dressed and with white gloves, to have reasonable and polite discussions with legislators in order to convince them to support reproductive choice and oppose the anti-abortion bills. She was highly effective, but I thought we needed to send a stronger political message to our adversaries, especially among the Democrats. Many of the Republican legislators were actually more openly pro-choice at that time. Dick Lamm's 1967 abortion reform bill, the first in the country, passed with total bipartisan support, was carried in the Senate by Republican senator John Bermingham, and was signed into law by Republican governor John Love.

At one point in our discussions about legislative strategy, Ruth floated the idea of having a Friday evening conference for legislators where we would discuss issues such as fetal viability, the ethics of abortion, legislating to support birth control programs, and fetal personhood. I told Ruth that I thought this would play into the hands of the anti-abortion people by accepting their premises, which focused on the fetus instead of the needs of the pregnant woman. I proposed having a national conference in Denver with participation of leading experts on the medical and public health aspects of abortion services and experts on the legal issues as well as inviting people like Sarah Weddington, who had argued and won the *Roe v. Wade* case, to be speakers. She reluctantly agreed, and I started putting together the ideas and invitations for this conference. Judy Widdicombe, a nurse who was the founder of Reproductive Health Services in St. Louis, told me about the Sunnen Foundation as a possible financial donor and put me in touch with Sam Landfather, the head of the foundation. Sam agreed to fund the conference.

Bonnie Andrikopoulous, the head of the Colorado chapter of the National Organization for Women, and I began arranging for a meeting place (the campus of the Colorado Women's College in Denver) and making calls to invite leaders from around the country. We set the meeting to occur at the end of February 1976. It was to be the Western Regional Conference on Abortion, the first national conference on this subject since the International Conference on Abortion Techniques and Services held in New York City in 1971.

Notes

1 Hern, W.M. Laminaria in abortion: Use in 1368 patients in first trimester. *Rocky Mountain Medical Journal* 72:390–95, 1975. PMID: 1198023; https://www.drhern.com/wp-content/uploads/2018/06/first-tri-laminaria-75.pdf
2 Hern, W.M. and Oakes, A.G. Multiple laminaria treatment in early midtrimester outpatient suction abortion: a preliminary report. Advances in Planned Parenthood 12:93-7, 1977.
3 Hern, W.M. The illness parameters of pregnancy. *Social Science and Medicine* 9:365–72, 1975 (England). https://doi.org/10.1016/0037-7856(75)90137-7

7   Abortion in the seventies

The response to my invitations to leaders in the abortion field across the country to participate in the Western Regional Conference on Abortion was beyond my expectations. Sarah Weddington accepted my invitation to be the keynote speaker. Cyril Means, a professor at New York Law School, who had drafted the 1970 New York law, agreed to discuss the origins of abortion laws in English and American traditions. Christopher Tietze, the leading expert on abortion health statistics, and who had advised the lawmakers in New York, agreed to come from New York City as did Dr. Jean Pakter, head of the maternal health division of the New York City Department of Health.

Judy Widdicombe, founder of Reproductive Health Services in St. Louis, who helped me with the Sunnen Foundation, agreed to speak on the challenges for nursing in abortion care. Dr. Louise Tyrer, with whom I had worked while at the Office of Economic Opportunity Family Planning Division, was now the vice president for Medical Affairs and medical director of the Planned Parenthood Federation of America. She agreed to be with us. My dear friend Ben Munson, who had been helping women have safe abortions in South Dakota since the mid-sixties, especially Native American women, agreed to speak about his experiences of performing abortions in one of the most conservative parts of the United States. Karen Mulhauser, head of the National Abortion Rights Action League, agreed to participate, as did Jeannie Rosoff, director of the newly formed Alan Guttmacher Institute.

Two brilliant young physicians from the Center for Disease Control Abortion Surveillance Unit, Ward Cates and David Grimes, came from Atlanta to discuss the public health impacts of the legalization of abortion in the United States. My mentor in medical school, Dr. Bill Droegemueller, spoke to us about new technologies in abortion services.

We had a star-studded cast from throughout the United States that included not only the national leaders but also local private practitioners such as Ben Munson, Dr. Lewis Koplik from New Mexico, and Dr. Bill Rashbaum, a nationally known OB/GYN specialist from New York City. I spoke about the public health aspects of abortion in Colorado. Jean Dubofsky from the Colorado Attorney General's office spoke to us about the legal aspects of abortion in Colorado.

Colorado governor Dick Lamm agreed to speak, and we received a letter of support from First Lady Betty Ford. The conference schedule included social workers, psychologists, and other social scientists. We had representatives from two federal government agencies, the Office of Management and Budget and the Equal Economic Opportunity Commission, discussing the economic and civil rights consequences of legalizing abortion. It was an amazing interdisciplinary collection of experts on many aspects of abortion

DOI: 10.4324/9781003514961-8

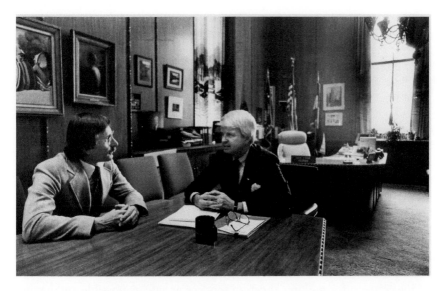

Figure 7.1 Dr. Warren Hern in conversation with Colorado governor Dick Lamm on July 31, 1976. Photo © Warren Martin Hern

ranging from the technical details of abortion procedures and prevention of risks to the national public health picture to participants in the political and legal controversies.

Colorado Women's College (CWC), which was modeled after and was very much like an exclusive Ivy League liberal arts college, was the ideal place for the conference. It had its own pleasant campus at the edge of Denver, the facilities were comfortable, and the college dorm facilities allowed us to have a large number of attendees from out of town. Several hundred people registered for the conference, many of them opposed to abortion. There were many students from CWC.

From the beginning, I decided to record the entire proceedings of the conference and have it transcribed, and I planned to publish the proceedings as a book, which I did. With more money from the Sunnen Foundation, I had 5,000 copies of the book published under the title, *Abortion in the Seventies*, with Bonnie Andrikopoulos and I as co-editors.[1]

The individual presentations were remarkable, and some of the panel discussions were particularly noteworthy. During one session that featured a discussion of the future of legislation that might follow the *Roe v. Wade* decision, I made the comment that the part of *Roe* referring to the ability of states to make "reasonable" regulations of second trimester abortion laid the groundwork for severe state restrictions on those procedures. Jeannie Rosoff from the Guttmacher Institute offered the opinion that such restrictions wouldn't be "reasonable" and that "reasonable people" wouldn't make them. My reply was that we are not dealing with "reasonable" people.

Notwithstanding my dim view of the anti-abortion fanatics that I had encountered so far in my limited experience in abortion services, the vocal opponents of abortion among those attending the conference were polite, respectful, argued their points calmly and clearly, and were treated with respect by the rest of us. How much things would change in the future!

One of the results of the Western Regional Conference on Abortion (WRCA) was the formation of the National Abortion Council, with Judy Widdicombe, Fran Kissling, and Karen Mulhauser as leaders of this initiative. The WRCA served as a stimulus and a spark of consciousness among pro-choice leaders that we needed a national organization of some kind to bring together the "issue" people, such as Karen, and the medical practitioners, such as Ben Munson, Lewis Koplik, and myself, in an effort to support both activities that were vital but very different.

One of the items high on the list was the development of standards for abortion care, a matter that had concerned me when I worked on the American Public Health Association Standards for Abortion Care with Chris Tietze when I was at OEO. It was not only vital to the health and safety of women seeking abortions to be protected by such standards, but it was also vital in order to win the confidence of the public in a medical practice that had a history of being highly stigmatized. The popular view was that "abortionists" – people who performed abortions – were incompetent, unscrupulous criminal butchers who exploited women and performed "botched" abortions in back-alley garages. Although this was sometimes true, historians Rickie Solinger and Leslie Reagan, among others, have shown that it was not always the case.[2]

But the negative view of abortion and those who performed them prevailed.

As a result of the concern for making abortion services as safe as possible and having them accepted as a normal part of women's health care, the National Abortion Council (NAC) was formed in the summer of 1976. I sent two of my staff members, Lolly Gold and Merideth, to attend the organizing meeting in Nashville, Tennessee. Later, the organizers asked me to be a member of the Standards Committee with Dr. Ken Edelin of Massachusetts, Dr. Ward Cates from the CDC, Dr. Bob Crist of Kansas, and Dr. Jane Hodgson of Minnesota.

At the same time, there was a separate organization being formed, the National Association of Abortion Facilities (NAAF), which was being organized by, among others, Margie Pitts Hames, who had argued the *Doe v. Bolton* companion case to *Roe v. Wade*, and Reverend Myron Chrisman, a Texas pastor who strongly supported abortion rights and access. Chris was setting up several abortion clinics in Texas. The primary focus of the NAAF was to support the abortion services as successful businesses in getting supplies and in supporting clinic administrators.

With different goals and somewhat different values, a degree of tension developed between the two groups even though members of both recognized the need for a national non-profit organization that could include and represent medical practitioners specializing in abortion services and the interests of clinics, focus on concerns about abortion as a public issue, and help with the nitty-gritty details of running clinics, such as where to get supplies of all kinds at what cost.

A joint meeting of the boards of both organizations was called. There was furious disagreement about whether there should be one organization, whether it would be possible to work together, and what the goals should be. The feminists wanted no part of NAAF, seeing it as a commercial operation for exploiting women. Some in the NAC thought the feminists were too radical.

By December 1976, the leaders of the two groups had agreed to form one organization, the National Abortion Federation. The first board meeting, in which I participated as a founding board member, met in Miami at the same time as the Association of Planned Parenthood Physicians (APPP) since many of us were attending that meeting, also. The purpose of the new organization was to promote safe abortion services and to support a highly professional approach to these services.

During the board meeting, I proposed that one of the first things to be developed should be standards of care for abortion services with member clinics being required to meet the standards in order to have a voting membership. Carole Dornblaser from Meadowbrook Women's Clinic (a NAAF founder) was asked to serve as chair of the Standards Committee, and I (a NAC member) was asked to be a member of it. Judy Widdicombe from the Reproductive Health Services clinic, one of the organizers of the National Abortion Coalition, was chosen as president of the newly formed National Abortion Federation, and Frances Kissling, also one of the organizers of NAC, was chosen as the new executive director. It was like putting together a small new government composed of conflicting factions in a power struggle. Not everyone was completely happy with the result.

Most unhappy were the feminists, who felt that the NAC issue people had sold out to the NAAF commercial approach to abortion services as a business. They also resented the presence of people like Dr. Bill Peterson, head of the OB/GYN services at the Washington (D.C.) Hospital Center, who, as a retired U.S. Air Force colonel, held and represented strong traditional views of women at the same time that he was a pioneer in making abortions available in a very traditional hospital. He carried off this daunting feat in spite of the hospital bureaucracy because of his personal charisma and forceful personality and his determination to make this happen for the right reasons, namely because women needed this help. Although personally charming and affable, this crusty, pipe-smoking bird colonel who was used to giving orders and having them obeyed was seen by the feminists as the paragon of male chauvinism, a view that amused him.

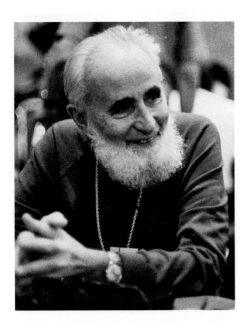

Figure 7.2 Dr. Christopher Tietze at 1978 National Federation meeting, San Francisco, California. Photo © Warren Martin Hern

Board meetings of the new organization were stimulating, to say the least, with radical feminists at one end of the table demanding to have their expenses paid for attending the cross-country meetings and Bill Peterson at the other end of the table, smoking a pipe, comfortable in his status as an objectionable alpha male. Chris Tietze, in his charming Austrian accent, did his white-bearded avuncular best to leaven the situation with gentle humor and wise advice.

Back in Boulder, I was having my own challenges with the anti-abortion demonstrators aggressively harassing my patients and staff by coming to the only entrance to my office at all hours. The other tenants on my "garden level" of the office building moved out because they didn't want to be next to or associated with my abortion practice, so I remodeled and occupied those spaces. When the internists upstairs offered to sell me the building, I took out three high-interest loans and made the deal with everything I had as collateral because it was clear that a new owner could put me on the street rather than have an abortion practice in the building. This was happening to colleagues all over the country.

In my practice, I kept thinking of ways to improve my serial multiple laminaria protocol for performing early second trimester outpatient abortions so that the women needing them would not have to go through the saline or prostaglandin injections that had become the standard methods for second trimester abortions. The results I was getting for the patients were excellent, and I submitted an abstract for the 1976 APPP meeting to be held that December in Miami. Louise Tyrer later told me that my abstract was met with opposition and strong arguments against it in the APPP program committee because my new procedure was considered so radical. Opponents were worried that someone would take this idea, make shortcuts, apply it in a less cautious way and have complications or deaths, and that APPP would be blamed for even permitting it to be presented at its meeting. Eventually, Louise and others prevailed and I was permitted to make my presentation. Ralph Wynn, the editor of *Advances in Planned Parenthood*, spoke to me at the meeting and offered to publish the paper in the next issue of the journal, which he did.[3]

Meanwhile, I finished editing the proceedings of the Western Regional Conference on Abortion, prepared the book manuscript with my photos and some x-ray images provided by Bill Rashbaum and had it printed as the first official publication of the new National Abortion Federation in early 1977.

The doctors who occupied the main street-level floor of the building, and from whom I bought the building, decided to move across the driveway to their new headquarters, so I took over the upper floor. This allowed me to separate the operating room area downstairs from the front office reception and counseling part of my practice.

Anti-abortion demonstrators, who had been coming through the back parking lot to the back door of my office, now picketed the new street-level front door of my office as well and harassed the patients as they walked by on the front sidewalk a few feet from the demonstrators. Patients would often come into my office in tears from the insults and verbal abuse they received from the demonstrators. The demonstrators parked their cars in the parking lot next to my building that I shared with the owners and occupants of the next building west of me, 1120 Alpine, and I couldn't do anything about it.

One time I went out with a clipboard to start writing down the license numbers of the cars of the demonstrators, and one of the demonstrators, a man named Zenon Raskowski, who had started the "Fight the Abortion Clinic" organization in 1973, tried to run me over with his car. As I was running several miles a day for exercise, I was able to get out of the way in time, but it was a close call. I called the police to report the incident, but nothing happened.

I resolved to buy the 1120 Alpine building if I had another opportunity so I could control the parking lot and keep anti-abortion fanatics out of that building for security reasons. It was offered as part of the deal when I bought the main building at 1130 Alpine, but I couldn't get the financing to buy both buildings. I could barely make the payments on the three loans I took out to buy the building in which I was already working. Anti-abortion fanatics all over the country were buying or leasing spaces next to abortion clinics and subjecting both patients and staff members to round-the-clock harassment. I worried about violence.

At one point, we saw the anti-abortion demonstrators parked in the middle of the internists' new parking lot and pointing a video camera at the back door of my office. I called the physician in charge and asked to speak to him in my office. When I told him about this and told him that he must not permit their parking lot to be used for this kind of harassment, he said, "We don't want to get involved." I said, "Well, you're involved if you let this happen, and you can't permit this violation of my patients' privacy. This has to stop now." It stopped, but I was furious that my colleagues had allowed it to happen in the first place – to say nothing of being alarmed and horrified by the aggressive intrusion of the anti-abortion fanatics, who appeared ready to violate any social norms of personal respect, especially for women experiencing a painful personal crisis in their lives.

Trouble in South Dakota

Meanwhile, a crisis erupted in South Dakota involving my friend, Dr. Ben Munson, who had performed abortions there beginning in the late 1960s. He had been prosecuted under state law for performing illegal abortions, but he had appealed the decision and eventually won. But a local district attorney who was supportive and sympathetic to Ben's work, Jim Abourezk, took Ben out in the country in his pickup one day so they could chat privately. "Ben, you have to stop performing abortions." "I can't help it," replied Ben.

Notwithstanding the controversy, Ben was beloved in the community, especially by the Native Americans, whom Ben had helped in many ways. But then came Bill Janklow, an ambitious politician who had started his career as a bartender working for Jim Abourezk. Janklow was now the attorney general of South Dakota.

Janklow's opportunity to exploit Ben's work for political purposes came (or was contrived) in 1977, when, the day before the statute of limitations expired, Janklow arrested Ben and charged him with manslaughter. A woman Ben had helped in 1973 died following an abortion, and Janklow had a sensational case to help his political career.

The patient, whom Ben saw in his office, was thought to be about 12 weeks pregnant. But after beginning the procedure, Ben determined that she was at least a month further along in her pregnancy, and he decided that it was not safe to try to continue the procedure without more preparation. He gave her antibiotics and instructed her to come back the next day from her hotel across the street when it would be safer to continue and complete the abortion procedure. Ben knew that this would be possible and safer. But the patient didn't return. She and her friend went to visit Mount Rushmore and then continued back home to the city of Pierre almost two hundred miles away. She didn't tell anyone what had happened. A couple of days later, she developed a fever and became septic. Her family took her to the local hospital where she told the doctors what had happened.

They called Ben, who told them that they must perform a hysterectomy immediately and give the patient intravenous antibiotics or she would die of sepsis. The doctors said she was too sick to operate on. She died. The family was distraught, but they didn't blame Ben for what had happened.

Janklow, preparing to run for governor of South Dakota, saw his opportunity and arrested Ben. The patient's family begged Janklow not to prosecute Ben. He had tried to help their daughter.

When I learned of Janklow's prosecution of Ben, I went to Rapid City for the trial and advised his attorneys as we listened to Janklow present his case against Ben. There were many flaws in the prosecution, and Janklow left out important facts such as the reasons for not trying to complete the abortion at first and the failure of the patient to return for completion of the abortion procedure the next day.

Janklow's prosecution was so poor that the judge instructed the jury to deliver a directed verdict of acquittal without hearing the case for the defense. Janklow was furious, but he got elected governor, and his political career blossomed. Ben was left bankrupt even though he was acquitted.

Jim Abourezk was elected U.S. senator from South Dakota and retired after one highly effective term, but not before he had organized a fundraiser in Washington to help Ben with his legal expenses. Both men were strong champions of the Native American people of South Dakota. Ben must be remembered as one of the lonely great champions of women's rights to have reproductive freedom in the United States.

First NAF meeting

The National Abortion Federation decided to have its first annual meeting in Denver in the fall of 1977. I was asked to chair and organize the meeting, which I set up at the Colorado Women's College since it had proved to be a friendly venue for us. We had good attendance and started the tradition of sessions devoted to scientific papers concerning abortion services. There were spirited discussions as there were strong differences in the approach to early abortion.

At a major clinic in New York where tens of thousands abortions were performed a year, the director, an anesthesiologist, used general anesthesia for all patients, whereas most of the rest of us, concerned with the higher risks associated with general anesthesia, used local anesthesia. The choice appeared for some of us to be either to make patients comfortable but to put them at higher risk of a fatal complication of general anesthesia or to help them get through a somewhat more uncomfortable brief procedure with a lower risk by using local anesthesia supplemented by narcotic analgesia. These were important choices that affected people's lives.

A more vigorous conflict presented itself in the meeting of the standards committee, of which I was a member. The feminist representatives from California were flatly opposed to standards of care that could be imposed. Their reasoning was that the application of standards of care would add to the cost of the procedure and that this was punitive for low-income women. My view was that high standards of safety and medical care were necessary not only to prevent complications or even death; but they were also necessary to maintain public confidence in our work. In my view, which I stated as clearly as I could, there were two different issues: necessary standards of care for patient safety and social justice. If poor women couldn't afford abortion services because the cost of making them safe put them out of reach for low-income people, the answer was not to lower standards of medical care but to find ways to help poor women get access to the service through financial assistance.

The Republican Party was active in opposing public assistance for safe abortion services as typified by the Hyde Amendment. Henry Hyde openly stated that his legislation was aimed at poor women since they were the most vulnerable and were a constituency with weak political representation. It was a cynical but effective strategy that punished poor women and their families. It helped Hyde get reelected in his anti-abortion district.

Two members of the standards committee were nurses working at abortion clinics (of whom one was Gail, who worked for me); both women considered themselves strong feminists. They resented the attitudes of the Feminists who were opposed to safe standards for abortion services. In one of our subsequent standards committee meetings, a feminist leader from a southern Feminist Women's Health Center, now allied with a similar clinic in Colorado, actively tried to disrupt the meeting in order to prevent standards from being adopted. Our next meeting was held behind locked, closed doors. We were working on standards for safe care that could be applied by all clinics and physician's offices in order to prevent complications. The Feminist leader from the southern clinic later became president of the National Abortion Federation, which gave her an opportunity for revenge.

My mountain home was my refuge and respite from all this. I would get home alone on a late Saturday evening, spend Sunday skiing or hiking around my house, go skiing or backpacking on Monday and Tuesday, depending on the season, and go back to Boulder to see patients on Wednesday morning. Some friends joined me from time to time to share these activities. It was also a good time to read, write, or play the piano or guitar. I liked the solitude and the beautiful view of the Continental Divide.

I worried about someone waiting to kill me there.

Notes

1 Hern, W.M., and Andrikopoulos, B. (eds.) *Abortion in the Seventies: Proceedings of the 1976 Western Regional Conference on Abortion*. New York: National Abortion Federation, 1977. Available from *Alpenglo Graphics*, Boulder, Colorado

2 Solinger, R. *The Abortionist: A Woman against the Law*. New York: The Free Press, 1994; Reagan, L.J. *When Abortion Was a Crime: Women, Medicine and Law in the United States, 1867–1973*. Berkeley: University of California Press, 1997.

3 Hern, W.M., and Oakes, A. Multiple laminaria treatment in early midtrimester outpatient suction abortion. *Advances in Planned Parenthood* 12:93–7, 1977. https://www.drhern.com/wp-content/uploads/2018/05/multiple-laminaria-elim.pdf

8 Abortion politics and public policy in Colorado

In 1976 I got a call from Ray Kogovsek, a member of the Colorado legislature, who said he wanted my help. He wanted to meet me for lunch at a restaurant across from the Colorado State Capitol building so we could talk about a problem that was bothering him. I had met Ray at a couple of Democratic political events, and we had a friendly relationship. But it was most unusual, it seemed to me, that a member of the legislature would want anything from me, a private medical practitioner specializing in abortion services. Ray had been elected to the Colorado Senate a few years before and was thinking about running for Congress from his southern Colorado congressional district, the center of which was Pueblo, a coal and steel town with many blue-collar workers. There were many Hispanic workers in the steel mills, and Ray's own family roots were in Yugoslavia in southeastern Europe. Pueblo was a Democratic town, but culturally it was very conservative, with many ethnic neighborhoods.

Over lunch, Ray explained to me that he was struggling with the abortion issue. People in Pueblo, especially Catholic working-class families like his own, were against abortion, and Ray himself was against abortion. He thought it was wrong. But he also felt uncomfortable with considering any bills in the legislature that would place restrictions on abortion. Colorado had been the first state in the country to reform its abortion law in 1967, but the restraints in that law were swept aside by the *Roe v. Wade* decision of 1973. Ray didn't think that the state should interfere with a woman's right to make that choice even though he was personally very uncomfortable with abortion. By the time he called me, I was becoming well known in Colorado as a physician who performed abortions and as someone who defended the right of women to have them.

The longer we talked, the more it was evident that Ray was struggling with his conscience and trying to resolve the conflict between his own personal and religious views and the views of his constituents over what he saw as an important issue of public policy. Should public policy about abortion be determined by the canons of the Catholic Church, to which not everyone belonged, or by what the community as a whole believed? What was best for the community and for women? He was asking fundamental questions about this difficult issue. He was worried about how to respect the views of his constituents – and get reelected – and yet do the right thing as a legislator for the whole state.

"Ray," I told him, "You are entitled to your own views and your own conscience about this, and you should be candid about those views with your constituents. There's nothing wrong with your saying that you are against abortion personally and that it violates your own religious beliefs but that the public policy needs to give everyone the

DOI: 10.4324/9781003514961-9

freedom to make their own decisions about abortion. That matters most for women. They have to be able to make those decisions."

Ray was grateful for the opportunity to speak with me candidly about his struggle. He followed my advice, answered questions from his constituents honestly, won their respect for his position, and won reelection to the Colorado Senate. He was later elected to three terms in the U.S. House of Representatives from the Third Congressional District, which covers the western third of the state of Colorado. He was a humble, honest man who served the people of Colorado and his country. He died a beloved man. Many of us thought of him as representing the best of the democratic tradition in American society. It is hard to imagine what he would have thought about the harsh politics and intractable conflict over abortion that we are experiencing today.

Ray Kogovsek's problem was symbolic of the national dilemma today. How do people who have a strong moral objection to abortion resolve the conflict between their own sincere belief and the essential work of democracy, which is to order society by laws that are just for many people with widely different views on the same subject? With many subjects in the public arena, compromise is necessary and essential, such as how to pay for public projects or which among competing legitimate needs gets priority. With abortion, what is the possibility of compromise? Either the woman, whose body and whose life are most profoundly and permanently affected by a pregnancy, is permitted to make this choice or someone else, who is unknown to her and has no stake in the pregnancy or life of the woman, is permitted to deny her that choice.

Due process is a vital element of our constitutional rights, but not permitting the woman to make that choice is a denial of due process. It also interferes with her right to privacy as a person, it interferes with her confidential relationship with her physician, and it interferes with her intimate relationship with her husband or partner.

Any law that restricts her access to safe abortion services interferes with all these protected rights and relationships. Finally, since pregnancy and childbirth have inherent risks of death for each woman, any legal restrictions on her access to safe abortion can deprive her of her life without due process. That is a fundamental violation of her own right to life under the U.S. Constitution.

Assuring that a woman has the protected right under the Constitution to make the decision about continuing the pregnancy does not deprive anyone else of their right to life, privacy, liberty, or anything else. Those opposed to abortion claim that her decision to end a pregnancy interferes with the fetus's right to life, but the fetus and pregnancy are a direct threat to the life of the woman, and, as stated in the Jewish tradition, she has a right to defend herself against that threat to her life. No one has the right to force her to continue the pregnancy and have a baby. There is no compromise possible on that point. That's why those who oppose abortion are willing to use lethal force to impose their view on the woman or on the physician who helps her, that's why those who oppose abortion will stop at nothing to impose their views on others whom they don't even know, and that is why those who oppose abortion seek to use the coercive power of the state to impose their views on the entire society without compromise.

The only compromise possible is that those who oppose abortion are free to speak their views and try to convince others not to have abortions. Also, if someone is against abortion, they shouldn't have one, and no one should force them to do so.

Tim Wirth's campaign for the U.S. Senate

In 1986 my friend, Tim Wirth, who had served in Congress for 12 years representing our congressional district, ran for the U.S. Senate. His opponent, Ken Kramer, was an extreme right-wing Republican who, of course, was opposed to abortion.

Helping Tim with his campaigns was routine. Our friendship went back to 1958 when he, his brother, and I worked together digging ditches and filling them up on a highway construction job south of Denver for our summer jobs. Tim and John were students at Harvard and I had just finished my sophomore year at the University of Colorado. Being bigger and stronger than John and I, Tim got the coveted assignment of ATO (air tool operator) – running the jackhammer – which paid 25 cents an hour more than our baseline $2.10/hour. John and I teased Tim mercilessly. Dirt clods were thrown (in jest).

I don't remember talking about foreign affairs or national politics on the job. I do remember our foreman, a nice guy who had a propensity to scratch himself in private places when he was instructing us on our work assignments.

Toward the end of the 1986 Senate campaign, Tim asked if he and his staff could use my office for phone banking since I had lots of phones, and we did. The election polls showed a close race. On the Sunday before the election, gory anti-abortion leaflets appeared on the windshields of all the cars parked near several churches a few blocks from my office. I grabbed some, and then I alerted TV reporter Lance Hernandez from Channel 7, whom I knew from his having reported on my work. Lance showed up and took a video of the anti-abortion leaflet on a car. His report on this was on the Sunday evening newscast.

Tim won, with the strong help of pro-choice women voters, in one of his squeaker "Wirth landslide" victories (49.9 percent – 48.4 percent).

Roy Romer for governor

That same year, Roy Romer, the Democratic state treasurer, ran for governor. Although I was keenly interested in supporting only Democrats for state office since nearly all were pro-choice, I was especially interested in helping Roy because of his reputation for integrity and my dislike of his Republican opponent, Ted Strickland, an oil-and-gas attorney who was anti-abortion.

Sue O'Brien, whom I had known as the news director at KOA-TV Channel 4, was Roy's campaign chairman. One day I got a call from Sue asking for some help. On a widely reported radio talk show segment, Strickland had made some volatile comments about America marching toward being a "Christian nation." Sue said, "If a tape of this broadcast should happen to fall into your hands, what do you think could happen to it?" "Well," I said, "I can't really predict what would happen, but it just might happen to fall into the hands of an enterprising newspaper reporter." "Check your mail," Sue said. The tape arrived at my office, I found a reason to drive to Denver, I found myself at the back door of the *Denver Post* on 15th and California Street that I knew well from my days as a *Post* free-lance photographer in the fifties, somehow walked past the big web presses turning out the day's newspaper, up the stairs to the second floor, and just happened to walk through the back door of the *Denver Post* city room. There I happened to run into Carl Miller, an old friend who had been Dick Lamm's press secretary, and the Strickland tape fell into Carl's hands. Who ever thought that would happen?

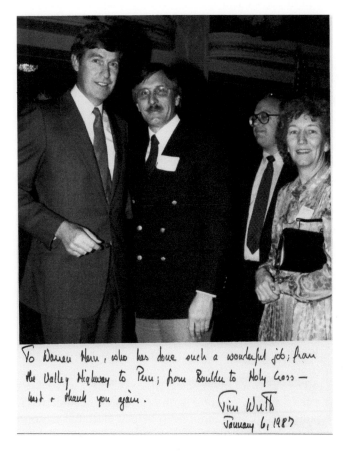

To Warren Hern, who has done such a wonderful job; from
the Valley Highway to Peru; from Boulder to Holy Cross —
best + thank you again.
                                        Tim Wirth
                                        January 6, 1987

Figure 8.1 U.S. Senator Tim Wirth and Dr. Warren Hern, January 6, 1987.

The next day, the *Denver Post* carried a headline article about Strickland's comments. I don't know whether this report had any influence on the election results, but Roy Romer won the election by 58.2 percent to 41.03 percent.

A political and constitutional catastrophe in Colorado

Ruth Steel was an admired, outstanding, and highly effective civic leader in Colorado in many ways during the mid-twentieth century, especially in the area of reproductive rights. Aside from being the founder and first director of Colorado Planned Parenthood, she held many leadership positions in education and on matters of social justice. She worked to protect the environment. She was a dear friend, included me in her circle, and I joined others on many occasions in her comfortable home for meetings about protecting and advancing abortion rights and services in Colorado.

Ruth played a key role in supporting legislators Dick Lamm and John Bermingham in passing the 1967 abortion reform bill that was signed into law by Republican governor John Love. We worked together on various projects.

She was a close observer of the political scene, especially the state legislature and its members. She tipped me off on critical occasions so I could testify against anti-abortion bills. I worked with her as I led the effort to host the 1976 Western Regional Conference on Abortion.

In 1984 opponents of abortion mounted a ballot issue campaign to change the Colorado constitution to prohibit the use of public funds for abortion services in Colorado. Ruth mobilized the pro-choice community and raised money to oppose the constitutional ballot measure. Her group produced several television ads featuring prominent "respectable" pro-choice physicians (not me!) and other community leaders to implore the voters to reject the measure. The TV ads were quite somber, were not convincing, and there was no substantial effort to organize the voters. The ballot measure was going down to defeat one week before the election, but the anti-abortion fanatics, who organized voters at churches and other community events, won by less than one percentage point. It became unconstitutional in Colorado to use public funds to help poor women have abortions in Colorado.

In 1988 Ruth and her colleagues decided to try to repeal the constitutional change approved by the voters in 1984. Early that year, her group called a meeting at Montview Presbyterian Church on 20th Avenue in Denver. Major national leaders such as Ellie Smeal, president of the National Organization for Women and founder of the Feminist Majority, spoke to a packed crowd of several hundred people. There was standing room only. The speakers implored the assembled pro-choice activists to fan out and gather the nearly 100,000 signatures needed to get the repeal measure on the Colorado ballot that fall.

One organizer, a professional hired by Ruth, said that a group that size with that much energy "could take over the state."

Soon after that, I made a trip to Denver from my medical office (where I was taking care of my abortion patients) to attend a brief meeting at the campaign headquarters. Stan Greenberg, the Democratic pollster and consultant who helped elect Bill Clinton president, asked me for a ride to Boulder so he could visit his brother Ed, a political science professor at the University of Colorado. We talked politics, including the need for a strong "ground game" organizing effort to win the election. As we rode up the Boulder Turnpike in my battered 1986 Subaru jalopy, he said, "You're a doctor. Where's your Maserati?" "You're ridin' in it," I said.

A few weeks after that, Ellie Smeal called me, tearing her hair out. "They have no field operation down there," she said. "We have to do something! They have to get out there and organize the voters!" "I agree with you, Ellie, but I can't do much about it. I'm just a doctor." She decided to put a member of her staff on loan at the Colorado pro-choice repeal office.

The pro-choice activists collected over 80,000 signatures and they got the repeal measure on the ballot. But they didn't get any names, addresses, telephone numbers, or other contact information. Nada. They had no voter lists or GOTV campaign. The anti-abortion people organized the living shit out of the Christian Evangelicals and defeated the abortion repeal ballot measure by a 20 percent margin: NO – 60.24 percent to Yes, 39.76 percent. We are still living with the consequences of these two elections.

The 1988 pro-choice campaign featured the same dismal, soporific TV ads that were in some ways worse as they depicted women suffering with no hope and featuring wooden appearances by local celebrities.

Jean Thulemeyer, one of Ruth's extremely competent but frustrated lieutenants, asked to have lunch with me to talk about trying again in 1992. "Please, no," I said. "We're losing by more each time." The ballot issue was a great organizing issue for the anti-abortion fanatics, and they had us down and out.

One morning after the election, Ruth called me and said, "Warren, the reason we lost is that the doctors who do abortions didn't give us enough money!" "Bullshit, Ruth, I just got through spending $30,000 to put in bullet-proof windows in my waiting room so my patients and the rest of us don't get killed by some fanatic with a high-powered rifle. My front windows were shot out in March!" It was a "spirited" conversation with what international diplomats call a "frank exchange of views," but we remained friends.

The Colorado pro-choice community is better organized now and there is a new campaign to enshrine abortion rights in the Colorado constitution.

More abortion politics

In 1990 my friend, Josie Heath, decided to run for the U.S. Senate. Her opponent, U.S. Representative Hank Brown (R-CO), was also a friend who I had known since our days as undergraduates at the University of Colorado in the 1950s. Hank and I were not close friends, but I admired him, thought highly of him in his public career, and disagreed with him on some basic issues such as abortion. Hank was not an anti-abortion fanatic by any means, but he had cast many votes against reproductive health care and abortion rights. So in the weeks before the election, I called a press conference at the state capitol and denounced Hank's candidacy on the basis of his anti-abortion votes. Since he had votes on both sides of the issue, my statement was, "Whatever your position is on abortion, Hank has a vote for you." I accompanied this written and spoken statement with a list of all the votes that Hank had cast in which the abortion issue was in play (amendments to the defense budget, amendments to the agriculture bills, etc.). A hostile reporter from the *Rocky Mountain News*, Peter Blake, was in the audience.

Within minutes after my press conference, I got a call from the current director of the Colorado NARAL group telling me that Hank had been on the phone with her, furious with my press conference, demanding that she stop me from making such remarks and demanding that I retract the remarks I had just made. "I can't do anything about Dr. Hern, and I didn't even know he was going to have a press conference," she told Hank. "I don't have any control over what he says. That's impossible."

Hank won the election, and a few years later, I was chosen as a delegate from the Colorado Medical Society (CMS) to lobby members of Congress on Medicaid funding or something. I was assigned to meet with Hank since I knew him personally. I was escorted into his office and given a frosty greeting, I was pleasant as possible to my old acquaintance (who I liked personally and still respected), and gave him my CMS pitch. It was like two old bulls bumping chests for a few minutes, but he didn't throw me out of his office.

Many years later, Hank became the distinguished president of our alma mater, the University of Colorado, and we exchanged friendly greetings every time we met. By current Republican standards, he is a flaming liberal as well as being a nice, decent person, qualifications that would no longer get him elected precinct captain in a Republican Party precinct meeting. He would be thrown out of the meeting.

In 2002 I tangled with a Republican governor of Colorado, Bill Owens, someone for whom I had no respect, when I had a press conference and denounced his policies that were hostile to reproductive health care, especially for the poor women of Colorado. During his first year in office, 1999, Owens cut off funding for Rocky Mountain Planned Parenthood and Boulder Valley Clinic, funds that were used for birth control and cancer screening. I said that Owens had brought the spirit of the Taliban to Colorado. Owens made a screeching denunciation of me to the press, and the chair of the Colorado Republican party, Dick Wadhams, announced that I was a "partisan pit bull." Thanks, Dick. I'll take the compliment. Sounds like I hit a nerve.

But as if to refute Wadhams, I took on Bill Ritter, a Colorado Democrat who decided to run for governor in 2006, and I publicly criticized Ritter for his opposition to abortion. Bill gave me the courtesy of a one-hour meeting to discuss the matter after I complained that he had refused to meet with me about this issue, but he was very clear that he was opposed to abortion. He refused to say that he would veto anti-abortion legislation. Although I had many reasons to admire Bill Ritter as a person and as a public servant, his opposition to safe abortion services and willingness to support anti-abortion legislation was not acceptable, and I let the public know that. As it turns out, Bill got a lot of static from other people about this, and, after he took office, he vigorously supported family planning assistance for poor families in Colorado. He had an excellent single term as governor, and we remain on friendly terms.

9 Doing something radical in the most conservative way possible

The best and safest way to perform a second trimester abortion continued to be controversial. Saline injection abortion continued to have relatively high major complication rates and death rates for the women who experienced them. The new prostaglandin injection abortions too often resulted in live births of fetuses that were not viable.

My own approach of using the serial multiple laminaria treatment of the cervix over several days followed by instrumental evacuation of the uterus was yielding very low major complication rates (of less than 0.5%), short procedure times, low blood loss, and, for most patients, little discomfort. What I was doing was arguably radical, but I was doing it in the most conservative way possible.

My first paper on this was published in early 1977, and Louise Tyrer invited me to make a presentation at a joint risk management seminar in Vail in the late winter where she and her husband and I could ski together after the conference. My presentation would be included in a panel that also featured a presentation by Dr. Dan Mishell, professor and chairman of the Department of Obstetrics and Gynecology at the University of Southern California School of Medicine. He was, and is, one of the most respected and distinguished persons in the field of reproductive medicine.

Due to a winter storm in the mountains, my late arrival occurred just as I was scheduled to speak, but just after Professor Mishell had finished his presentation. Unbeknownst to me, Professor Mishell had just stated a few minutes earlier that the only way to perform a second trimester abortion was, as was the classical tradition, to wait until the 16th week of pregnancy and only then perform the abortion by injection of hypertonic saline solution or prostaglandin. The idea of doing a dilation and evacuation (D & E) abortion with instruments instead of via the injection procedure followed by vaginal delivery of the fetus and placenta was to be condemned as unacceptably dangerous and irresponsible.

Ignorant of this injunction and his stern advice because I missed his presentation, I presented my research in an expanded version of what I had presented a few months earlier and what had just been published.[1]

The reports that I received later were that Professor Mishell was furious with me because I contradicted and embarrassed him in public with my unexpectedly favorable clinical results. After all, who was I, a small town doctor in a small private practice with not even an OB/GYN residency training to prepare me or university teaching faculty position to show I had professional knowledge of the subject? How could I possibly be taken seriously? He never forgave me.

At the same time, all of us at my office were experiencing serious emotional stress in performing these procedures. In the first place, I was concerned for the risks to the patient

DOI: 10.4324/9781003514961-10

since all the conventional advice was against what I was doing, but it appeared to be safer for the patients.

I was clear that it was safer and better for the patients than the traditional alternative saline injection followed by induction of labor and delivery of the fetus and placenta, sometimes without medical personnel available in the hospital ward setting, but viewing larger fetal parts was unnerving to many of us including me.

Some of us had dreams that were disturbing. In one dream of mine, the fetus was being delivered intact and the heart was still beating, as had happened in the operating room. In my dream, I tried to shield my staff assistants from the view of this.

The ethical dilemma remained: this was much safer for the patients, but the emotional cost of the operation was transferred from the patients to the medical and counseling staff. With the conventional injection/induction/delivery protocol, the emotional anguish and distress were experienced by the patient, often alone, and the nursing staff. The doctors performed the injections but were not present when the fetus was delivered, sometimes with agonal movements or more.

In 1978, with my head counselor, a psychiatric nurse, as my co-author, I presented a paper at the annual meeting of the Association of Planned Parenthood Physicians in San Diego with the title, "What about us? Staff reactions to D & E abortion." In the paper I stated that "We have reached the point in this technology where there is no possibility of denying an act of destruction. It is before one's eyes. The sensations of dismemberment flow through the forceps like an electric current. It is the crucible of a raging controversy, the confrontation of a modern existential dilemma. The more we seem to solve the problem, the more intractable it becomes."

The paper was then published in *Advances in Planned Parenthood* in 1980.[2] There were negative reactions among my own colleagues. I was criticized for discussing this sensitive issue in public. It made people uncomfortable that anyone outside our operating rooms was aware of this issue. The anti-abortion fanatics picked up the paper as presented in San Diego and quoted it widely (without the attribution, to my annoyance, of the correct journal citation). It amounted to right-to-life porn in the hands of our adversaries.

My idea was that this was an authentic experience that had important ethical implications for our clinical practice. Should we choose a procedure that was easier on us but more dangerous and stressful for the patients (and their nurses on the labor wards) or a procedure that was clearly safer for the patients but stressful for us, the health practitioners? My clear choice was the latter. The patients' safety and interests must be first.

The second thing is that I am a human being with ethical concerns and sensibilities. What I do as a physician occurs in an ethical context. I am not an automaton or an abortion-dispensing machine. I have feelings about what I am doing. I am a writer. I write about my experiences. This was an important experience in my life, and it had wider implications.

The anguish and stress that I experienced in performing these procedures had important consequences for my personal life.

In addition to the stress of removing the fetus and other uterine contents with instruments and managing that operation, I was deeply concerned about the patients' safety in general and acutely aware that any failure on my part that resulted in serious injury or death for the patient would have catastrophic implications for what we were doing for women's health care everywhere.

I was out on a limb, and I couldn't expect any support from the medical community locally or in general. It was up to me not to fail and to show the medical community that what I was doing was safe and beneficial for my patients. Without any other physicians in my practice, I was on call 24/7/365, which added to the stress, although there were several physicians who would always take calls for me if I were going to be out of range for a few days while I was backpacking in the mountains. My friend, Dr. Sherburne Macfarlan, was always there for me, and he gave me freedom that I otherwise would not have had.

In many ways, Mac saved my life. He is gone now, and I miss him.

During this time, I met and became acquainted with a wonderful young woman who worked part time at the hospital during the summer and who was a highly qualified teacher for children with disabilities during the school year. As we spent more time together, we enjoyed a wide variety of activities, including cross-country skiing, hiking, fishing, and backpacking in the Colorado mountains. We explored wilderness areas in Colorado and made a trip together to the Canadian wilderness. As much as we enjoyed each other's company, we had different needs At the end of a week seeing patients, on Saturday evening, I wanted to retreat to my home in the mountains for the solitude and natural beauty and time it afforded me for reflection. I was in emotional pain or, at least, stress from the procedures that I was performing, including the stress of the public controversy, my concern for the safety of my patients, and the sense that I was developing something important and new that was potentially a breakthrough in abortion services. It was a little frightening. And I was worried about my physical safety because of the threats. I also needed time alone to think about what was happening and what I was doing.

My friend had a wide circle of friends in Boulder, a wonderful family of her own, and she enjoyed spending time with them on the weekends. I needed her love and company, which was especially healing for me after a week of emotional stress and pain. She needed to be with her friends and her own large family. It certainly was not strange that she did not find the idea appealing of trudging up the side of a mountain in the middle of the night on a steep trail on snowshoes or skis in the night through deep snow and freezing wind to my empty house perched on top of a hill. The view in the morning of the Continental Divide was beautiful, but city life was easier and, in many ways, more attractive. She had a wonderful family that I enjoyed, and I was welcome in the family circle.

In spite of this, my needs for reprieve in the mountain solitude were too great. I could not resolve these conflicts. I did not have the emotional maturity, insight, or sufficient self-awareness to discuss these issues in order to meet both her needs and mine and to work things out. With great misgivings, I ended the relationship. It was painful for me, and I am sure it was painful for her, but I didn't know what else to do. There were times later in my life when I would have given almost anything to have such a relationship. In retrospect, that choice meant that I would not have – at that time – the family and relationships that I wanted in my life. I was giving up having a "normal" life in town with all of the connections, experiences, and obligations that would entail. I stayed in my mountain house, went skiing and backpacking by myself, read books, wrote papers and books, played music, and listened to the exquisite song of the hermit thrush singing from a treetop in front of my house.

The work continued. A friend and colleague from my OEO days, John Wells, started a publishing company featuring a series of pocket-sized handbooks for health-care workers having to do with various aspects of reproductive health care such as oral contraceptives and abortion. He asked me to prepare an *Abortion Services Handbook*, which I did, and which was published in 1977.[3] (I literally sketched out the basic outline of the book on the back of an envelope while I was driving home from skiing one day). It was successful and in demand until the explosion of new abortion technology made most of it obsolete. But it was clear that I needed to make a record of what we were doing and share it with my medical colleagues whether or not they were interested. Some of them were.

I began submitting a series of clinical reports to major medical journals to this end, and they were published. There followed invitations to publish my work in various monographs, and I was invited to prepare the first of several chapters for a multi-volume textbook, *Gynecology and Obstetrics*, edited by Dr. John J. Sciarra of Northwestern University School of Medicine.

This was a singularly important opportunity, and I began preparing this manuscript as I was entering the first year of my program for a Ph.D. in epidemiology at the University of North Carolina School of Public Health, where I had studied for my Master of Public Health degree. I began thinking about writing a textbook on abortion practice.

Since my treasured copy of *Gray's Anatomy* textbook from medical school was published by Lea and Febiger in Philadelphia, one of the most respected publishers of medical textbooks, I went to their office when I was in Philadelphia. The office was in the old center of Philadelphia, probably where it was when Ben Franklin was around. I immediately felt I was in an eighteenth-century environment with clerks wearing green visors on high stools reading hand-written manuscripts written by famous authors, but there was no cigar smoke. I spoke to one of the editors, and he brusquely dismissed my request on the grounds that abortion was not an important enough topic for a textbook.

The next target was Appleton-Century-Crofts, which had published one of my monographs on second trimester abortion. They politely turned me down. Then I had a break.

One of the editors of my new manuscript, which was a chapter for Sciarra's textbook, told me that she thought I was a good writer, and she asked if I would be interested in preparing a textbook for that publisher, J.B. Lippincott Company, also a highly respected publisher of medical textbooks. "Sure," I said. Since I was now in the middle of my first year of classwork for my Ph.D. course (fall of 1980), I could not work on it then, but I began accumulating notes for the project.

By the spring of 1980, I was completing my second term as a founding member of the board of directors of the National Abortion Federation (NAF), and I was now chair of the standards committee. As I had been accepted for graduate school for my Ph.D. in epidemiology, I resolved to end my official responsibilities at NAF and concentrate on my graduate work, which began that fall in Chapel Hill.

My goal for years had been to earn a Ph.D. in epidemiology in order to have a career in teaching and research in that subject, which I found endlessly fascinating. I intended to base my dissertation research on my previous research results among the Shipibo of the Peruvian Amazon. In the course of my M.P.H. research, I found that the Shipibo had the highest fertility of any human group and that this constituted a profound change from previous reports of Amazonian tribal groups having very low fertility (few children born to each woman).[4]

The hypothesis that I wished to test was that cultural change, especially as the result of the influence of Christian missionaries, was highly associated with the abandonment of traditional family structures among the Shipibo. Shipibo tribal custom, as was common among native Amazonians, was to prefer sororal polygyny, in which several women, all sisters, were wives of one man.

The hypothesis was that this family arrangement permitted and favored post-partum sexual abstinence for the women, which resulted in long birth intervals and fewer total live births per woman during her reproductive years. This tribal custom was disrupted by Christian teaching that polygyny was immoral and must end. The result was that women could no longer practice post-partum sexual abstinence, and this resulted in short birth intervals, more frequent childbearing, higher fertility, and rapid population growth.

These results, in turn, had negative consequences for maternal health and infant survival. This pattern has been seen in other parts of the world, including West Africa. One of the consequences that I learned about in my earlier studies of the Shipibo in 1964 and 1969 is that women had a very extensive and sophisticated culture concerning the use of herbal contraceptives to limit and space births and to end fertility.

Unfortunately, the effectiveness of these remedies appeared to be dependent on the simultaneous observance of post-partum sexual abstinence, which was disrupted by the loss of the custom of sororal polygyny.

One of the most important points was that Shipibo women were determined, and even desperate, to control their own fertility, and they used methods that were sometimes dangerous or potentially fatal to do so.[5]

Political problems

At the national level, abortion opponents were becoming more energized, and President Jimmy Carter tried to pacify the National Council of Catholic Bishops.[6] At the same time, he showed important deference to women's concerns by including, for example, Sarah Weddington as an advisor in his White House staff. Sarah played a critical role in the appointment of Ruth Bader Ginsberg, a strong supporter of women's rights and equality, to the federal bench.

The 1980 Republican National Convention marked a turning point as the Republican Party nominated Ronald Reagan on an aggressively anti-abortion platform thanks to Jesse Helms and the New Right. The pro-choice leaders in the Republican Party, starting with Mary Dent Crisp, were vanquished.

Jesse Helms was elected to the U.S. Senate from North Carolina in 1972, representing a racist, anti-union, anti-abortion philosophy that was consistent with the broad Republican strategy for making the South a bastion of Republican power by drawing white supremacists away from the Democrats and bringing them into the Republican Party. Helms was backed up by the tobacco industry and his own television broadcasting station. As a graduate student in North Carolina in 1968–1970, I watched as he announced his rabid right-wing TV editorials and brought tobacco-stained Klansmen on his programs to discuss civil rights. It was clear what kind of constituency he was cultivating for national office.

After entering the Senate in 1973, Helms took up the cause against abortion and sponsored the Helms Amendment that outlawed the use of federal funds for abortion services.[7] The act prohibits the use of foreign aid funds to pay for abortion "as a method of family planning or to motivate or coerce any person to practice abortion."

Jesse Helms was now a major leader in the U.S. Senate and a major hero to the anti-abortion movement. Having been reelected by an overwhelming majority in 1978, Helms played a key role in expelling pro-choice women, such as Mary Dent Crisp, from the 1980 Republican National Convention and placing the strident anti-abortion plank in the party platform that year.

NARAL meeting in Washington

On the fifth anniversary of *Roe v. Wade* in 1978, the National Abortion Rights Action League held its annual meeting at the Shoreham Hotel in Washington, D.C. The featured event of the meeting was a panel composed of courageous physicians who had been performing abortions illegally, some for ten years or more. The group included Dr. Henry Morgentaler of Canada, a survivor of Auschwitz and Buchenwald, who had been openly performing abortions in defiance of Canadian laws for years and who had been imprisoned in Canada for doing so; Dr. Ben Munson of Rapid City, South Dakota; Dr. Edward Keemer, an African-American physician in Detroit; and Dr. Kenneth Edelin, an African American physician in Boston.

Dr. Edelin had been charged with manslaughter and prosecuted in Boston by a Catholic, anti-abortion district attorney, who accused Dr. Edelin of purposefully killing a 20-week fetus that he had delivered by hysterotomy from an adolescent patient whose attempted induction abortion had failed. Ultimately, Dr. Edelin's prosecution failed, but it placed him at the center of the maelstrom of anti-abortion politics and racial injustice in conservative Boston, and the prosecution threatened to derail his promising career as an expert obstetrician/gynecologist.

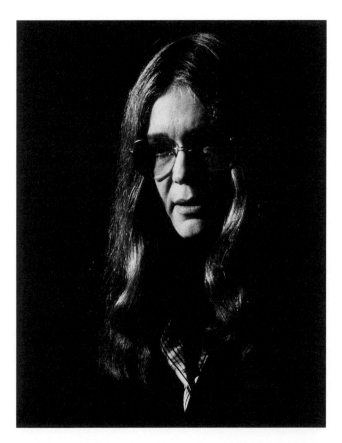

Figure 9.1 Gloria Steinem during a TV interview at the 1978 meeting of the National Abortion Rights Action League, Shoreham Hotel, Washington, D.C. Photo © Warren Martin Hern

Dr. Keemer, who had served the African American community as an obstetrican/gynecologist for decades, had been charged with performing illegal abortions and was fighting for his own survival.

Dr. Munson, who was beloved by the Native American community in South Dakota and who had also served all the women of South Dakota for decades, had been prosecuted the year before by South Dakota's politically ambitious attorney general, Bill Janklow, who used his persecution of Dr. Munson effectively in his campaign for governor of that state. Janklow's prosecution of Dr. Munson failed, but it left Dr. Munson bankrupt.

Dr. Edelin joked on the stage that his mother had told him never to "hang out with known criminals," but here he was among them.

A star of the meeting was Gloria Steinem, whose informal photo portrait I made while she was talking with TV reporters.

After the session with the physicians was over, I approached Dr. Morgentaler, who happened to know who I was, and we had a wonderful visit over coffee in the hotel cafeteria. It was the beginning of a long warm friendship that lasted for the rest of his life.

Except for Dr. Keemer, who I did not see again, I remained in contact with the other three for the rest of their lives. Henry, in particular, was like a brother. He invited me to stay at his home in Toronto, he invited me to speak at conferences he organized, he visited me in Boulder, and he invited me to join him and his family on their vacation trips. He was an extraordinary person and I treasured his friendship.

While in Washington for the NARAL event, I had an opportunity to visit with my friend Pat Schroeder in her congressional office. She was a strong supporter of women's health and reproductive freedom from long before she was elected to represent Denver in Congress and throughout her career.

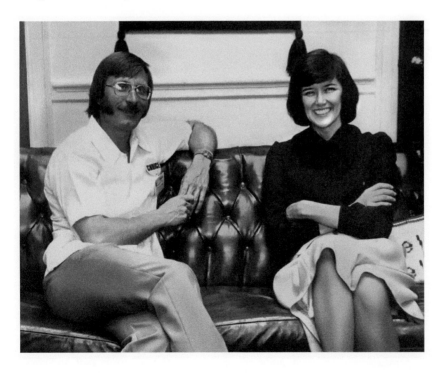

Figure 9.2 Dr. Warren Hern meets with Rep. Pat Schroeder (D-CO) in 1978.

The commute

In September 1980, I began my course work for my Ph.D. at the UNC School of Public Health in Chapel Hill, and I commuted each week between Colorado and Chapel Hill. I would catch Eastern Flight 1026 from Denver to Atlanta on Sunday afternoon and then on to Raleigh-Durham, attend classes from Monday until Thursday afternoon, catch an evening flight to Denver, see patients on Friday and Saturday, then fly back to Chapel Hill on Sunday. It was a good year to have airline stock. When my travel agent asked me how the commute was going, I told her, "I don't know what hell is going to be like, but I think that Eastern Flight 1026 to Atlanta on Sunday afternoon is a good preparation." Another physician who had started working for me saw my patients earlier in the week. On different trips through the Atlanta airport, I did meet Bobby Unser, the Indy 500 race driver, and Caspar Weinberger, who held several cabinet posts under Nixon and Reagan and who was sued by the Southern Poverty Law Center for his malfeasance concerning the OEO Sterilization Guidelines that I wrote – small world.

I can't report any interesting conversations at this time.

The election

On Wednesday morning, November 5, 1980, the election returns showed that Ronald Reagan had just been elected president. In my cabin in the Colorado mountains, I watched on my small black-and-white TV as Reagan spoke to the press for the first time

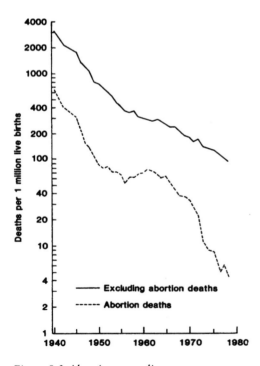

Figure 9.3 Abortion mortality rates.
Source: Cates, W. Jr. *Legal abortion: The public health record.* Science 215:1586, 1982. DOI: 10.1126/science.7071579.

as president-elect. Reagan's first words to the press were, "I'm going to make abortion illegal." The next day, at his first formal press conference, Reagan repeated this pledge.[8]

The following day, on Friday, on the *TODAY* show, I watched as Senator Strom Thurmond (R-SC) stated that he was going to ask for the death penalty for doctors who perform abortions.

Reagan and Thurmond made their statements on a day just before I left to see patients in my office and perform their abortions.

Thurmond's statements, in particular, sent chills down my spine. As I watched his statement, a coyote walked by the window where I was sitting. I reflected on how much I loved my life, my family, my friends, backpacking in the Colorado wilderness, reading by the fire, watching wildlife, skiing in the winter, and enjoying music. Thurmond was ready to take that away from me and end my life because I was helping women. Reagan, who signed the law liberalizing abortion laws in California, was ready to make me a criminal and lock me up in a prison. It was an intense moment in my life.

The anti-abortion leaders had seized the high moral ground by claiming to "defend life." It was clear to me that the only way for those of us who were helping women to keep the moral high ground was by placing our own lives on the line by doing our work to help them. It was a frightening and sobering moment of moral clarity. We were facing powerful forces from the president of the United States on down.

Nothing else would do. And it might cost us our lives.

The next week, I was back in Chapel Hill for a few days to attend classes. At a local coffee shop, where I went to have some of their famous pecan pie, I ran into one of my fellow tenants of Mrs. Poe, a dignified Southern widow who owned our rooming house for bachelor graduate students. As he was a Brazilian, we spoke Portuguese, which pleased him, and I enjoy the language. After I sat down and we exchanged friendly greetings, I told him of Reagan's election. "*Ja voceis tem um governo tão ruin que nois,*" he exclaimed ("Now you have a government just as lousy as ours!").

That fall, while attending a medical conference on abortion in Los Angeles and making a presentation, I met Linda, an OB/GYN nurse practitioner, who moved from Arizona to be with me in the spring of 1981, and we were married that fall.

On the day of his inauguration on January 20, 1981, after the ceremonies, Reagan welcomed the most radical anti-abortion fanatics into the Oval Office for a nice chat. This included Joseph Scheidler, a defrocked monk who was head of the anti-abortion Chicago "Pro-Life Action League" and who flew around the country in a Learjet organizing anti-abortion rallies at abortion clinics and doctors' offices.

The anti-abortion leaders meeting with Reagan in the Oval Office demanded the head of Dr. Ward Cates on a platter.

Reagan's newly appointed secretary of the Department of Health, Education and Welfare (HEW), Richard Schweiker, addressed the anti-abortion rally outside with a statement that this would be a "pro-life administration."

Pediatric surgeon Everett Koop had written an inflammatory anti-abortion book and made a film against abortion, and Reagan appointed him Surgeon General. For many Reagan appointees, the only essential qualification that was necessary for a high public office in the new administration was fanatic opposition to abortion.

Marjorie Mecklenberg, the person appointed by Reagan first as director of the adolescent pregnancy programs and then as Deputy Assistant Secretary for Population and Family Planning, a post first occupied by distinguished obstetrician Louis Hellman, was known principally for her opposition to contraception and abortion.

From that point, political attacks on abortion rights and women's reproductive health rights from the Reagan administration and its allies such as Jerry Falwell were relentless.

A principal goal of Ronald Reagan and his administration was to make abortion a political crime against the state. A major consequence of these public attacks on abortion by the most important public officials in the country was to inflame anti-abortion fanatics to the point of violence against doctors and clinics.

A few months after Reagan took office, a paper by Dr. Ward Cates of the Centers for Disease Control in Atlanta was published in *Science* showing a dramatic decline in maternal deaths due to abortion resulting from the legalization of abortion in the United States starting in 1967 and culminating in the *Roe v. Wade* decision of 1973.[9]

Soon after the publication of this article, Dr. Cates was removed from his official duties as a medical scientist and head of the Abortion Surveillance Unit of the Centers for Disease Control and Prevention (CDC) on orders of the White House.

Under the direction of Cates and his immediate predecessor, this unit had become the most trusted and reliable source of factual information about abortion morbidity, mortality, and other statistics in the world. It was a blue-ribbon outfit that Reagan attempted to decapitate by shuffling Dr. Cates off to a bare desk in a closet space in CDC.

Research in Peru

The course work I took for my epidemiology graduate work not only prepared me for formulating my research project in Peru, but it also helped me with the statistical analysis skills that I needed to understand my own medical practice research results. As a result, two of my clinical reports and research papers were submitted for publication in the spring of 1983 as I was preparing to go to Peru to conduct my Ph.D. dissertation research. They were both published in *Obstetrics and Gynecology* in the spring of 1984 when I was in Peru.[10] My textbook, *Abortion Practice*, was also published that year when I was in Peru.[11] My first copy of the book was delivered to me by dugout canoe in the village of Sharasmanan on the upper Pisqui River. Since abortion was illegal in Peru, I couldn't show it to anyone but Linda, who promised not to turn me in to the Peruvian authorities.

For 16 months, from June 1983 through October 1984, I conducted a household census in eight Shipibo villages on the Ucayali and Pisqui Rivers. The goal was to compare community polygyny rates and individual and community fertility rates in communities in different states of cultural change. This involved gathering fertility histories from every female from adolescence to old age, and these were done in each household, usually with the whole family in attendance. The interviews were conducted in Shipibo with some help from family members who spoke some Spanish. Linda conducted her own research on maternal/child health in the process.

An important discovery that I made in this research was that the Shipibo had ways of controlling their fertility by the use of herbal contraceptives and the family arrangement of polygyny (multiple wives), which allowed women who had just had a baby to observe a period of post-partum sexual abstinence that increased the time interval between births. These customs were disrupted by Christian missionaries, who regarded polygyny as immoral. One of the consequences of this cultural change introduced by Christian missionaries was more frequent childbearing and a larger number of live births

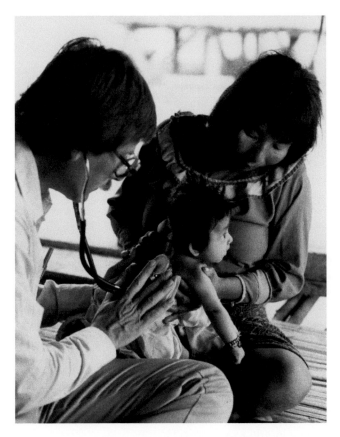

Figure 9.4 Dr. Warren Hern examines a Shipibo baby in the village of Paoyhän, 1984. Photo by
Linda Hodge. Photo © Warren Martin Hern

per woman. Each woman had more children and they were born closer together. This
resulted in a much higher rate of population growth in the village and an increased rate of
cultural change. It also appeared to result in higher infant and maternal mortality rates.

These results were significant because they stood in conflict with the "demographic
transition theory" advanced by demographers, who asserted that birth rates as well as
death rates would drop in traditional societies as cultural change and economic development occurred in the so-called Third World.

This prediction proved not to be true for the Shipibo, whose fertility rates (number of
live births per woman) went up as the result of this cultural change. As this also happened
in other traditional societies around the world, this helps explain the "population explosion" that occurred in the post–World War II years when the world rate of population
growth exceeded 2 percent per year for a time. A 2 percent growth rate means that the
population is doubling every 35 years.

Although the world population was about 2 billion at the beginning of World War II,
the human population has quadrupled to over 8 billion since then. Many of the global
ecological crises we face are the result of this fact.

My research in the Peruvian Amazon constitutes a microcosm of how this has happened.[12]

The assassination of Alan Berg

In June 1984 I interrupted my research in Peru to attend a family wedding, and, while I was back in Boulder, I received a call from the producer for Alan Berg, a radio talk show host who specialized in criticizing and ridiculing the right-wing fanatics who were threatening domestic terrorism.

Alan was Jewish, and he was especially hard on the anti-Semites among the right-wing belligerents. He challenged the ideology and beliefs of the Christian Identity movement. He was funny, and I liked Alan's outrageous commentary, but his humor was scathing, and he took no prisoners. I was afraid for him as I had come face to face with some of these people. I turned down the invitation because I thought Alan was playing with fire. I thought that the militant right-wingers were dangerous. I also felt I had enough enemies as I had been receiving death threats from anti-abortion fanatics and right-wing groups for almost 15 years – even before I began performing abortions.

On June 18, 1984, Alan was assassinated as he arrived at his home that evening by members of the neo-Nazi white supremacist group, The Order, who were determined to kill Jews and send Black people back to Africa. I was horrified by Alan's assassination, but I was not surprised. He was shot 12 times at close range with an automatic rifle as he was getting out of his car.

It was not difficult for me to imagine this happening to me.

Violence and conflict in 1984

In the fall of 1984 the physician who was helping me in my practice became ill, so I ended my research in Peru and returned to Colorado to see patients.

It was a time of increasing anti-abortion violence. During that year, anti-abortion terrorists bombed or burned 24 abortion clinics or doctor's offices. William Webster, the head of the FBI, said that the bombings weren't terrorism "because we don' t know who it is." My op-ed piece, "The anti-abortion vigilantes," was published on the op-ed page of the *New York Times* on December 21.[13] Newspapers in Boulder and Denver carried versions of this piece during the same time. Among other things, I stated that Reagan planned to make abortion a crime against the state.

1984 was also the year in which the anti-abortion video *The Silent Scream* was published and broadcast throughout the country.

This video was produced by Dr. Bernard Nathanson, who was by now the favorite "prodigal son" of the anti-abortion movement. He was a board-certified obstetrician/gynecologist who, in 1969, was a co-founder with Larry Lader and Betty Friedan of the National Association for the Repeal of Abortion Laws (NARAL). He was also a co-founder and director of one of first major abortion clinics in New York City. He performed tens of thousands of abortions. He worked together with these and other pro-choice leaders to legalize abortion in New York and elsewhere, laying the groundwork for the 1973 *Roe v. Wade* decision.

But sometime in the 1970s, he saw a real-time ultrasound image of an early abortion being performed and imagined that the embryo was crying out in pain and fear. From this viewing, he turned against abortion and became a leading opponent of the availability of safe abortions for women. One of the results was "The Silent Scream," which claimed to portray the distress of the embryo during the abortion procedure. The video featured Nathanson as the priestly interlocutor of this horror movie. It reminded me of something I had seen before.

The following is an excerpt from an article of mine on the video that was published in the Denver Post *on July 6, 1985*:

In the 1950s, several of my Englewood High School classmates and I heard that a "sex education" movie was going to be shown at the South Drive-in near Littleton. Since none of us knew anything reliable about sex and were desperately curious about it, we couldn't resist the opportunity to go. The first film was about venereal disease. The movie showed men whose genitals were in various stages of horrifying putrefaction. The message was clearly to avoid kissing girls or doing anything more serious. The second film was about abortion. It portrayed a handsome young couple, an athletic hero and a cheerleader, who kissed during a walk through the woods. The next thing you know, she was entering a seedy, back-alley place to have an abortion; the shades were down and screams issued from within. Next, she appeared, clutching her abdomen, whereupon she staggered onto a trolley car and collapsed in a pool of blood. The families and community were scandalized; the couple's lives were ruined. Heavy implications of sin and shame permeated the narration. Message for the evening: don't have sex. The lucky ones will be struck by lightning and killed instantly.

"The Silent Scream" reminded me of nothing so much as those "sex education" films made in the 1940s and designed to scare the wits out of high school boys with sexual fantasies. It is a horror movie complete with scary music and somber intonations. There are wooden portrayals of weeping young women who have no thoughts to express or connections with the subject. There are dark innuendos at the end of the film about mutilations and sterility from abortion and criminal control of the "abortion industry;" no evidence is given.

In one part of the movie, its narrator, Bernard Nathanson, dons the ritual white coat of medical priesthood and gives a pseudo-clinical description of abortion technique complete with the chilling sound of forceps locking shut on an imaginary fetal skull. He moves then to a misleading narration of an abortion procedure viewed by ultrasound. The murky view of the fetus is speeded up for effect when the abortion procedure begins. The film allegedly portrays abortion of a 12-week fetus, but the model Nathanson holds in his hand is that of a fetus of 20 or more weeks. The ultrasound image is highly magnified. His narration is accompanied by soothing pastoral music when he speaks of the fetus "moving serenely in its sanctuary" and by funereal music when he describes it as a victim.

The fetus and uterus are not attached to any woman who is a person, who has thoughts, feelings, plans, reasons, needs or medical risks resulting from pregnancy itself. The woman, in this film, is not important; she counts for nothing. The fact that abortion has become an indispensable component of health care for American women is irrelevant to the narrator.

Experts on fetal development, neurophysiology and ultrasound state that Nathanson's narrative is flat wrong. A 12 week old embryo that is two inches long does not have the neurological development to feel pain much less fear. Many of the effects that Nathanson attributed to the fetal movements were produced by speeding up the video at certain moments. Even his allies against abortion concede that the film exaggerates the dangers of abortion and is "overdramatized." The film is propaganda, pure and simple. It is sophistry, and it is dishonest. It is not intended to inform but to deceive, to inflame opinions, to create feelings of guilt, horror and anguish, and to create sympathy – for the fetus.

The fetus becomes a demigod, a fetish object to be protected against evil. Strangely enough, the film has no other goal but the imposition of guilt. Nathanson does not ask for abortion to be made illegal. He merely requires that the film be shown to any woman seeking an abortion – a requirement for indoctrination and mental abuse of women that has already been struck down by the U.S. Supreme Court.

The goal of the film is sadistic, and it is sadistic toward women. The issue is not whether abortion or any other surgical operation is aesthetically pleasing – it isn't. The issue is not whether propagandists can manipulate the magical symbols of science to inflict guilt and inflame the ignorant – they can. The issue is whether the propagandists and zealots will succeed in destroying women's rights as citizens in our society. If they succeed, we are all diminished.

Local anti-abortion harassment

In 1985 a man named William Woodley, whose day job was as an atmospheric scientist in Boulder, became head of the Colorado Right to Life Committee and put me at the top of his hate list. Although he started by picketing the front door of my office, and we affectionately referred to him as "Elmer Fudd" because of his strong resemblance to this cartoon character, he began coming to the back door of my office to harass me and my patients. This included stationing himself and his accomplices at 6 AM outside the door of a small sleeping quarters in an outlying addition to my office where my wife and I stayed when I was on night call and we had to stay in Boulder. This was very hard on our relationship. It was maddening, to say the least.

At about this time, a pro-choice organization in Boulder invited me to speak at an event at a local junior high school. Woodley was there and tried to interrupt my presentation. As the meeting closed, Woodley shouted that I was "creating an atmosphere of violence and confrontation." "You're fulla shit, Woodley," I gently explained to him.

A few weeks later, Woodley made an announcement during an anti-abortion rally on the anniversary of *Roe v. Wade*, and the local newspaper carried an article reporting that Woodley was suing me for $6 million, which was about $5.9873 million more than I had. His planned penalty for me was mysteriously reduced to $2 million for some reason.

Woodley's complaint was that I had "damaged his reputation." I replied that his reputation was already so bad that I couldn't possibly damage it. We took Woodley to court, his suit was dismissed, we filed for legal fees, and Woodley was forced to pay my attorneys $31,000. It was the last we heard of Woodley.

Notes

1 Hern, W.M., and Oakes, A. Multiple laminaria treatment in early midtrimester outpatient suction abortion. *Advances in Planned Parenthood* 12:93–7, 1977. https://www.drhern.com/wp-content/uploads/2018/05/multiple-laminaria-elim.pdf

2 Hern, W.M., and Corrigan, B. What about us? Staff reactions to D & E. *Advances in Planned Parenthood* 15–38, 1980. https://www.drhern.com/wp-content/uploads/2018/05/staff-reaction-de.pdf

3 Hern, W.M. *Abortion Services Handbook*. Chicago: Interfacia, 1978.

4 Hern, W.M. High fertility in a Peruvian Amazon Indian village. *Human Ecology* 5:355–68, 1977. https://www.jstor.org/stable/4602425 ; https://www.drhern.com/wp-content/uploads/2019/10/High-fertility-in-a-Peruvian-Amazon-Indian-Village.pdf

5 Hern, W.M. Knowledge and use of herbal contraceptives in a Peruvian Amazon village. *Human Organization* 35:919, 1976. https://doi.org/10.17730/humo.35.1.b7h6706718u56412

6 Shannon, W.V. Jimmy Carter and the Catholic bishops. *New York Times*, September 5, 1976. https://www.nytimes.com/1976/09/05/archives/jimmy-carter-and-the-catholic-bishops.html; United States Conference of Catholic Bishops statement on *Roe v. Wade* decision. January, 1973. http://www.usccb.org/issues-and-action/human-life-and-dignity/abortion/roe-v-wade.cfm

7 Barot, S. Abortion restrictions in U.S. foreign aid: The history and harms of the Helms Amendment. *Guttmacher Policy Review* 16(3), September 13, 2013. https://www.guttmacher.org/gpr/2013/09/abortion-restrictions- us-foreign-aid-history-and-harms-helms-amendment

8 President-Elect Reagan's Press Conference, November 6, 1980, Los Angeles, California.pdf Courtesy of Ronald Reagan Presidential Library and Museum. Received May 9, 2019.

9 Cates, W., Jr. Legal abortion: The public health record. *Science* 215:1586, 1982. DOI: 10.1126/science.7071579

10 Hern, W.M. Correlation of fetal age and measurements between 10 and 26 weeks of gestation. *Obstetrics and Gynecology* 63:26–32, 1984. PMID: 6691014 https://www.drhern.com/wp-content/uploads/2018/05/correlation-fetal-1026.pdf; 12. Hern, W.M. Serial multiple laminaria and adjunctive urea in late out patient dilatation and evacuation abortion. *Obstetrics and Gynecology* 63:543–49, 1984. PMID: 6700903.

11 Herrn, W.M. *Abortion Practice*. Philadelphia: J.B. Lippincott Company, 1984.

12 Hern, W.M. Polygyny and fertility among the Shipibo of the Peruvian Amazon. *Population Studies* 46:53–64, 1992.; Hern, W.M. Shipibo polygyny and patrilocality. *American Ethnologist* 19(3):501–22, 1992.; Hern, W.M. Cultural change, polygyny and fertility among the Shipibo of the Peruvian Amazon. In *Demography of Lowland South American Indians: Case Studies from Lowland South America*, Kathleen Adams and David Price (Eds.). *South American Indian Studies* 4:77–86, 1994.

13 Hern, W.M. The antiabortion vigilantes. *New York Times*, Op-ed page, Friday, December 21, 1984. https://www.nytimes.com/1984/12/21/opinion/the-antiabortion-vigilantes.html

10 Know the tree by its fruit

"Know the tree by its fruit"

Matthew 7:15–20

From the beginning of my time performing abortions in Boulder, Colorado, in November 1973, there have been demonstrators and protests in front of the first clinic I helped establish and then my own private practice from January 1975 onward.

At the beginning, I saw them sort of like ants at a picnic. They were bothersome and annoying but pretty harmless. In fact, sometimes I would go out and talk to them to see if I could understand why they were doing what they were doing.

"What are you doing?" I asked. "We're praying for you, Dr. Hern." "Why don't you pray for somebody who's not beyond redemption?" I asked. "We don't think you're beyond redemption, Dr. Hern." "Well, you just don't have enough information. You don't know how bad it is. It's hopeless. No way will I get into Heaven." "We don't think you're hopeless, Dr. Hern." "If you believe that, I have a bridge to sell you," I said.

But it got worse. Patients would come in shaking and crying from the verbal assaults. One couple discovered they had left their insulin supplies back in Wyoming so they crossed the street to the hospital to go to the emergency room to get some insulin. The protesters followed them all the way over and all the way back telling the couple that they were murderers and shouldn't kill their baby. The couple had a wanted pregnancy that had terrible complications and they were grieving. No matter. The demonstrators wanted them to feel worse.

The anti-abortion protesters feel good by making other people feel bad.

They are out there standing in the cold of winter and the blazing heat of summer to suffer and save their own souls at the expense of my patients. They bring their toddlers to suffer also and to inflict guilt on the patients entering my office to have an abortion. It is exploitative child abuse. They are using their own children for a political purpose that the kids can't possibly understand much less give their consent. They are pawns in psychological warfare and in a political death struggle.

On numerous occasions, protesters would show up with a ram's horn that made a terrible racket that made it difficult to have a conversation with a patient inside my office. On many other occasions, someone would show up with a microphone and loudspeaker and turn it up as high as possible while directing vile language, insults, and shouts of "Mommy, don't kill me!" against the patients.

We could hear this racket in my operating room, recovery rooms, and counseling rooms.

DOI: 10.4324/9781003514961-11

Patients repeatedly told me that being assaulted psychologically and audibly by the protesters was the worst part of the whole experience.

Deliberate violation of the cultural norms of distance

Anthropologist Edward T. Hall studied the social and cultural norms of approach and appropriate distances in different cultures and pioneered the field of *proxemics* (the social and cultural use of space).[1] Hall made some important observations and conclusions that directly apply to anti-abortion demonstrations.

Every culture has its "normal" or "acceptable" space or distance between persons depending on the situation, social status, and relationship between the persons involved. An "intimate" space of 1 ½ feet includes personal touching, affection, grooming behavior, and sexual behavior. A "personal" space between 1 ½ – 4 feet is an appropriate distance for a conversation with a close friend or known person. A "social" distance of up to 12 feet is set by, for example, a conversation with someone who is an acquaintance but not personal friend, seats at the dinner table, and the spaces people observe between each other at a cocktail party or a business discussion. A "public" distance of up to 25 feet includes a lecture, sales pitch at a business meeting of more than a few people, a political rally, or some formal event. These distances vary from culture to culture. An excellent diagram can be found in Morgen Jahnke's paper, "Proxemics."[2]

Professor Hall's work has given rise to, and scientific understanding of, the expression, "my personal space."

Notice how far apart people are when they are standing in line to vote, for example. The distances are pretty regular. Other animals display this characteristic. It's organic. We're wired for it. That's one of the reasons why aggressively violating the cultural norm causes so much stress for abortion patients. It's a deliberate anti-abortion strategy to impose pain.

Cultural differences in proxemics

People in northern European cultures have a "personal" distance that may be two or three feet, but, in Brazil, such a person would be regarded as "cold" or unsocial.

Brazilian men get very close to each other, fondle the other man's jacket lapel, or give a hug and kiss on both cheeks to an old friend (also seen in Middle Eastern and Mediterranean cultures). An American man used to a greater personal or social distance may feel inexplicably uncomfortable with this at first and unconsciously sense it as a homosexual advance, which it is not. Once the American man understands that this is part of normal friendly interaction between two adult men in Brazil, the discomfort evaporates. But then the American man experiences culture shock going back into American or northern European society where people keep their distance. This brings a certain amount of confusion and sense of emotional deprivation or social isolation after having experienced the spontaneous warmth of Brazilian or other Latin American cultures.

I speak of this from personal experience from having gone back and forth over the past 60 years between the United States and various Latin American countries, where I have lived, worked, and done research. I have close friendships and professional relationships with both men and women. With many people I know in Latin America, I am treated as part of the family. It's wonderful. It feels normal.

My Brazilian medical colleagues treated me as a brother, a member of the family, and it took me a while to understand that this was a normal treatment for someone for whom they simply had warm affection and respect.

Back home, some of my American friends and associates may find my now normal Latin American comfort zone unusual or uncomfortable, but it depends on the person's ethnic background. Latino and Mediterranean people find it normal.

Anti-abortion protesters consciously and deliberately violate these unspoken norms of American culture by pressing closely to women entering abortion clinics or doctors' offices in order to make the women (and their partners) extremely uncomfortable. This is accompanied by shouting highly personal and emotionally laden admonitions of guilt, punishment, sin, and such pleas as "Please, Mommy, don't kill me!" The combination of ignoring cultural norms of intimate, social, and public distance and shouting vile epithets delivered at inapproriate distances make women feel guilt, shame, fear, humiliation, and violates their personal space. That is exactly the purpose and goal of the anti-abortion demonstrators. They make the women entering my office experience unwelcome and painful feelings. It is cruel and sadistic. It is pitiless. This is their Christian message:. It is part of God's plan – some religion. These "Christians" don't bother reading *1 Corinthians 13*.

Boulder Buffer Zone Ordinance

By 1986 the anti-abortion demonstrations had become so aggressive that Cynthia Pearson, head of the Colorado NARAL organization at that time, decided to try to get the Boulder City Council to do something about it. The ordinance was designed to protect two clinics in Boulder, my office, the Boulder Abortion Clinic, and the Boulder Valley Women's Health Center (new name for the clinic I helped begin in 1973). The process proceeded over a couple of years, beginning with our presentations to the Boulder City Council.

The Buffer Zone ordinance aimed to create a space around the entrances to the two clinics within which the demonstrators could not approach patients closer than a certain distance. In my argument, I recommended that the demonstrators be required to stay in the Boulder city park, in western Kansas, or somewhere in New Jersey.

The American Civil Liberties Union (ACLU) argued that they had to be allowed to be closer than that to be able to exercise their First Amendment right to free speech. My view was, and is, that the demonstrators' purpose is not to express an opinion, which they could do with complete freedom anywhere, but to harass patients by exposing them to feelings of guilt, shame, and fear, thereby discouraging them from having an abortion. They could do this only at my office to my patients who arrive for private medical care. It is a deliberately planned psychological assault. It is psychological rape, and its intent is the same for women who *have* been raped and who are coming to see me end the pregnancy caused by the hideous previous violent assault. The deliberate cruelty of the demonstrators pours acid into this wound.

Christian charity, anyone? What a despicable lie.

The "buffer zone" isolates and captures victims for the demonstrators' predatory behavior.

The unsatisfactory result of the law, which was still an important and welcome expression of community sentiment in Boulder, was that, within 100 feet from the entrance to the clinic in question, the demonstrators could not approach closer than eight feet of the patient to speak to them or shout at them. If the message or the degree of proximity bothered the patient, she could call the police. I argued that the patients were too terrified by these frightening people to call the police or do anything else but get away from them as soon as possible.

Forty years later, this is still the case. The ordinance is unenforceable, and it gives clear permission for unconscionably cruel harassment by the so-called Christians.

In my testimony before the Boulder City Council, I argued that the close proximity of the demonstrators as well as the verbal abuse inflicted intolerable physical and emotional stress on my patients who were coming to me for private medical care.

Following adoption of the Boulder Buffer Zone Ordinance, anti-abortion organizations filed suit in Denver Federal District Court (*Buchanan v. Jourgensen*), and the case was heard by Judge Zita Weinshienk in Denver Federal District Court on March 6, 1987.[3]

I arranged for Dr. Hall to come to Denver to be a witness for us as well as a social psychologist, Marianne LaFrance. They both testified that the deliberate violation of the customary space distances as well as the accompanying threats were extremely stressful for the patients. I was also a witness and testified about the damaging and dangerous effects on the physical and mental health of the patients by the aggressive demonstrators.

Dr. Hall, who began studying this cultural phenomenon in the 1960s, gave a lucid description of how the anti-abortion protesters deliberately violate these subliminal cultural norms in order to influence the patients' feelings and behavior. Both scientists were

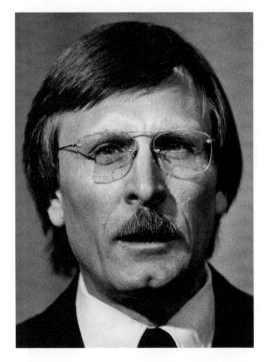

Figure 10.1 Dr. Warren M. Hern testifies before the Boulder City Council, 1986. Photo for the *Denver Post* by Duane Howell

explicit in their assessments of this situation. I described the wide variety of signs and symptoms exhibited by my patients as the result of these psychological assaults.

These phenomena and testimony by the two experts as well as my testimony are provided in my paper, "Proxemics: The application of theory to conflict arising from anti-abortion demonstrations," published in *Population and Environment* in 1991.[4]

The court ruled in favor of upholding the ordinance.

State representative Diana DeGette sponsored a similar bill, the Colorado "bubble" bill, that would be applied throughout Colorado. Her bill was co-sponsored by Colorado senator Mike Feeley (D-Lakewood), the bill passed, and it was signed into law by Governor Roy Romer on April 20, 1993.[5]

The final passage of the Colorado bill into law was accelerated by the cold-blooded assassination of Dr. David Gunn by "peaceful" "pro-life" anti-abortion fanatic Michael Griffin in Pensacola, Florida, one month earlier on March 10, 1993.

The law was challenged (*Hill v. Colorado*) and was heard before the U.S. Supreme Court on January 19, 2000.[6] The court ruled 6–1 in favor of Colorado. My article, "Bubble law goes to the Supreme Court," appeared in the Sunday Camera on June 11, 2000, when the Court was about to hear several other abortion-related cases.[7]

The American Civil Liberties Union, which forced the adoption of the close 8-foot limit rather than a more realistic one during the negotiations in Boulder, argued for the anti-abortion plaintiffs before the Supreme Court on the grounds of the First Amendment. The ACLU contradicted itself in this case. So much for women's rights to privacy and safe abortion.

Canadian law requires anti-abortion demonstrators to stay a minimum of 100 meters (a little more than 300 feet) from the entrance to the clinic or doctor's office. They may not approach the patients at all. This is a much more reasonable regulation that respects the needs for privacy of the patients.

When the U.S. constitutional right to freedom of speech conflicts with the U.S. constitutional right to cast a secret ballot, political actors and messages are required to be at least 100 feet from the entrance to the polling booth.

The same decision can be made to protect women seeking personal private medical care by keeping anti-abortion fanatics 300 feet from the entrance to a private medical office. Eight feet is too close, and 100 feet is too close.

Fast forward to the present

In 2023 one of the volunteer escorts who came to protect the patients gave me the following (unredacted) report:

From Rose

Event 1

A nurse comes outside of the clinic to tell the volunteer escorts that there is a woman and her partner on Broadway at the bus stop. They are afraid to walk down the street, through the protesters, to go to their appointment. Myself and another volunteer then start walking east on Alpine Ave. to look for them. Immediately the protesters send their elementary age children to run after us and in front of us. One of the children reached these people before we did. It was very confusing for them.

I talked with the young couple to explain who I was and we began heading west on Alpine back to the clinic.

I had my arm around the shoulders of this petite, pregnant Black woman as we approached an office near the clinic. The protesters have been yelling this whole time and the woman is sobbing, holding onto me. My fellow volunteer was being equally supportive of the young Black man who had accompanied her. She is begging me for a different way to get into the clinic that would not require going through the protesters. At that moment there was no other option to offer her, so we continued walking up the street.

Now imagine this, two young Black people from out of state exercising their legal rights to go to a health appointment. They are facing being surrounded by a hostile group of mainly white people who are yelling at them, shaming them…this is threatening to them.

At this moment, as we are approaching the protesters, a tall woman steps into the sidewalk and blocks our way. I had never seen this woman before and I have not seen her since. I pushed forward without hesitation using my shoulder, as this is a public sidewalk, and she was pushed off balance so stepped to the side. She then stepped back onto the sidewalk and blocked the other volunteer with the woman's partner. The other volunteer had to do the same thing I had done and pushed her aside to walk by.

By this time another escort could see that we needed a different option and had driven her car onto Alpine, turned around, and pulled up near us in the middle of the street. We carefully hustled the woman and her partner into the car. The main moment of fear that I experienced was in this moment. She was so panicked and wanting to get away from the protesters that she almost ran to get in the car. She tripped on irrigation pipes that the city has sticking up next to the sidewalks there! Luckily I had one of her arms and her partner had the other so we kept her from falling…barely. They were driven the 20–30 feet to get through the driveway to the clinic.

The woman who had blocked the sidewalk proceeded to ask to file charges against myself and my fellow volunteer for assault. This brought the police out to the clinic to follow up. They soon left when they realized she had blocked a public sidewalk. The woman never filed charges.

Event 2
Everything that goes on outside of the clinic gets escalated for the whole neighborhood and local businesses, including Boulder Mental Health Center, a few doors down, when the protesters use electronic amplification units that they wear on their chests. They are very, very loud to where people inside businesses can hear the words that are being said. These men focus on the patients most of the time but are now focusing on the volunteers. They are calling us out by name, throughout the neighborhood, saying terrible things. There used to be only one man doing this but as of December 5th there are now two men from the Rose's Society harassing us and the patients at 80–90 decibels. This is well above the decibel limit in the municipal code but the police are unable to ticket them because there is only one person in the police department that is certified to read a decibel reader! Meanwhile, this man is yelling into the neighborhood our names, asking us questions like "have

you had an abortion?", "I was in law enforcement for 15 years!", "what you are doing is illegal," and "You are murderers...how do you sleep at night," etc. It goes on and on and, yes, there are 1st amendment rights but this moves from protesting to individual harassment. Especially when it is being amplified through the neighborhood.

The women who are inside the clinic recovering hear every word of this vitriol. This is incredibly stressful to these women who have every right to heal and recover in peace. In fact, there is a part of the city municipal code that says that.

These people with the amplifiers are breaking at least two codes...the city needs to enforce the decibel noise ordinance and the health center protection ordinances.

Event 3

Once again, when two of us went off private property to find someone who was afraid to walk through the protesters, we were followed by one particular woman who is a regular member of the protest group. I was further ahead but this woman walked close enough to the other volunteer that she was singing "follow the leader" in a whispery voice right behind her. This scared her and she stopped and the woman was so close she ran into her. This is very threatening, creepy behavior. The woman crossed down the alley and left. The volunteer that this happened to has filed charges.

From Nancy

An ongoing harassment by the protesters (via microphone) directed at entering patients is "Wouldn't you rather have your sick baby die in your loving arms than kill it now."

Sometime this fall, after an African American woman entered the clinic, one of the protesters yelled out to us that we were racists because we were killing Black babies and keeping down the Black population.

We, the escorts, have been asked why we hate babies, how can we live with what we are doing, etc. In general, they try to provoke us.

Another concern is for passersby. When there is a large group of protesters on the sidewalk, people, including disabled folks and people from the mental health center, walk out onto Alpine to avoid them.

From Susan

For the past year and a half, I've been volunteering at the entry to the Boulder Abortion Clinic in order to provide a tiny bit of support to women who come there for help. There appear to be two protesting organizations with "members" at work in front of the clinic at least 1 day every week, regularly on Tuesday mornings and occasionally other afternoons. The larger group, associated with an organization called "40 days for Life," according to their signs, is made up of older men and women and one or two families with several toddlers and young children. Their practice is to pray aloud, recite the rosary, call out to the patients offering help with adoption, diapers, and conversation to change the decision of the patients. The volume of their voices elevates whenever a patient arrives at the clinic and the shouting continues until we can get the patient into the front entry.

The second organization (the Rose Society) has been represented by one older man, who now seems to have "acquired" a partner during December, because they both say their name is Kevin and they both use speech amplification devices to shout at arriving patients and the people who accompany the patient. They offer New Testaments with inserted printed materials to any pedestrian brave enough to walk on the same side of the street. The older Kevin always puts out a variety of signs proclaiming the mothers who did not choose abortion or showing a bloodied infant body and what appear to be dismembered legs. He always claims "the love of his life had an abortion and was haunted by it for the rest of her life" at a very high volume. A cell phone app registered above 80 decibels on more than one week when I have been present.

The second "Kevin" arrived with his own, handmade sign which states "BABIES ARE STILL MURDERED HERE." He ceaselessly tried to engage me in conversation, and I slipped up by telling him my first name, which he then used to accuse me of sinning as well as to offer me an opportunity to join him for coffee or use him as my pathway to God, etc. He also employed his amplifier while badgering me and one of our youngest volunteers, asking if we'd had abortions or if we had children, if we believed in God or thought murder was good, etc. Both Kevins have "disappeared" from the street during a couple of occasions on which the police were called about the loudspeakers and patient harassment.

The groups used to appear by 9:00 AM and leave by 10:30 or sometimes noon and were smaller when the weather was severe, although they still brought the little ones. The belief was that a Catholic church in south Boulder provided free lunch on Tuesdays. We volunteers stayed until they were gone. In the last few months there appears to be an effort to have "shifts" of the various individuals and families to stay longer, stretching to 1:00 or 1:30. An additional five-person group of students from CU have begun showing up with their signs proclaiming them to be the "Pro-Life Generation". Fortunately, they join the prayers for 10 to 15 minutes and then depart again.

The second "Kevin" and the longer duration of the groups presence suggests an intensification of efforts to shame the patients and now even the escorts, at this time of intensified efforts to interfere with abortion access where it is still lawful. It seems to our volunteer group that the city codes cannot protect the existing patient and health clinic rights to privacy at the same time as the existing rights to free speech of the protesters. First enforcing the city's existing safety and noise ordinances and then allowing construction of better barriers at the entry to the property might avoid physical harm.

The free speech protection already exists although the distance ordinances are being ignored.

From Faith

This happened sometime early in the summer of 2023:

A trans person, wearing a skirt and with a beard, was walking up Alpine, across the street from the protesters. One of the protesters (younger guy with a mullet) yelled across the street to this person, saying "Put on pants!" The trans person then turned around and walked back past the protesters on their side of the street. I don't know if they engaged with the protesters initially, but this same person followed him, taunting, and saying that they "should kill himself."

The protesters left soon after that. We discussed it among ourselves (we were quite shocked), and finally one of us went to talk to the last protester, who was still getting into their car (not the person who had yelled at the trans person). That person did apologize for the incident.

New volunteer escort report on January 30, 2024
Hello Dr. Hern,

We thought we should report a few things that happened yesterday.

The young guy with a mullet haircut and a MAGA hat was there, and it seems like whenever he shows up things get more heated.

He tends to get into conversations with women who are walking down the sidewalk. He tries to engage with them by complimenting their appearance, or their dogs if they have one. Usually they disagree with his ideas and get into arguments with him. Twice today he told women, who were white and who support abortion, that they must be Jewish, and that they should go back to Israel. (very anti-Semitic comments). (one of the women was Ann, from our group, who was raised Catholic. The other was a woman on the street). He also got into an argument with a lovely young woman who really held her own against him, and argued back very effectively. He finally told her that in 30 years she was going to be like those ugly old witches (us!) who were trying to prevent him from talking to the patients. She told him that she certainly hoped she would be just like us, and then came over to talk to us.

By the way, he has been filming the limo driver every time he drops someone off. He also has been filming us, which just seems like an attempt to intimidate us. He's creepy.

[*End of volunteer escorts report*]

***

Comment on escorts' observations

In Nazi Germany, the Jews were demonized, and they were increasingly treated in insulting, discriminatory, humiliating, and marginalizing ways. They were first called names, they had to wear a yellow star, they were ordered about, they had to get off the sidewalk, they lost jobs, and, ultimately, they were cruelly massacred. It was a gradual but inexorable process.

Christian anti-abortion demonstrators are treating women who seek personal medical care in these hideous ways. Women suffer and die as a result. What are the next steps?

How are the white Christian Evangelicals and MAGA hoodlums different from the brown-shirted Nazi thugs?

The young Black woman in the Event #1 was a very young adolescent (younger than 15) who had been raped and was 25 weeks pregnant. Her father, also Black, was with her to help her and protect her. They had flown across the country from the Deep South, where they face daily racism, to an unknown community to see a doctor they didn't know to have a controversial operation for a very intimate personal problem.

In addition to the racism displayed by the white anti-abortion protesters, how could this father and daughter coming to my office for help with this deep family tragedy cope with the terror and horror of their abuse by the demonic white protesters? It was unimaginable cruelty.

An important part of our counseling support is to help patients cope with the insults and guilt trips inflicted on the patients by these merciless people. They care nothing about the women as persons who are experiencing the most difficult and vulnerable times in their lives.

They feel good by making other people feel bad.

It's about power. Make somebody feel something they don't want to feel is painful.

The fanatic Christians are unbelievably self-righteous, punitive, and cruel. What kind of a religion is this that leads them to treat others who they don't even know in this way?

It is certainly the opposite of what I thought I learned about Christianity as a young person.

Jesus said, "Know a tree by its fruit." The fruit of this Christian tree is bitter, nauseating, poisonous, punitive, and dangerous.

It is the face of fascism in America. It is evil.

Soon after these incidents occurred, which had signaled an ominous increase in the violence and aggressiveness of the anti-abortion demonstrators, I retained a private limousine company at considerable cost to pick up the patients and bring them to the door of my office so they would not have to be subjected to the systematic psychological rape imposed by the fanatics in front of my office. I also hired a uniformed, armed off-duty police officer to stand in front of the entrance to my office between the patients and the demonstrators.

I cannot assume that my patients can safely walk to or ride the bus to my office, get off, and walk undisturbed up the public sidewalk to the front door of my office. I must protect them from these unconscionable assaults by people who call themselves Christians. I will do so. But what other physicians have to do this to protect their patients? None.

These are not normal costs of a medical practice, but they are necessary to protect the patients from the outrageous abuse by the self-righteous Christians who don't have anything better to do with their lives than to interfere with the lives of other people they don't know. Their self-inflicted spiritual, emotional, moral, intellectual, and social poverty is pathetic.

Christians should be ashamed. They are not. They know they are right. They talk to God and carry Guns. Do what they say.

"*The principal feature of Christianity is the manufacture, assignment, maintenance, management and exploitation of guilt*"[8] (from Holland, *Tiny You*, op.cit.).

A daily threat to me

The anti-abortion protesters do not confine their attacks and threats to patients and volunteer escorts.

To reduce the risk of my being assassinated by someone who is on a three-story building to the east of my office and has an unobstructed view of my staff parking lot, I created a special parking place for myself so I would be less exposed to gunfire while moving from my car to one of the back doors of my office. I made it so the car door on the driver's side was just by the building door. I get my keys ready so I can move quickly to get through the door before a sniper could get me in his sights.

But this special spot to reduce that risk has me parking at the bottom of a driveway leading to the street in front of my office and looking through the controlled access steel

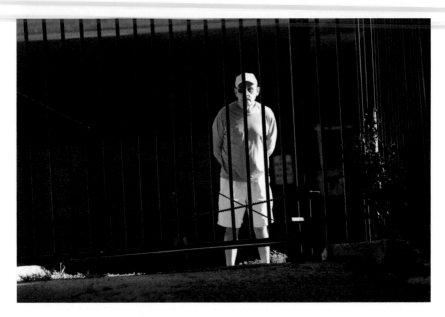

Figure 10.2 Tuesday stalker R____ C____ watching me arrive and get out of my car. Photo ©
   Warren Martin Hern

gate across the top of the driveway. Someone standing on one side of the gate can see me
directly in my car.

   One of the demonstrators (not always the same person) routinely stalks me by standing by the front steel gate in a position where he can look directly at me when I park my
car on arriving at my office. This is unnerving because I don't know if this person will
pull out a gun and shoot me as I am parking or as I get out of my car to enter my office.
I must assume that the person is armed and dangerous. This is harassment and attempted
intimidation.

   I can never walk out of the front door of my office or drive out of the front gate of
my parking lot when the protesters are there. It's too dangerous. Think about that. I'm a
doctor helping women. Why should someone want to kill me for doing that?

Lingering effects of anti-abortion demonstrators on patients

It is often difficult to tell how much effect the anti-abortion demonstrators have on individual patients. Some, like the adolescent young woman mentioned earlier in this chapter, come into the office crying, shaking with fear, and report that the verbal assaults of
the demonstrators are the worst part of the experience of having an abortion. Others take
it in stride. Nothing will deter them from getting the medical care they need.

   For some patients, the effects are long-lasting. An example is a woman who I helped
over 40 years ago when she was very early in her pregnancy. She called us 15 years later
to ask for her medical records. We sent them, but she called again asking to speak to me
as she wanted more than had been sent. Here is my file memo after that conversation:

   In our conversation, M. constantly referred to her "child," and she wanted to know
how I could kill "children." I replied to her that we do not kill "children." She was

hostile, provocative, combative, rude, and accusatory. She said that the aborted "child" was not a "blob of tissue," and I pointed out to her that we never described it to her as that. She wanted to know what we do with the "children" after we "kill them." I replied that the embryo or fetus is inspected after the abortion to determine the length of pregnancy and whether there are any pathological conditions that could affect the woman, then the tissue is cremated along with other surgical tissue. After each of my answers, she would pause, as though she were writing down my answer.

At one point, she asked me if I had children. I asked her at that time if she called me to ask me personal questions. She was hostile and didn't answer. I stated that I am a physician and that I responded to her request for help at one time and provided her with medical care, and that I wished to help her if she needed that, but that it was not appropriate for me to answer personal questions. She accused me of being angry at her. The tone of her voice and conversation was extremely combative and belligerent. When I recommended that she seek professional counseling, she stated that she "became a Christian six years ago," and that her personal counselor is now "Jesus Christ." I stated that I supported whatever means she wished that would give her comfort and support.

I promised to send her medical records and ended the conversation.

It is uncommon but not rare for patients to blame me for their decision to have an abortion or end a pregnancy. Somebody has to be guilty. *Why?*

Somebody has to be guilty. Who's got the guilt?

Even though I am the principal target of the anti-abortion assassins, everyone who works in my office is at constant risk. My staff knows this, but they show up to help the patients anyway. The patients show up anyway. They need our help.

They are all very brave.

Notes

1 Hall, E.T. *The Silent Language*. Garden City, NY: Doubleday, 1959.
2 Jahnke, M. Proxemics. Interesting thing of the day, February 15, 2007. https://itotd.com/articles /6277/proxemics/
3 *Buchanan v. Jorgensen*, 1987. U.S. District Court, Denver, March 6, 1987.
4 Hern, W.M. Proxemics in the abortion debate: The use of anthropological theory in conflict arising from antiabortion demonstrations. *Population and Environment* 12(4)379–88, 1991. https://www.jstor.org/stable/27503211
5 McAvoy, T. Romer signs abortion-patient "bubble" bill into law. *Pueblo Chieftain*, April 20, 1993. https://www.chieftain.com/story/special/1993/04/20/romer-signs-abortion-patient-bubble/8809895007/
6 *Hill v. Colorado*, 530 U.S. 703 (2000); https://supreme.justia.com/cases/federal/us/530/703/#tab -opinion-1960804https://supreme.findlaw.com/static/fi/images/efile/supreme/briefs/98-1856/98 -1856fo9/brief.pdf ; Amicus brief of the American College of Obstetrician/Gynecologists before the SCOTUS, *Hill v. Colorado*.
7 Hern, W.M. Abortion "bubble bill" going before U.S. Supreme Court: Law has origins to buffer zone rule enacted by Boulder City Council. *Sunday Camera*, Guest Opinion, June 11, 2000. https://www.drhern.com/wp-content/uploads/2019/10/abortion-bubble-bill.pdf
8 Holland, J. *Tiny You: A Western History of the Anti-abortion Movement*. Berkeley: University of California Press, 2020.

11 Anti-abortion violence

Assassinations and stochastic terrorism

On January 22, 1982, the ninth anniversary of the *Roe vs. Wade* decision, the office of Dr. Hector Zevallos, the Hope Clinic for Women, near Granite City, Illinois, was firebombed. That August, Dr. Zevallos and his wife, Rosalie Jean, were sitting in their home watching television one evening when three armed men wearing masks entered their home, blindfolded them at gunpoint, and took them hostage. The three men took the couple to an abandoned underground National Guard ammunition bunker left empty after World War II.

The doctor and his wife were bound hand and foot, blindfolded and gagged, and kept there on the dirt floor for eight days.[1] The kidnappers, who called themselves the "Army of God," threatened to kill both of them if Dr. Zevallos refused to stop performing abortions and unless President Ronald Reagan denounced abortion (he already had, but the kidnappers didn't know this). Dr. Zevallos resisted this demand, but, finally, he was persuaded by his wife to say that he would close his clinic if the kidnappers let them free. One of the kidnappers received a message from God that they should not kill the doctor. The couple was released.

Dr. Zevallos, an obstetrician/gynecologist who was 53 years old at the time of this incident, was a tall, congenial, move-star handsome man whose Andean Inca ancestors are apparent in his appearance and his courtly manners. He was a graduate of the distinguished University of San Marcos in Lima. He opened the Hope Clinic for Women in Granite City in 1979, where he had delivered many babies in his obstetrical practice, and his patients came from throughout northern Illinois, Missouri, and Indiana.

All three of the kidnappers were arrested, found guilty, and sentenced to long prison terms.

The kidnapping of Dr. Zevallos and his wife was the first assault on a physician by anti-abortion fanatics. They were released without physical harm, but they were severely traumatized by the experience.

Abortion clinics attacked

In 1984 two dozen abortion clinics or physicians' offices were bombed, burned, or otherwise attacked. William Webster, director of the FBI, said in an interview that it wasn't terrorism "because we don't know who did it." "Bombing an abortion clinic is not an act of terrorism."[2]

The bombers were caught, prosecuted, and convicted. One of them said that the bombings in Florida were a "Christmas present to Jesus."

DOI: 10.4324/9781003514961-12

On December 21, 1984, after the most recent anti-abortion firebombing of a physician's office, my op-ed article, "The anti-abortion vigilantes" was published in the *New York Times*.[3] NBC News sent a crew to interview me for the *NBC Nightly News*. At the end of the interview session, the producer said, "Well, I now know everything there is to know about abortion." The next evening, the segment on abortion aired in the newscast. My interview and the information I gave was not included. The segment ended with the camera focused on blood spattering into a bottle as a first trimester abortion was being completed.

The woman, a person, who was having the abortion, was nowhere to be seen. She was irrelevant to the story. The last image was of Tom Brokaw contemplating that image of the blood-spattered bottle.

I was profoundly relieved that we were not included in that program, and I was more relieved that my interview had not been included. I thought it was a despicable, sensational, and inflammatory way to end the nationally broadcast TV report on abortion. It contributed to the growing anti-abortion hysteria and violent crimes, which began in 1979 with the firebombing of Bill Baird's clinic in Hempstead, New York.[4]

From the time of the anti-abortion violence at Baird's clinic in 1979 through 1988, there were 110 violent attacks on abortion clinics and doctor's offices in the United States.[5] We were under siege. Our worst fears were being realized. The anti-abortion fanatics were becoming more and more violent. I became increasingly worried about fatal violence.

Encouraged by his enhanced status under Ronald Reagan, Joe Scheidler went around the country in a Learjet leading demonstrations against doctors and abortion clinics with a bullhorn shouting obscenities at women entering clinics. On national television programs, he would repeatedly intone, "I have yet to shed a tear over the smoldering remains of an abortion clinic." His book, *Closed: 99 Ways to Stop Abortion*, was a best-selling handbook on anti-abortion violence.[6,7]

Scheidler was a defrocked monk who was the leader of the Chicago "Pro-Life Action League." He was, incredibly, permitted to attend the 1985 annual meeting of the National Abortion Federation and harass speakers. I was horrified, but I decided to try to understand him and express my concern about the threats he was making. I went up to him and spoke to him in person. He was wearing his trademark white suit and hat. He looked down on me from his 6'4" height with steely blue eyes as I said, "The language you are using is going to get someone hurt and even killed. I think there is room to disagree about this issue and still be civilized."

Scheidler looked me in the eye and said, very slowly and ominously, "I'm coming to destroy you." The encounter was frightening. I shuddered and thought, "Here's the enemy. This man will stop at nothing. This isn't about abortion; it's about power." He looked like a Nazi, he thought like a Nazi, he talked like a Nazi, and he acted like a Nazi. He was a thug. I decided then that he was an extremely dangerous person who was the greatest threat to our work for women.

Scheidler in Boulder

A few months later, it was announced that Scheidler was coming to Boulder to speak to a student rally against abortion and to lead demonstrations against me and my office. Since my textbook, *Abortion Practice* had been published in 1984, Scheidler and other antiabortion leaders had put me in their crosshairs. His pending arrival and planned rally against me at the University of Colorado was announced in the newspapers.

Berlin

Just before this, I was invited to make a presentation at the Christopher Teitze Symposium in Berlin that was designed to highlight current knowledge about abortion techniques and services and honor our beloved colleague, Chris Tietze. My friend and colleague, George Tiller, was there with his wife, Jeanne. George and Jeanne decided to rent a car and drive over into East Berlin through Checkpoint Charlie in the Berlin Wall. I had no idea this was possible, but they invited me to go with them, and I went.

One of the saddest and most moving experiences in my life was standing across the street from the Jewish Community Center and synagogue and looking at the flame marks on the buildings from *Kristallnacht*, which happened in my lifetime on November 9–10, 1938, when I was five months old. I reflected on the millions of Jews who lost their lives in Hitler's gas chambers and the tens of millions of others who died in World War II, and I wept.

It is one of the great tragic landmarks in human history that signaled the brutality of Hitler's Nazi regime and the potential for inhumanity by humans against other humans.

On my way back to the United States my seatmate was my friend, Dr. Louise Tyrer, who was the medical director and vice president for medical affairs for the Planned Parenthood Federation of America. Louise and I chatted about what we had seen in Berlin.

On arriving at my office, I immediately left for a medical meeting in Seattle. The next day, a Saturday, my office manager, PJ (who was herself Jewish) was alone in my office taking phone calls from women who needed appointments for the next week. A stone came crashing through one of the front windows of my office. PJ was terrified. It was *Kristallnacht* in a small place. She called me, and a message was brought to me during the luncheon meeting. I needed to return immediately to Colorado, so I left.

By the time I reached my office, PJ had arranged for the broken window to be boarded up and had scheduled for new glass to be placed on Monday.

This event had been preceded by the announcement that Joseph Scheidler was coming to Boulder to speak at an anti-abortion rally directed toward me and my office. Since my textbook, *Abortion Practice*, had been published the year before, Scheidler decided that I should be the prime target of his machinations.

A dentist next door had seen the perpetrator take a rock from a stone flower planter in front of my office window and heave it through the window. The police caught him and prosecuted him. He was a supporter of Scheidler who had been inflamed to take this action because he was encouraged by Scheidler's rhetoric.

That night, I woke up and decided to do something else before replacing the glass. I went to my photo workshop, cut out a large piece of foam core board used for mounting photos, and wrote on it in large letters, "This window was broken by those who hate freedom." I was outraged. My situation was trivial by comparison, but I had just seen some of the results of Nazi hatred of Jews in Berlin, and the broken glass in my office front window was the small-scale result of the same hateful mentality.

Scheidler arrives

The following Monday, October 25, 1985, Scheidler led a demonstration against me and my clinic with his bullhorn and rabid followers. But my sign was visible at his back as he spoke to the assembled TV cameras and reporters. As usual, we had no patients scheduled for that day, a Monday. He claimed that no patients were coming in because I had closed my office because I was afraid of him. Members of the press came in to interview me. One reporter said, "Scheidler says you're afraid of him. Is that true?" "I am afraid of three things," I said. "Lightning, grizzly bears, and sharks. Scheidler didn't make the cut."

I decided that if a man like Scheidler, who was in league with all the tyrants of history, would come all the way from Chicago to try to stop me from what I was doing, I must be doing something very important for the cause of human freedom.

Scheidler's campaign against me continued for months. At one point, I took out a full-page ad in the local paper with the headline, "Pledge a Picket For Choice." In the ad, I offered to match a pledge of $1 per anti-abortion picketer per day with $5 of my own as a contribution to a pro-choice candidate for public office.[8] When a newspaper reporter called Scheidler to ask for his reaction to my offer, he said, "It's *diabolical*." Bingo!

In 1986 the National Right to Life Committee had its annual convention in Denver, Colorado. All of the Republican candidates for president were invited, all accepted, and all attended except George H.W. Bush.[9] One of the candidates, evangelist Pat Robertson, was quoted in the *Denver Post* as telling the assembly, "We can't permit abortions because if we do, we won't have enough people to fight the wars and pay the taxes." There could not have been a more eloquent statement of the authoritarian exploitation of women as reproductive machines for purposes of the fascist state.

George H.W. Bush, who had supported Planned Parenthood and family planning legislation as a member of Congress, went on to secure the Republican nomination for president. His son, George W. Bush, was his emissary to the fundamentalist evangelical Christians. The younger George Bush assured the Christians that his father was against abortion. The elder Bush won the election.

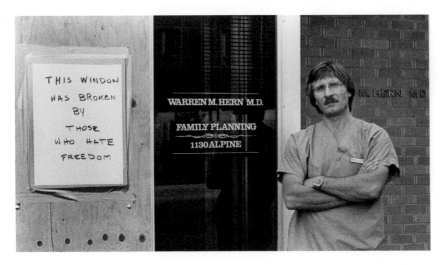

Figure 11.1 Dr. Warren Hern stands next to a window broken Friday at the Boulder Abortion Clinic. The *Daily Camera*, October 22, 1985. Photo for the Daily Camera by Brian Lincoln

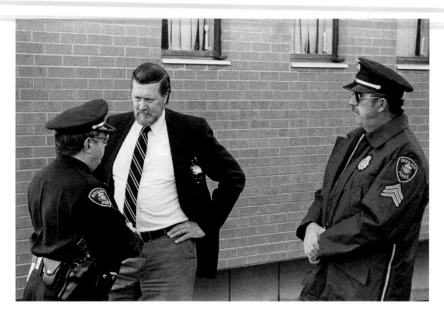

Figure 11.2 Joe Scheidler, trespassing on the author's property, receiving instructions from Boulder police officers, October 23, 1985. Photo © Warren Martin Hern

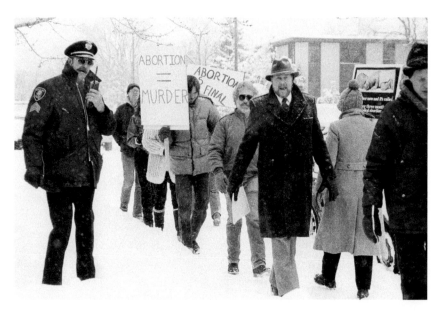

Figure 11.3 Joe Scheidler in anti-abortion protest in front of my office, December 1985. Photo © Warren Martin Hern

On the same weekend that the Right to Life convention took place, the National Organization for Women (NOW) held its annual meeting in Denver and celebrated its 20th anniversary. NOW planned to hold a major rally on the steps of the state capitol. Ellie Smeal was the president of NOW at the time and asked me to be one of the speakers. We marched in a parade from the Hilton Hotel in downtown Denver to the state capitol steps. There were hundreds of people in the crowd.

Ellie presented me with the "Unsung Hero Award" from the National Organization for Women.

The group was addressed by Ellie; Pat Blumenthal, who was the head of NARAL Colorado; Congressman David Skaggs; and me. It was a high point. At one point, I called out Reagan on the abortion issue and said he should be impeached. The crowd started chanting "*Im-peach, Im-peach, Im-peach....*etc." It was exhilarating and an intense moment, and it helped me to understand how politicians – especially demagogues – can get addicted to getting crowds fired up.

When I got through speaking, Skaggs said to me, "Wow! That was amazing! Have you done this before?" "Nope," I said, "but it's fun."

After the big event of the day was over, there was a big party with dancing at the Hilton, but Linda and I left to go home to the mountains.

My op-ed article, "Must Mr. Reagan tolerate abortion clinic violence?" was published that day in the *New York Times*.[10]

Throughout the eighties, there were countless anti-abortion demonstrations, clinic invasions, and violent anti-abortion incidents. Doctors were called "baby killers," "child killers," and various other invectives. Scheidler, evoking the Nazi gas chambers, called abortion clinics "abortoreums."[11]

I had so many death threats I thought about setting up a death threat hotline modeled after the "sex talk" hotlines. "You want to threaten Dr. Hern's life? Easy. Give the operator your name, address, telephone number and credit card number for quick relief. Only $5 a minute, talk as long as you like!" Nah. Too much trouble.

Shots fired

On February 4, 1988, five shots were fired through the front windows of my office into the patient waiting room.[12] I had just walked through the room. A member of my staff was almost hit by the bullets. There were cars in the parking lot. The shots were intended to kill someone.

The next day, I stood on the lawn in front of my office, held a press conference, and offered a $5,000 reward for information leading to the arrest and conviction of the person who fired the shots. I installed bullet-proof windows at a cost of thousands of dollars. The case is still open. The reward stands.

The gunshots fired into my office occurred the same week that my divorce from Linda was final. The two events were not unrelated because the antiabortion harassment had a disastrous effect on my marriage of seven years. The juxtaposition of the two events did nothing positive for my self-esteem. They were clear signs of disapproval. The message from many sources was: "Go away."

At this moment, I began to think seriously about closing my medical practice and going to live with the Shipibo Indians in the Peruvian Amazon, who had appreciated my efforts to understand them and to help them since 1964.

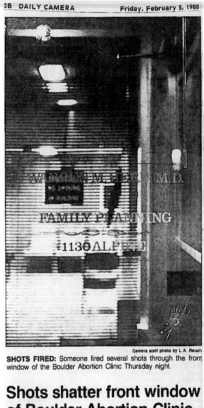

2B   DAILY CAMERA   Friday, February 5, 1988

Camera staff photo by L. A. Rauch

SHOTS FIRED: Someone fired several shots through the front window of the Boulder Abortion Clinic Thursday night.

Shots shatter front window of Boulder Abortion Clinic

Figure 11.4 News clipping showing a window broken by gunshots at the Boulder Abortion Clinic.

The sense of isolation was compounded later when I increasingly had the feeling that I was an undesirable person from a woman's point of view because of my work and notoriety performing abortions. After beginning to get acquainted with one young woman who made it clear that she really liked me, she said, "I really want to be with you, but I can't take you home to my parents." This happened more than once.

In the middle of all this, for years before, and for year afterward, we received hundreds of hang-up calls, hundreds of obscene tirades and insults on the reception telephone line, bomb threats with evacuations, unwanted deliveries of merchandise, and vandalism. The janitor's tires were slashed while he was working at night to clean the building. One counselor owned a car that was exactly like mine – the same make, year, model, color, and perfectly anointed dirt patterns. One evening when she came out to go home, all the lug nuts on the wheels were loosened so the wheels would fall off. This was potentially deadly for her, but if it had been my car, I would have been driving on treacherous mountain roads – a normal activity for me – to get home. If a wheel came off, I could go over the cliff and die. This was not a subtle threat. Staff members were stalked and harassed as they went about their errands to the beauty shop, to get groceries, or to go to the bank. Babysitters turned them down.

Randall Terry, a high school dropout, failed rock musician, and unemployed used car salesman, found his calling as a radical anti-abortion leader calling for increasingly aggressive and disruptive demonstrations. He and his followers seriously disrupted the Democratic National Convention in Atlanta in 1988.[13]

He formed Operation Rescue, an organization committed to physical disruption of abortion services, harassment of patients, and obstruction of clinic entrances. The term "Rescue," of course, referred to the group's intention to "rescue" the "innocent" fetuses about to be destroyed by the evil "guilty" women and even more evil "guilty" physicians. Anti-abortion fanatics assumed the moral high ground of rescuing an "innocent" victim for whom all observers could have only sympathy.

On September 25, 1988, while campaigning for the presidency, Vice President George Bush expressed the view that doctors who do abortions should be imprisoned. He was elected by a comfortable margin.

On October 10, 1990, Randall Terry stood surrounded by his followers in front of my office in Boulder, Colorado, calling me a "human hyena," a "child killer," and other epithets and praying for my death by a vengeful God. CBS's *60 Minutes* showed a video of Terry's prayer on their broadcast concerning the "Lambs of Christ" on February 2, 1992.[14]

In 1991 Terry led the "Summer of Mercy" in Wichita, Kansas, for six weeks resulting in the arrests of 3,000 people.[15] He was welcomed by the governor of Kansas and the mayor of the city of Wichita. The focus of the anti-abortion demonstrators was Dr. George Tiller's office, Women's Health Care Services, where he performed abortions. Terry constantly referred to physicians who performed abortions as "baby killers" and "child killers." During the Wichita demonstrations, anti-abortion picketers surrounded Tiller's clinic with signs that said, "Babies Killed Here" and "Tiller's Slaughter House."

On December 28, 1991, a man wearing dark glasses and a ski mask and carrying a sawed-off shotgun entered the Central Health Center for Women in Springfield, Missouri.[16] Hearing the screams of her daughter, Claudia Gilmore, the office manager, ran to the front office where she found the man, who slowly asked, "Where's the doctor?" As Gilmore and her daughter tried to push the man against a wall, he hit Gilmore on the head with the shotgun, which discharged into the ceiling. The screams and shotgun blast were heard by Don Catron, the building's owner, who ran to help and tried to push the gunman out the door. Gilmore tore off the man's mask; he then shot Catron in the abdomen. As Gilmore turned to help the disemboweled and bleeding Catron, the gunman shot Gilmore in the back, severing her spinal cord. The shooter was never found. The clinic closed.

As of March 1, 1993, there had been 1,285 acts of violence against abortion clinic facilities and doctors' offices. Over 100 facilities had been completely destroyed.

Assassinations

Anti-abortion terrorists began adopting the tactic of placing a doctor's image on a **WANTED** flyer made to resemble the kind of poster placed in post offices by the police looking for criminals in the 1940s and 1950s. One of these featured Dr. David Gunn, a Florida physician.

On March 10, 1993, Michael Griffin waited for three hours outside a Pensacola, Florida, abortion clinic for Dr. David Gunn to arrive for work. When Dr. Gunn stepped out of his car, Griffin shot him three times in the back, saying "Don't kill any more babies."[17,18]

Griffin, a fundamentalist Christian, called himself "pro-life." Outside the clinic, anti-abortion protesters held up signs saying "David Gunn kills babies" and "Execute Baby Killers." During the year before Dr. Gunn's assassination, the Associated Press reported that Randall Terry had "an old-fashioned 'wanted' poster of Gunn distributed at a rally for Operation Rescue leader Terry." The poster reportedly included a picture of Gunn, his home phone number, and other identifying information.

Michael Griffin was defended *pro bono* by Joe Scarborough, an anti-abortion local attorney. Scarborough later ran for and was elected to Congress with the strong support of anti-abortion groups, receiving $15,210 from the National Right to Life Committee.[19] He represented the Pensacola district, where the first two assassinations of abortion doctors occurred. In Congress, he voted against two 1995 bills intended to protect abortion clinics from violence.[20]

After leaving Congress. Scarborough, having become a darling of the political right, became the host of a lucrative MSNBC morning talk show, *Morning Joe*, where his income is $8,000,000 per year.[21]

Although it was national headline news, reported and discussed on every other MSNBC program, it took five days for Scarborough to allow any mention of Dr. George Tiller's brutal assassination by an anti-abortion fanatic on Sunday, May 31, 2009, much less express any disapproval.[20]

In August 1993, a few months after Dr. Gunn was assassinated, Pope John Paul II came to Colorado. He was followed by anti-abortion fanatics. On the morning of August 12, my op-ed article, "The pope and my right to life – Wearing body armor to the abortion clinic," appeared in the *New York Times*.[22]

In the article, I discussed the relationship between religious fanaticism, opposition to abortion, and anti-abortion violence.

That morning, Randall Terry went on the National Christian Radio Broadcasting program. Quoting scripture and mentioning me by name, he invited his listeners to assassinate me. We got phone calls from around the country.

That week, the *Mobile Register* refused to run an ad designed by Rev. David Trosch, a Catholic priest in Magnolia Springs, Alabama, showing a doctor being shot under the heading, "Justifiable Homicide." An article including an interview with Trosch appeared in the *Register* on Sunday, August 15, and his views became national news.[23]

The following week, on August 19, Shelly Shannon, attempting to assassinate Dr. George Tiller, shot him in both arms as he drove his vehicle out of his own parking lot.[24]

The *New York Times* headline two days later was "An Abortionist Returns to Work after Shooting."[25]

An abortionist. Not a skilled and dedicated physician helping women in spite of his injuries, but an "abortionist" – the term used for incompetent, avaricious butchers exploiting women in back-alley abortion clinics.[26]

That same day, on August 21, Dr. George Patterson, who owned four abortion clinics in Alabama and Florida, was shot and killed in downtown Mobile.[27]

There was no evidence of robbery. The police said they could not determine the motive for the murder. Quoting the *Orlando Sentinel*, "Although police said the killing occurred in the course of a robbery and was not abortion-related, it drew praise from an anti-abortion activist. 'Regardless of who killed Dr. Patterson, he definitely deserved to die because of the many children he killed,' said the Rev. Paul Hill of Pensacola, who represents the anti-abortion group Defensive Action."[28]

"The killing has stopped, and so it had the desired result," said Hill.[29]

One month later, on September 3, 1993, Father David Trosch, Reverend Paul Hill, and 33 other people gathered to prepare a "Defensive Action Statement" of "justifiable homicide" for abortion doctors.[30]

This was published under the aegis of the Army of God. One of the signers was Reverend Paul Hill, a Christian minister.

At about this time, I received a personal note from the woman who shot Dr. Tiller in 1993, Shelly Shannon, from her cell in the Kansas state prison. The note did not contain a direct threat, but the message was clear: *You're next.* Shannon was released from prison in May 2018.[31]

In November 1993, both houses of Congress passed legislation making it a federal crime to assault patients and health workers at abortion clinics. President Clinton signed it into law. My invitation to be at the signing ceremony was canceled by White House staff members who did not want the president to be seen next to a doctor who performs abortions.

Less than a year after that, Reverend Paul Hill assassinated Dr. John Britton and his bodyguard, retired Air Force colonel James Barrett on July 30, 1994, as Dr. Britton was preparing to enter the same Pensacola abortion clinic at which Michael Griffin assassinated Dr. David Gunn.[32]

Colonel Barrett's wife was seriously injured. With a shotgun, Hill shot the doctor, Colonel Barrett, and his wife at point-blank range as they were sitting in a pickup truck in front of the clinic. The clinic was owned by Dr. George Patterson up until the date of his murder.

Anti-abortion terrorists had distributed **WANTED** flyers with pictures of Dr. Britton prior to his assassination by Paul Hill.

On November 8, 1994, Dr. Garson Romalis was mortally wounded when shot twice in his kitchen with an AK-47 military rifle from a distance of about 20 meters.[33] Dr. Romalis nearly died in this attack. The suspected assailant was James Kopp.

On December 30, 1994, John Salvi, a known "peaceful" anti-abortion demonstrator, walked into a Planned Parenthood clinic in Brookline, Massachusetts, and shot and killed Shannon Lowney at point- blank range. He then went to the Preterm clinic a short distance away and shot and killed Leanne Nichols. Five others were wounded at the two clinics.[34]

During most of 1994, a man named Ken Scott began parking his van painted with lurid images of dismembered fetuses in front of my office and conducting aggressive demonstrations, terrifying my patients.[35]

In November 1994, Scott, a survivalist, marksman, and anti-abortion fanatic, began stalking me. He tried to come to my house in the mountains, but he made the mistake of calling the sheriff's office to ask for directions. On one occasion when he was arrested, he told the police that he had two goals in his life: to kill his ex-wife and to kill me.

One day, as I was on my way to speak to the Boulder county attorney about Scott's actions against me, he started following me in his van a few feet from my rear bumper. Using my knowledge of the hills and side streets in Boulder, I drove an evasive route and lost him, but I was shaking by the time I got to the county attorney's office. There was a court order to place him under psychiatric observation that I needed to sign. Scott was placed under court order in the Fort Logan Mental Health Center as a threat to the community, but the psychiatrist in charge, bending to pressure from Scott's anti-abortion supporters, released him. My attorney later obtained a restraining order, but I had to be protected from him by armed officers.

Scott sued me for $10 million claiming that I had used my medical license and standing to have him placed in the psychiatric institution.[36]

I was defended by Howard Bittman, the attorney who obtained the restraining order, who defeated Scott in court and obtained court costs and attorney's fees from Scott. But my life was still in danger from Scott. It still is.

I appealed to the U.S. Department of Justice for help. I wrote a report about 20 years of anti-abortion activity at my office for the Criminal Division of Department of Justice and presented it in person to Joann Harris, the director, on January 6, 1995. At the conclusion of my report, I said,

> The classic problem of democracy is that it grants great liberty to those who hate freedom. The anti-abortion movement, and especially its appropriation of legitimate religious expression for sinister and basically seditious, terrorist purposes, is testing our commitment to free speech to the limits. In fact, the use of free speech and freedom of religion by anti-abortion demagogues is dangerous to the lives and liberty of many peaceful U.S. citizens.
>
> There is no deterrence at present for anti-abortion demonstrators since they do not respect either civil or criminal laws or basic assumptions of Western culture. There being no deterrence, civil authorities must recognize that the only protection at this point is self-defense, and many of us are prepared to shoot back. This is a prescription for civil war, which is what is happening, except that one side is still holding its fire.
>
> Every anti-abortion demonstrator must now be considered armed, dangerous and a potential assassin until proven otherwise. *The anti-abortion movement must be considered the source and spawning ground of a violent, terrorist movement which threatens the social fabric and civil society of laws of the United States. It is a greater threat to personal security than any foreign enemy of the United States.* That it is intimately connected to a larger political movement and benefits a particular political party is a separate issue.[37]

At about this time, I got a call from Janet Benshoof, who had headed the ACLU Reproductive Freedom Project and then founded the Center for Reproductive Law and Policy in New York, to warn me about a plan to kill me. Janet had a "mole" at the anti-abortion "White Rose Society" banquet held around the end of 1994. The participants, Janet told me, had discussed the assassinations of doctors that had already occurred, and then the conversation turned to "who's next?" Janet's informant reported to her that the White Rose people had discussed killing me as the next primary physician to be assassinated and discussed the details of how this should be done. It was chilling. We reported this to the FBI, but we didn't have enough information for it to be pursued.

Also during this time, a Colorado Bible radio talk show host, Bob Enyart, focused on me in his regularly broadcast anti-abortion tirades. One day, I got numerous calls from people all around the country who had heard his last rant and called me to say, "This guy wants you killed."

The same pattern was established by James Dobson, a psychologist and Christian leader who founded the "Focus on the Family" ultraconservative religious indoctrination center in Colorado Springs, Colorado. He had a national radio broadcast audience in the millions and spewed anti-abortion poison every week about me, my colleague Dr. George Tiller, and others. We called his outfit "Focus on the Fetus."

On January 22, 1995, the "National Coalition of Life [sic] Activists" held a press conference in Virginia and announced their hit list of the first 13 doctors they wanted eliminated. They called it "The Deadly Dozen." One of the 13 physicians -was just a woman. Both Dr. Tiller and I were on the list to be assassinated. I was put under 24-hour armed guard for a time by U.S. federal marshals. It was a terrifying experience.

The Mafia has the decency to keep its hit lists private.

The federal marshal protection was withdrawn that summer when the new Republican-led Congress decided that killing doctors who do abortions is not a crime.

During this time, the same group put up a "Nuremberg" website with the names, addresses, and personal information of all the doctors in the country who were performing abortions. It constituted a national hit list. The doctors who were assassinated had lines drawn through their names; those who were just injured were shaded in grey.

That spring, as I was on my way to speak at a conference in Europe, I was requested to stop in New York City for a meeting at the law firm Paul, Weiss to discuss a lawsuit its attorneys were being asked to carry against the "American Coalition of Life [sic] Activists'" website listing the doctors to be assassinated. The plaintiffs were to be me, several of my medical colleagues who were listed on the hit list, and Planned Parenthood of Williamette County in Oregon. A brilliant young lawyer named Maria Vullo was to be our lead attorney. In our meeting, the senior leaders of this top New York law firm listened along with Ms. Vullo as I described the terror we were experiencing on a day-to-day basis.

On November 10, 1995, Dr. Hugh Short was shot in his home in Canada by James Kopp. Dr. Short lost the use of his arm in this attack.[38]

On November 11, 1997, Dr. Jack Fainman, an obstetrician who also performed abortions, was shot in the shoulder in his home in Winnipeg, Canada. The suspected assailant was James Kopp. The injury ended Dr. Fainman's medical career.[39]

On January 29, 1998, Eric Rudolph exploded a bomb at a Birmingham, Alabama, abortion clinic, killing a police officer, Robert Sanderson, and critically wounding nurse Emily Lyons.[40]

Officer Sanderson, who was moonlighting as a security guard at the New Woman, All Women Health Care Clinic in Birmingham, Alabama, was inspecting the front entrance to the clinic when a remotely controlled bomb hidden in a flower pot exploded at 7:33 AM, killing him instantly. Nurse Emily Lyons was critically injured, losing her sight in one eye.[41]

The bomb was set off by Eric Rudolf, who evaded authorities for five years before he was apprehended in North Carolina. He is now serving four consecutive life sentences at the federal ADX Supermax Florence prison in Colorado.

On October 23, 1998, Dr. Barnett Slepian was shot in the back through his kitchen window as he was preparing soup for his family.[42]

James Kopp, a well-known anti-abortion demonstrator, fired the shot and then fled to France, where he was arrested. Dr. Slepian's assassination had been preceded by the **WANTED** flyers circulated in western New York where he worked and lived. He was the fourth doctor who performed abortions to be assassinated in the United States.

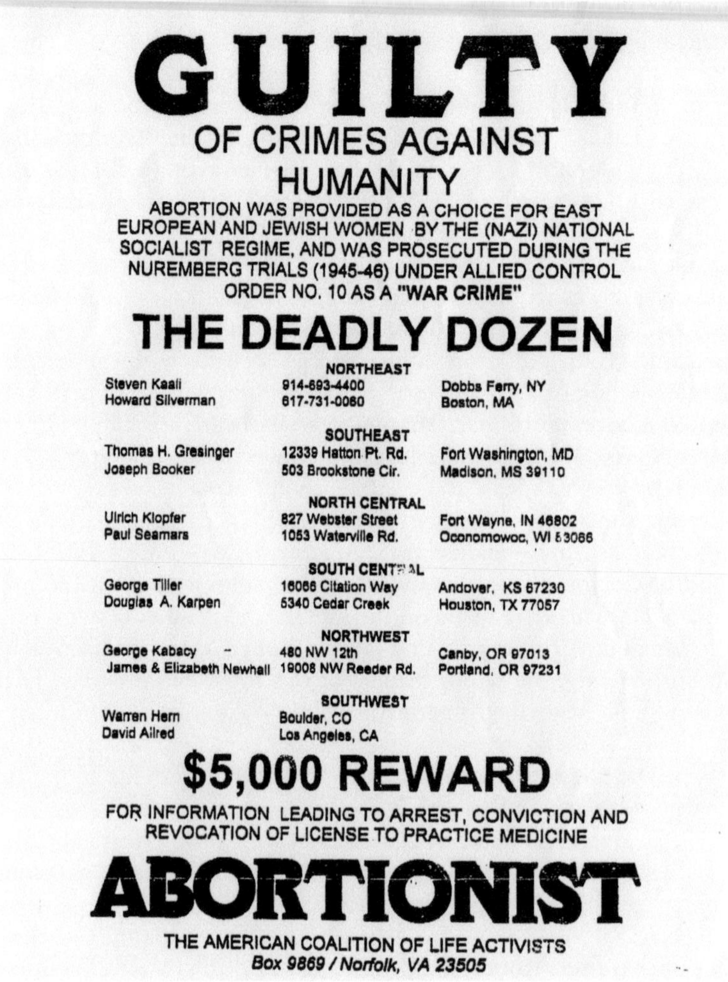

GUILTY

OF CRIMES AGAINST
HUMANITY

ABORTION WAS PROVIDED AS A CHOICE FOR EAST
EUROPEAN AND JEWISH WOMEN BY THE (NAZI) NATIONAL
SOCIALIST REGIME, AND WAS PROSECUTED DURING THE
NUREMBERG TRIALS (1945-46) UNDER ALLIED CONTROL
ORDER NO. 10 AS A "WAR CRIME"

THE DEADLY DOZEN

NORTHEAST
Steven Kaali	914-693-4400	Dobbs Ferry, NY
Howard Silverman	617-731-0080	Boston, MA

SOUTHEAST
Thomas H. Gresinger	12339 Hatton Pt. Rd.	Fort Washington, MD
Joseph Booker	503 Brookstone Cir.	Madison. MS 39110

NORTH CENTRAL
Ulrich Klopfer	827 Webster Street	Fort Wayne, IN 46802
Paul Seamars	1053 Waterville Rd.	Oconomowoc, WI 53066

SOUTH CENTRAL
George Tiller	16058 Citation Way	Andover, KS 67230
Douglas A. Karpen	6340 Cedar Creek	Houston, TX 77057

NORTHWEST
George Kabacy	480 NW 12th	Canby, OR 97013
James & Elizabeth Newhall	19008 NW Reeder Rd.	Portland, OR 97231

SOUTHWEST
Warren Hern	Boulder, CO	
David Ailred	Los Angeles, CA	

$5,000 REWARD

FOR INFORMATION LEADING TO ARREST, CONVICTION AND
REVOCATION OF LICENSE TO PRACTICE MEDICINE

ABORTIONIST

THE AMERICAN COALITION OF LIFE ACTIVISTS
Box 9869 / Norfolk, VA 23505

Figure 11.5 Guilty poster produced by the American Coalition of Life Activists.

Kopp is thought to be the would-be assassin who shot Canadian physician Garson Romalis with an AK-47 from a distance of about 50 feet through the back window of Dr. Romalis's Vancouver home in 1994.[43]

Dr. Romalis almost bled to death on his kitchen floor. He knew that his femoral artery was severed, and he was trying to press his thumb on it, which was gushing blood, to stop the bleeding, but he was aware that he was about to lose consciousness. He told his wife, who was terrified, to call an ambulance.

Kopp was later charged with the attempted assassination of Dr. Hugh Short, another Canadian physician who performed abortions. The bullet that Kopp fired shattered Dr. Short's elbow, ending his surgical career. By that time, Kopp was already serving a prison sentence in the United States for the assassination of Barnett Slepian.

Six years after the first assassination attempt, Dr. Romalis was seriously wounded again when an assailant stabbed him just outside his office.[44]

Court case against "American Coalition of [Life] Activists"

Our court case against the American Coalition of Life Activists was prepared by Ms. Vullo over four years, and the trial began in Federal District Court in Portland in January 1999.[45] All of us plaintiffs were present as were all of the several defendants who had created this terror.

Ms. Vullo made an eloquent and spirited presentation of the evidence, which included showing the posters containing the doctor's name and photo that had been circulated prior to the assassination in each case. "The sequence is crystal clear," she said. "The doctor to be killed is listed on the website, then a poster is distributed in the neighborhood of the clinic, and this is followed by the assassination. Poster, murder, poster, murder, poster, murder." "This is a campaign of terror backed up by lethal violence. These people must be held accountable, and this must stop!"

The trial lasted for three weeks. At the end, the jury found the anti-abortion organization guilty, and the judge ordered the defendants to pay $108 million in damages to the plaintiffs.[46] The defendants responded that they only followed God's law, not civil law. After a series of appeals, they were forced to pay.

But the threats and assassinations didn't stop.

In 2004, U.S. Senator Tom Coburn (R–OK) advocated the death penalty for doctors who perform abortions. He is in favor of capital punishment and thinks it should be applied to "abortionists" who "take innocent lives." "I favor the death penalty for abortionists."[47]

Operation Save America

In 2005, "Operation Save America" came to Colorado, and after demonstrating against abortion and gay rights in Denver for a few days, the group came to Boulder. They made a flyer with my picture on it together with an inflammatory message about my work performing abortions.

The flyer was distributed in neighborhoods for blocks around my office and where they thought I lived. I purchased full-page ads in local papers with a copy of the flyer included and denounced the group as fascist thugs. I received hundreds of letters of support, and I published them all in another full-page ad in two newspapers the following week. Having completed their target identification of me as the person to assassinate, the group left Colorado.

Assassination of Dr. George Tiller

As George Tiller became increasingly famous, his work caught the attention of Bill O'Reilly, a Fox "News" broadcaster who specialized in sarcastic, cutting, derogatory comments about many people. He began attacking Dr. Tiller as "George Tiller, The Baby Killer" on his highly successful nightly commentary program. From 2005, O'Reilly

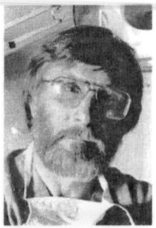

Abortionist Warren Hern

A baby killer lives in your neighborhood.
Abortionist Warren Hern is the owner and operator
of Colorado's first free-standing killing center.
Over the past three decades he has profited from the
the slaughter of thousands upon thousands of
innocent children. Please tell him that you are
uncomfortable with a murderer in your neighborhood.
Lev 19:17 You shall not hate your brother in your
heart. You shall surely rebuke your neighbor,
and not bear sin because of him.

Figure 11.6 Poster depicting the author.

invoked Dr. Tiller's name in his attacks on abortion 42 times, and he used this epithet of "George Tiller, The Baby Killer" 24 times.[48]

On May 31, 2009, Scott Roeder, who had stalked Dr. Tiller for years, walked into the lobby of the Reformation Lutheran Church in Wichita, where Dr. Tiller worshiped with his family, on a day when Dr. Tiller was serving as an usher for his fellow worshipers. He walked up to Dr. Tiller, who was having a doughnut and cup of coffee with his fellow ushers, and shot him in the temple. Dr. Tiller died instantly.[49]

Bill O'Reilly has Dr. Tiller's blood on his hands.

Shooting in Colorado

On November 27, 2015, Robert Dear Jr., muttering "No more baby parts," arrived at the Planned Parenthood clinic in Colorado Springs, Colorado. Before he was finally captured by the police, one police officer and one civilian were dead, and nine other people were injured including five police officers and four civilians.[50]

Dear described himself as a "warrior for babies." The event followed a sequence of hearings conducted by Representative Marsha Blackburn (R–TN) during which fraudulent anti-abortion videos were shown and false accusations were made that Planned Parenthood clinics were "selling baby parts."

Stochastic terrorism

This is called "stochastic terrorism" – the outbreak of unpredictable random terrorism and directed violence as the result of encouragement of it by a celebrity or widely known public figure such as Bill O'Reilly – or Donald Trump.[51] The violence is psychologically legitimized by the authority of the public figure. In Dr. Tiller's case, and others, it was a political assassination of a dedicated physician who helped women.

My friend is gone

The following is the text of a speech I was invited to give at the Temple Emanuel in Denver on Thursday, June 4, 2009, four days after Dr. Tiller was assassinated. The speech was published as an editorial in the *Colorado Statesman* on June 19, 2009:[52]

Dr. George Tiller's political assassination is result of rabid anti-abortion harassment

Editor's Note: Dr. Warren Hern delivered the following address at Temple Emanuel in Denver on June 4 at the invitation of Rabbi Steven Foster, Betty Serotta, NARAL Colorado Pro-Choice and the Religious Coalition for Reproductive Choice.

George Tiller, my friend and medical colleague for over 30 years, is dead of an assassin's bullet. George was shot at point-blank range with a handgun in the foyer of his Lutheran Church in Wichita, Kansas. He was acting as an usher for the congregation at the time. The church service had started, his wife was in the choir, and George was welcoming his fellow worshipers to the service.

The last time I was in that church with George was at his daughter's wedding.

The assassination of George Tiller in his place of worship is horrifying, despicable and tragic for his family, friends and colleagues. He was a dedicated, conscientious and courageous physician who had endured one assassination attempt in 1993 — when he was shot in both arms — and endless harassment at his home, office and church. Kansas authorities used the coercive power of the state to hound and persecute Dr. Tiller with a variety of unconstitutional and specious charges.

For those of us who knew him, a man who served his country as a Navy flight surgeon, who provided medical care for tens of thousands of women and their families and who loved his family, this loss is incomprehensible. Those of us who were his friends and colleagues will miss his easy good humor, unfailing generosity and graciousness, and willingness to share and exchange the kind of clinical information that doctors cherish.

George took over his father's family practice in Wichita when his parents, sister and brother-in-law were killed in a plane crash in 1970. He had planned to close his father's practice and continue his plans for a residency in dermatology.

He soon found that women had come to his father for help to have safe abortions — illegal at that time. Women appealed to George to continue his father's compassion and service. At first, he refused — and one woman died from a badly done abortion. George changed his mind. He became not only a skilled family practitioner, he became highly skilled in difficult late abortion procedures. His patients came from around the world with tragically complicated pregnancies for his help.

In the highly specialized world of late abortion for women with desperate needs, George and I were each other's only peers. We talked a lot and often about our patients, families, and political struggles. We skied together in the Colorado Rockies. We both had trouble staying on the trail. Somehow, we both had a tendency to resist supervision.

George Tiller was kind, gentle, considerate and compassionate. He was funny. He was devoted to his family and friends. He was not vengeful in spite of the opprobrium, violence, and hatred heaped upon him by opponents of abortion. He was generous in every way to his friends, community, and good causes. He was an outstanding asset to our society, and he was a joy to those who knew him. He was a man of peace.

But this is not just the personal tragedy of one abortion doctor, one honorable physician who took over his late father's family practice. This brutal, cold-blooded, premeditated political assassination is the inevitable and predictable result of over 35 years of rabid anti-abortion harassment, hate rhetoric, violence, and intimidation.

I have some experience with this subject.

Within two weeks after starting to do abortions at Colorado's first freestanding, nonprofit abortion clinic in Boulder in 1973, I started getting obscene death threats in the middle of the night. I slept with a rifle by my bed at my house in the mountains, and I expected someone to try to kill me.

In 1982, Dr. Hector Zevallos and his wife were taken captive by the "Army of God" in Granite City, Illinois, because of Dr. Zevallos' work in performing abortions.

After two dozen clinic bombings in 1984, FBI Director William Webster said that the incidents weren't terrorism because "we don't know who's doing it."

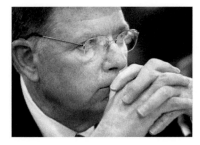

Figure 11.7 Dr. George Tiller.

Since those times, the anti-abortion rhetoric has been filled with descriptions of doctors as "baby killers," "mass murderers" and "child killers." The antiabortion fanatics call themselves "pro-life" while they are killing doctors and other health workers who help women. This despicable phrase implies that those of us who save women's lives are "pro-death" and "anti-life." "Pro-life" is not a neutral, descriptive term. It is a dagger of psychological warfare that is backed by hate and terror. It is a profound libel and insult to those who help women. Words kill, and the phrase "pro-life" is an obscene and grotesque sophistry. It is a cruel and vicious fraud.

Fox News TV host Bill O'Reilly, who calls himself "pro-life," made an obsession of obscenely referring to Dr. Tiller as "George Tiller, the baby killer." He repeated this epithet dozens of times. He demonized and vilified Dr. Tiller on the public airwaves. This is called "target identification." This is electronic fascism.

It is only one of many examples, others supplied by Dr. James Dobson, the former head of Focus on the Family located in Colorado Springs. In August, 1993, Randall Terry, head of Operation Rescue, went on National Christian Radio Broadcast Network and, referring to me by name and citing Scripture passages, invited his listeners to assassinate me.

How can you defend yourself against this?

Dr. David Gunn was assassinated in 1993. Dr. John Britton was assassinated in 1994. Dr. Bernard Slepian was assassinated in 1998.

Dr. Tiller is the fourth American abortion doctor to be assassinated by known "pro-life" anti-abortion fanatics, and at least three other people have been murdered for the same reasons. Others, such as nurse Emily Lyons, have been maimed for life.

Dr. Tiller's assassination is the latest event in the historic pattern of anti-abortion violence. This movement says to those of us who help women: "Do what we tell you to do, or we will kill you." And they do.

We don't have to invade other countries to find terrorists. They are right here, killing abortion doctors.

What does Dr. Tiller's assassination mean? Why was he chosen by the assassin for death in the church on a quiet Sunday morning in Wichita?

What did Dr. Tiller represent to the anti-abortion fanatic who killed him?

He represented freedom. He represented individual dignity. He represented opportunity for women to become full citizens and participants in our society. He represented social change. He represented the value of the individual adult human being as opposed to state control of individual lives. He represented a thought. The man who killed Dr. Tiller tried to kill a thought.

The idea that an embryo or fetus is equal to, or more important than, the life of a cantankerous adult doctor is no longer a sick private delusion. It is a collective psychosis masquerading as religion that has become a political force threatening democratic society. Dr. Tiller's crime was not that he killed children — which he did not — but that he brought liberty and health to women. He saved their lives and futures. That's why every doctor in America who does abortions lives under a death threat.

As I said in 1993, after the assassination of Dr. Gunn, we can only hope that Dr. Tiller's tragic and senseless murder will wake up the American people to the radical Christian right's determination to take absolute power in our society and to control its vital institutions.

The main difference between the American anti-abortion movement and the Taliban is about 8,000 miles. Also, the Taliban wants a fascist Islamic theocracy, whereas the American anti-abortion movement wants a fascist Christian theocracy.

The main difference between the American anti-abortion movement and the Salem Witch Hunts is 300 years.

Last week, we observed the 65th anniversary of the Normandy Invasion. The difference between those of us who help women by performing abortions and the guys who hit the beach in 1944 is that we get to choose and we have a better chance of surviving. It's the same issue, the same adversary, the same clash of values, the same struggle, but different weapons.

All of these historical convulsions are about power.

The question is not, "When does life begin?" but, "Who is best prepared to make the decision to transmit life to a new generation: the individual or the state?"

In this matter, the individual woman is more competent than any government. To its eternal disgrace, the Republican Party has exploited the abortion issue since 1974 to get power. It has been a conscious, deliberate, cynical choice of political strategy by this party, and its leadership was captured long ago by the most radical elements in the religious right. It is a mutual exploitation. The Republican agenda is about money and power. The radical religious right's agenda is about power and money. Working together, they gave us eight years of George W. Bush.

In 1994, following the assassination of Drs. Gunn and Britton and the attempted assassination of Dr. Tiller in 1993, and following the declaration of an Alabama Catholic priest named David Trosch that killing doctors who do abortions is justifiable homicide, I was being stalked by Ken Scott, a local survivalist, marksman and anti-abortion fanatic. I went to the Department of Justice and asked for help. In a report that I prepared in the fall of 1994 for the Civil Rights division of the U.S. Department of Justice, which is dated January 6, 1995, I stated:

The classic problem of democracy is that it grants great liberty to those who hate freedom.

The anti-abortion movement, and especially its appropriation of legitimate religious expression for sinister and basically seditious terrorist purposes, is testing our commitment to free speech to the limits. In fact, the use of free speech and freedom of religion by anti-abortion demagogues is dangerous to the lives and liberty of many peaceful U.S. citizens.

There is no deterrence at present for anti-abortion demonstrators, since they do not respect either civil or criminal laws or basic assumptions of Western culture.

Two weeks after I submitted my report, the "American Coalition of Life [sic] Activists" held a press conference in Virginia, home of the Moral Majority, on January 22, 1995, and announced its hit list of the first 13 doctors they wanted eliminated. I was on the list, and so was George Tiller.

The Mafia has the decency to keep its hit lists private.

George was assassinated last week. I am now, once again, under the 24-hour protection of heavily armed U.S. marshals. They risk their lives for me. The U.S. Attorney General made that happen.

Why is it necessary for an American doctor who helps women to be protected from assassins?

What does this mean for American society? What does it mean for freedom in the United States?

When the anti-abortion fanatics finish killing off all the abortion doctors, who's next? People who read newspapers? People who write for newspapers? People who read books? Federal judges? Homosexuals? Women who don't wear veils? Members of Congress? People who preach from the wrong part of the Bible?

The American anti-abortion movement is opposed to the rule of law, a secular society, the American Constitution, representative government, personal freedom, democracy and thought.

The spirit of true freedom, the security of its citizens, the peace of civil society, and the soul of America is at stake here. Dr. Tiller's assassination is the latest blow to that freedom.

Wake up, America.

Warren M. Hern, a physician, is director of the Boulder Abortion Clinic.

Notes

1 Sheppard, N., Jr. Doctor's abduction stuns steel town. *New York Times,* August 23, 1982. https://www.nytimes.com/1982/08/23/us/doctor-s-abduction-stuns-steel-town.html
2 Clarkson, F. Anti-abortion terrorism threatens all Americans. *WE News*, February 13, 2002. William Webster, on abortion clinic bombings, *Face the Nation*, 1984. https://womensenews.org/2002/02/anti-abortion-terrorism-threatens-all-americans/
3 Hern, W.M. The antiabortion vigilantes. *New York Times*, op-ed page, Friday, December 21, 1984. https://www.nytimes.com/1984/12/21/opinion/the-antiabortion-vigilantes.html
4 McFadden, R.D. Abortion clinic set afire on L.I. *New York Times*, February 16, 1979. https://www.nytimes.com/1979/02/16/archives/abortion-clinic-set-afire-on-li-suspect-is-held-scene-of.html
5 Grimes, D.A., Forrest, J.D., Kirkman, A.L, and Radford, B. An epidemic of antiabortion violence in the United States. *American Journal of Obstetrics and Gynecology* 165(5), part 1:1263–68, 1991. https://www.sciencedirect.com/science/article/abs/pii/000293789190346S
6 Schudel,M. Joseph Scheidler, a major architect of the anti-abortion movement, dies at 93. *The Washington Post*, January 20, 2021. https://www.washingtonpost.com/local/obituaries/joseph-scheidler-dead/2021/01/20/2b794640-5a83-11eb-8bcf-3877871c819d_story.html
7 Scheidler, J.M. *Closed: 99 Ways to Stop Abortion*. Lake Bluff, IL: Regnery Books, 1985.
8 Hynes,M. Hern to donate $1 for every picket to Amendment #3 repeal. *Daily Camera*,March 5, 1988.
9 Obmasik,M. Robertson, Kemp blast ruling. *The Denver Post*, June 14, 1986.

10 Hern, W.M. Must Mr. Reagan tolerate abortion clinic violence? *New York Times*, op-ed page, June 14, 1986. https://www.nytimes.com/1986/06/14/opinion/must-mr-reagan-tolerate-abortion-clinic-violence.html

11 Schudel, M. *ibid.*

12 Daily Camera. Shots shatter front window of Boulder Abortion Clinic. *Daily Camera*, February 5, 1988; Robey R: Shots fired at Boulder Abortion Clinic. *The Denver Post*, 6 February 1988.

13 Associated Press. Abortion foes jailed in Atlanta. *New York Times*, July 30, 1988. https://www.nytimes.com/1988/07/30/us/abortion-foes-jailed-in-atlanta.html

14 Stahl, L. The Lambs of Christ. *60 Minutes*, February 2, 1992. WorldCat® https://www.worldcat.org/title/lambs-of-christ-february-2-1992/oclc/26466475

15 Wilkerson, I. Drive against abortion finds a symbol:Wichita. *The New York Times*, August 4, 1991. https://www.nytimes.com/1991/08/04/us/drive-against-abortion-finds-a-symbol-wichita.html

16 Schmitt, W. The Springfield abortion clinic shooting of 1991. *Springfield News-Leader*, December 17, 2016. https://www.news-leader.com/story/news/politics/2016/12/18/springfield-abortion-clinic-shooting-1991-injured-two-and-made-history/95016376/; Associated Press. Gunman wounds two inside abortion clinic. *New York Times*, December 29, 1991. https://www.nytimes.com/1991/12/29/us/gunman-wounds-two-inside-abortion-clinic.html?searchResultPosition=1

17 Rohter, D. Doctor is slain during protest over abortions. *New York Times*, March 11, 1993. https://www.nytimes.com/1993/03/11/us/doctor-is-slain- during-protest-over-abortions.html

18 Booth,W. Doctor killed during abortion protest. *Washington Post*, March 11, 1993. https://www.washingtonpost.com/wp-srv/national/longterm/abortviolence/stories/gunn.htm

19 Roth, Z. Report: Before congressional run, Scarborough represented killer of abortion doctor. *TPM Talking Points Memo*, June 5, 2009. https://talkingpointsmemo.com/muckraker/report-before-congressional-run-scarborough-represented-killer-of-abortion-doctor

20 Barrett, W. Morning Joe finally breaks his silence about defending abortion-doc killer. *The Village Voice*, June 5, 2009. https://www.villagevoice.com/barrett-morning-joe-finally-breaks-his-silence-about-defending-abortion-doc-killer/

21 Clapchowder, G. Morning Dough: Joe Scarborough's salary and the ways he spends his millions. *The Richest*, November 1, 2021. https://www.therichest.com/rich-powerful/morning-dough-joe-scarboroughs-salary-and-the-ways-he-spends-his-millions/; Paywizard.org https://paywizard.org/salary/vip-check/joe-scarborough

22 Hern, W.M. The Pope and my right to life. *New York Times* , op-ed page, August 12, 1993. https://www.nytimes.com/1993/08/12/opinion/the-pope-and-my-right-to-life.html?searchResultPosition=4

23 Associated Press. Priest is scolded in abortion ad. *New York Times*, August 18, 1993. Also reported in the *Mobile Register*, August 1993. https://www.nytimes.com/1993/08/18/us/priest-is-scolded-on-abortion-ad.html

24 Faison, S. *Abortion doctor wounded outside Kansas clinic. New York Times*, August 20, 1993. https://www.nytimes.com/1993/08/20/us/abortion-doctor- wounded-outside-kansas-clinic.html

25 Johnson, D. An abortionist returns to work after shooting. *New York Times*, August 21, 1993. https://timesmachine.nytimes.com/timesmachine/1993/08/21/713993.html?pageNumber=5

26 Hern, W.M. 'Abortionist' carries a charged meaning. *New York Times*, Sept. 7, 1993. https://www.nytimes.com/1993/09/07/opinion/l-abortionist-carries-a-charged-meaning-856193.html?searchResultPosition=6

27 Mitchell, G. Suspect sought in killing of doctor who performs abortions. Associated Press, August 23, 1993. https://apnews.com/d547d5edbb2bae250e9ef7d3976e22ae

28 Suspect in doctor's death on parole from life term. *Orlando Sentinel*, September 8, 1993.

29 Smothers, R. Abortion doctor's slaying is baffling police in Mobile. *New York Times*, August 29, 1993. https://www.nytimes.com/1993/08/29/us/abortion-doctor-s-slaying-is-baffling-police-in-mobile.html

30 Defensive Action Statement by The Army of God, https://www.armyofgod.com/defense.html

31 Thomas, J.L. Abortion clinics on edge after woman who shot Kansas doctor is released from prison. *Kansas City Star*, November 7, 2018. https://www.kansascity.com/news/local/crime/article221194600.html

32 Smothers, R. DEATH OF A DOCTOR: THE OVERVIEW- Abortion doctor and bodyguard slain in Florida; Protester is arrested in Pensacola's 2nd clinic killing. *New York Times*, July

30, 1994. https://www.nyes.com/1994/07/30/us/death-doctor-overview-abortion-doctor-body-guard-slainin-florida-protester.html

33 Reuters. Canada tightens security at abortion clinics after shooting. *New York Times*, November 10, 1994. https://www.nytimes.com/1994/11/10/world/canada-tightens-security-at-abortion-clinics-after-a-shooting.html

34 Kifner, J. Anti-abortion killings: The overview; Gunman kills 2 at abortion clinics in Boston suburb. *New York Times*, December 31, 1994. https://www.nytimes.com/1994/12/31/us/anti-abortion-killings-overview-gunman-kills-2-abortion-clinics-boston-suburb.html

35 Jackson, S. The fight of their lives. *Westword*, February 13, 1997, https://www.westword.com/news/the-fight-of-their-lives-5057143

36 Court Listener. *Scott v. Hern*, 98-1320 (10th Cir. 2000).

37 Hern, W.M. Report to Department of Justice, November 1994

38 Nolan, D. Hamilton doctor Hugh Short was a victim of sniper shooting by anti-abortion radical in 1995.*The Hamilton Spectator*, March 25, 2019. https://www.thespec.com/news/hamilton-region/obit-hamilton-doctor-hugh-short-was-a-victim-of-sniper-shooting-by-anti-abortion-radical/article_e343bf2d-e252-5202-a016-89da058a32fc.html

39 CJN admin Survivor of anti-abortion shooting pens memoir. *Canadian Jewish News* November 24, 2011. https://thecjn.ca/arts/books-and-authors/survivor-anti-abortion-shooting-pens-memoir/

40 Bragg, R. Bomb kills guard at Alabama abortion clinic. *New York Times*, January 30, 1998. https://www.nytimes.com/1998/01/30/us/bomb-kills-guard-at-an-alabama-abortion-clinic.html

41 Lyons, E., and Lyons, J. *Life's Been a Blast: The True Story of Birmingham Bomb Survivor Emily Lyons*. Washington, DC: National Abortion Federation, 2005.

42 Yardley, J., and Rohde, D. Abortion doctor in Buffalo slain; Sniper attack fits violent pattern. *New York Times*, October 29, 1998. https://www.nytimes.com/1998/10/25/nyregion/abortion-doctor-in-buffalo-slain-sniper-attack-fits-violent-pattern.html

43 Reuters. Canada tightens security at abortion clinics after shooting. *New York Times*, November 10, 1994. https://www.nytimes.com/1994/11/10/world/canada-tightens-security-at-abortion-clinics-after-a-shooting.html

44 CBC News. Abortion doctor attacked again. *CBC News*. July 11, 2000. https://www.cbc.ca/news/canada/abortion-doctor-attacked-again-1.203379

45 Sanchez, R. Abortion foes Internet site on trial. *The Wahington Post*, January 15, 1999.https://www.washingtonpost.com/wp-srv/national/longterm/abortviolence/stories/website.htm

46 CNN. Anti-abortion activists ordered to pay damages. *CNN.com*. February 2,1999. http://edition.cnn.com/US/9902/02/abortion.web.verdict.01/index.html

47 Coburn, T. *On The Issues: Tom Coburn on Abortion*. https://www.issues2000.org/Social/Tom_Coburn_Abortion.htm

48 Holan, A.D. Bill O'Reilly called George Tiller a "Baby Killer" without attribution. *Politifact*, June 5, 2009. https://www.politifact.com/factchecks/2009/jun/05/bill-oreilly/bill-oreilly-called-george-tiller-baby-killer/

49 Stumpe, J., and Davey, M. Abortion doctor shot to death in Kansas church. *New York Times*, May 31, 2009. https://www.nytimes.com/2009/06/01/us/01tiller.html

50 Lowery, W., Paquette, D., and Markson, J. "No more baby parts,'\" suspect in attack on Colo. Planned Parenthood clinic told official. *New York Times*, November 28, 2015. https://www.washingtonpost.com/politics/no-more-baby-parts-suspect-in-attack-at-colo-planned-parenthood-clinic-told-official/2015/11/28/e842b2cc-961e-11e5-8aa0-5d0946560a97_story.html

51 Angove,J. Philosophic and public security implications of "Stochastic Terrorism." *Max Planck Institute for the Study of Crime, Security and Law*. https://csl.mpg.de/en/projects/philosophical-and-public-security-law-implications-of-stochastic-terrorism

52 Hern, W.M. Dr. George Tiller's political assassination is result of rabid anti-abortion harassment. *Colorado Statesman*, June 19, 2009 (Text of invited speech at Temple Emanuel, June 4, 2009). https://www.drhern.com/wp-content/uploads/2018/05/statesmen-tiller-assasination.pdf

12   The illness of pregnancy

The woman sat across from me at my desk. She told me that she wanted to carry her pregnancy to term because she wanted so much to have a baby, but she couldn't go on any longer. "I don't feel pregnant. *I feel poisoned.*" She was in her 16th week of pregnancy and vomiting constantly. She retched all day and all night even at the sight and smell of food. She couldn't do her work. She couldn't take care of her children. She had *hyperemesis gravidarum* – uncontrolled vomiting of pregnancy.

Another patient was brought to me by air ambulance from Rapid City, South Dakota, for the same reasons. She almost died during the flight. She was diabetic before pregnancy, and the constant vomiting of pregnancy caused her electrolyte balance to be so out of order it threatened her vital functions. This, too, was a desired pregnancy, but at 18 weeks, her doctors advised her to end the pregnancy and referred her to me. After starting her treatment, I had her hospitalized across the street from my office in order to stabilize her electrolytes and vital signs. Then I brought her back to my office and performed the abortion.

In his book, *Liberty and Sexuality: The Right to Privacy and the Making of Roe v. Wade*, David Garrow quotes a woman named Marsha who said, after discovering that she would have to continue a pregnancy because of the laws against abortion, "My feeling about the pregnancy was that a horrible canc*er* was growing in my body that would ruin my life."[1] She had serious medical issues that were exacerbated by the pregnancy.

A woman from northern Colorado, also with a desired pregnancy, was referred to me by her doctors because they discovered that the fetus was afflicted with Trisomy 13, which is lethal for the fetus, and it can cause malignant hypertension in the woman carrying the pregnancy. This patient had slightly elevated blood pressure when she arrived in my office, but soon after we started preliminary procedures, her blood pressure began to rise. I admitted her to Boulder Community Hospital, where she went to the intensive care unit, but by 1 AM, her blood pressure continued to rise and she stopped producing urine. At 3 AM, I performed the emergency abortion procedure with the chief of obstetrics looking over my shoulder. There was no one else on the OB/GYN staff who had experience with or was trained to perform a mid-second trimester D&E abortion. The patient recovered, but only after several more days in the intensive care unit.

On numerous occasions, we received patients from other states and from Canada who had a history of ruptured membranes at the 18th or 20th week of a desired pregnancy. Some patients were given antibiotics and some were not. Some were referred to me, and some found me with the help of family members. All these patients needed an immediate D & E abortion, which I performed. One woman from Canada was several weeks from the time of her ruptured membranes until she reached me. She became septic immediately

DOI: 10.4324/9781003514961-13

following the abortion procedure, which meant that she had a lethal infection brewing in her uterus before I began. I admitted her to the hospital where she received intravenous antibiotic treatment and survived what could have been a fatal sepsis.

In Ireland a few years ago, there was a famous case of a young Indian dentist who had ruptured membranes at about 20 weeks into a desired pregnancy, but she was denied an abortion there because the doctors could detect a fetal heartbeat. In spite of the fact that there was no hope of having a live birth and survival of this fetus, the woman's pleas for treatment were ignored. Irish laws based in medieval Catholic religious beliefs would not permit her doctors to help her. She died.

In 1990, while on one of my research trips to the Peruvian Amazon where I have studied, lived with, and provided medical care for the Shipibo Indians since 1964, I arrived at a remote village on the upper Pisqui River to get some very bad news. A young woman who was 14 years old was taken down the river from the most remote village to another one where there was a traditional midwife to deliver her baby. But the girl had twins, and she died trying to deliver them. Both of the babies died, also. This young woman suffered the fate of hundreds of millions of women all over the world who have died from pregnancy.

The Shipibo women are especially vulnerable because, for most of the time I have known them, they have lived under essentially prehistoric conditions that most humans have experienced in tribal societies for hundreds of thousands of years. But the danger for women is not confined to those living in pre-industrial societies.

The great French physician François Mauriceau, who founded the medical specialty of obstetrics, called pregnancy "le maladie de neuf mois" (the disease of nine months) in his classic 1668 treatise, *Des maladies des femmes grosses et accouchées* ("The diseases of women who are pregnant and in childbirth").[2] It is the first textbook on obstetrics, and it is an extraordinary work in both the literary and the medical sense. Childbirth has been a chamber of horrors for many women. Mauriceau led the way to modern obstetrics.

Mauriceau's great compassion and historic contribution to the welfare of women was impelled by his grief in watching his sister die in a pool of blood from a placental abruption as she was about to deliver her fifth child.

Eighty years later, Émilie du Châtelet, a French aristocrat and a brilliant scientist who was Voltaire's lover, discovered at the age of 42 that she was pregnant. She knew she would die in childbirth. She worked frantically to complete her great work on mathematical physics and calculus by the end of her pregnancy. She finished her book and died a week later after delivering her baby.[3]

In my private medical practice specializing in abortion services, I see women every week who are at high risk of dying from pregnancy, including those who are ending a desired pregnancy for reasons of catastrophic complications.

A woman with a highly desired twin pregnancy came to me from another state following failure of her skilled physicians to succeed in treating the twin-to-twin transfusion syndrome that was likely to kill both twins and the woman as well. A week later a woman with an advanced pregnancy and nearly complete placenta previa like the one I attended in medical school came to me from Texas because the fetus she was carrying had no kidneys and could not survive. Before I could complete all the preparations for her procedure, she began hemorrhaging and could have died in a few minutes. I stopped the bleeding and completed her procedure quickly with minimal blood loss. What if she hadn't been in my operating room with my experience, an intravenous line already in place, special instruments that I have designed for this purpose, and my skilled staff ready to save her life? She could have died in a few minutes.

Who is ready to tell me I can't do this?

For hundreds of thousands of years, women have been at the mercy of their own biology as they faced the risk of death and catastrophic injury with each pregnancy.

The death rate due to pregnancy is called the "maternal mortality ratio." This is the number of deaths of women who die while pregnant, during childbirth, or within 42 days after delivery per 100,000 live births. At the end of World War I, the U.S. maternal mortality ratio was about 900 per 100,000 live births. In 1920 it was 680 per 100,000 live births. By 1960 it was 38 per 100,000 live births.[4] The improvement was due to the development of modern obstetrics, the availability of blood transfusions and antibiotics, and the successful management of problems like pre-eclampsia and other potentially fatal complications of pregnancy.

While the U.S. maternal mortality ratio was as low as 7 by the late 1990s, it is now almost 33 per 100,000 live births.[5] We are going backwards. The U.S. maternal mortality ratio is the highest of all Western industrialized countries. It is twice as high as Canada's and ten times as high as the same ratio in New Zealand.

The maternal mortality ratio for Black women in the United States is three to four times higher than for white women. In Alabama, it is five times the ratio for white women.[6]

Why?

There are many contributing factors, but restricted access to safe abortion services must be considered one of them. Women with high risk pregnancies are more likely to seek abortion, especially to have pregnancies terminated at a late stage due to medical conditions.

Restrictions on access to abortion have been increasingly severe in red states, especially in the Southern states. Women in Texas and states in the deep South are more likely to die from pregnancy than in other states. Living in a red state is a threat to your health, especially if you are a woman who is pregnant.

It is not just that it is impossible to get a safe abortion in a red state. It may be more difficult to have a safe delivery for your baby in a hospital. An Idaho hospital closed its doors to deliveries because half of the doctors who specialize in the management of high-risk pregnancies have left the state due to Idaho's restrictive abortion law. No doctor wants to risk prison to help women who are pregnant.

As of Friday, January 5, 2024, it is a crime punishable by prison if a physician performs an emergency abortion on a woman in Idaho.[7]

This is madness. It is a set of conditions now being imposed on half of American states and all of American women because of the religious and philosophical views of women as livestock whose purpose it is to have babies for the greater glory and political power of certain groups, especially white people and especially white men. Having babies is what women are *for*.

This madness denies that pregnancy can threaten a woman's life and denies that abortion is a vital component of health care for women in the twenty-first century. It denies that pregnancy has anything in common with other medical conditions or illnesses.

But pregnancy *is* an illness whether the woman chooses to be pregnant or not. It has all the classic characteristics of an illness. It has an etiology (cause); diagnosis; pathogenesis; pathophysiology; signs (objective evidence such as enlargement of the uterus and *hyperemesis gravidarum*, or uncontrollable vomiting of pregnancy); symptoms (such as nausea experienced by the patient); laboratory findings; physiologic changes that are often life-threatening such as hypertension of pregnancy or pre-eclampsia; duration (nine months or less); epidemiology (number of pregnancies at a specific moment in time or over a set period of time); distribution (by geographic area or social group); susceptibility (women in the "child-bearing" age range from 13 to 53 years); fatality rate (maternal mortality ratio); sequelae (uterine prolapse, vesicovaginal fistula, or rectovaginal fistula); and recovery rate (miscarriage, giving birth). As are many other illnesses, pregnancy can be prevented (by abstinence, contraception, or sterilization). Women who are pregnant display illness behavior and sick role behavior as defined by medical sociologists. There is a recovery period (post-partum period, usually defined as six weeks after parturition). There are cultural responses in traditional societies to the mortality risk of pregnancy such as *couvade*, in which the pregnant woman's male partner imitates the labor and pains of childbirth as a kind of sympathetic magic to help the woman survive the experience of delivering her baby. In parts of Latin America, a woman who is pregnant is referred to as "enferma" (sick); when she is delivering her baby at the end of her pregnancy, she is said to be "sanando" (healing). An entire branch of medicine, obstetrics, is devoted to helping women survive the risks of pregnancy by managing the problems that can kill a woman when she is pregnant, delivering a baby, or recovering from pregnancy.

Insurance companies classify pregnancy as an illness.

Pregnancy is not a benign condition. Women die from being pregnant. *The treatment of choice for pregnancy is abortion unless the woman wants to be pregnant and have a baby.* Then she deserves the best medical care possible to help her survive the pregnancy and have a healthy baby.

A subject as controversial as abortion invites both confusion and narrow partisanship among medical practitioners and in the public at large. Sometimes the debate centers on whether abortions should be performed or whether women should seek them; sometimes it focuses on the circumstances under which abortions should be performed.

Doctors conduct intense debates on the techniques of abortion and the qualifications of those who perform them. It is sometimes difficult to capture a broad view of the problem in any philosophical, historical, or medical sense. However, abortion is a subject that has concerned human beings for thousands of years and appears to become more complex and controversial each day.

It may be helpful to remember that pregnancy, first of all, is a biologic event happening to an individual woman; that induced abortion, or operative abortion, is a medical/ surgical event happening to an individual woman at her initiative; that it is possible only in the presence of an intrauterine pregnancy occurring in an individual woman; and that pregnancy is a biologic condition with a risk of death. It is true that pregnancy and abortion may have certain philosophical, moral, emotional, or social consequences and that the practice of abortion has an identifiable history in human affairs. All of these are valid and important subjects, and anyone who purports to provide abortion services should be aware of them.

The context of abortion practice, while it may occur with a backdrop of social and political controversy, is eminently medical. It is medical because women can die from pregnancy, and it is medical because they can die from abortion. The context is epidemiologic, also, because pregnancy is a community as well as an individual phenomenon; so is abortion.

Pregnancy as a condition being experienced by individuals can directly affect half the human species, women, and it indirectly or directly affects the rest. Not all women become pregnant, but most are susceptible to pregnancy. Women who are in the reproductive ages (generally regarded as ages 15–45, inclusive) comprise the population at risk. This includes those who have only sporadic sexual activity.

Susceptibility and *risk* are examples of epidemiologic terms. Epidemiology may be defined as *the study of the distribution and determinants of health and illness in the human community. Population epidemiology* relates the effects of fertility on the distribution and determinants of health and illness, and vice versa.[8] The study of the health effects of pregnancy and abortion is within the province of population epidemiology.

From an epidemiologic point of view, we may say that a woman who is *fecund* (capable of becoming pregnant) and who engages in coitus with a fertile man at the time of maximum *susceptibility* (shortly after ovulation) is *"exposed to the risk"* of pregnancy. Looking at the community in general, the women in the reproductive ages who are fecund and exposed to the risk of pregnancy constitute a *population at risk* in the same way that, for example, a group of people who have not been vaccinated against smallpox constitute a population at risk for smallpox (or a group of people who have not been vaccinated against Covid-19 constitute a population at risk of contracting Covid-19 with a *higher risk* of *fatal complications* than those who have been vaccinated).

Among the population at risk, we can describe an *incidence* of pregnancy (the number of new "cases") and the *prevalence* of pregnancy (the number of cases at any particular time). A *case-finding* technique for pregnancy can include a urine screening test, a pelvic examination, or an ultrasound exam just as we might give someone a tuberculin skin test or take a chest radiograph for tuberculosis. A *screening examination* may lead to a *diagnosis* of pregnancy. In fact, pregnancy may have certain *signs* and *symptoms*, just as do mumps and measles. *Laboratory studies* can be done that establish the diagnosis of pregnancy and document certain *physiological changes* that accompany pregnancy. There may be certain complications specifically associated with pregnancy. Many of these can be fatal.

Pregnancy can be *prevented* by a wide variety of methods of variable effectiveness. However, *prevention* usually involves *health behavior*, a kind of behavior described by sociologists that involves anticipation of illness and the search for methods of prevention. *Illness behavior*, on the other hand, is the result of someone searching for medical or surgical treatment of an existing condition, in this case, pregnancy. Illness behavior includes the request for or acceptance of *treatment* of the condition.

The *treatment* of pregnancy can take various forms. The *medical management* of pregnancy is usually called *prenatal care*; the physician does not intervene surgically in the pregnancy but monitors certain aspects of the woman's health, including blood pressure, blood sugar levels, and kidney function. Following the introduction of the drug mifepristone, *medical management* of early pregnancy now includes "medication abortion." *Surgical intervention* may occur early if the woman desires to terminate the pregnancy or if her life is in immediate danger; it may occur late, as in cesarean delivery, if the pregnancy is desired. The woman may benefit from or require *supportive psychotherapy;* for example, she may benefit from *problem pregnancy counseling* if she has difficulty deciding what to do about the pregnancy, *abortion counseling* if she wishes to terminate the pregnancy, and *psychiatric treatment* if she experiences a *post-partum psychosis*.

If this analysis seems to veer uncomfortably close to suggesting that pregnancy is a kind of illness, it does: Many, if not all, aspects of pregnancy can be understood best in terms of the cognitive framework of illness.[9] It helps us understand, for example, why women all over the world seek some form of treatment of pregnancy whether they are happily pregnant or not.[10] It helps us understand why the Cuna Indians of San Blas Island, the Tikopia of the South Pacific, the inhabitants of Tepoztlán, the Araucanian Indians, and many other tribal peoples regard pregnancy as an illness.[11] The people of

Tzintzuntzan, among others in Latin America, say that a woman who is pregnant "esta enferma" (is sick) and that when she is delivering her baby she "se alivia" (gets well) or (in the Peruvian Amazon Basin) "esta curando" (is healing).[12] It helps us understand why Devereux found abortion practiced in 450 societies, leading him to conclude that "abortion is an absolutely universal phenomenon."[13] It helps us understand why women will subject themselves to violence in order to interrupt pregnancy, and why this has been observed in many cultures.[14] It helps us understand why Western society has invented an entire medical specialty, obstetrics, devoted to the intensive medical care of women who are pregnant, so as to assure their survival. Modern obstetrics is also concerned with assuring that women with desired pregnancies have healthy babies, but the first emphasis has been on saving the woman's life and minimizing her impairment from the risks and complications of pregnancy.

Curiously, American obstetrics has held a paradoxical view of pregnancy in spite of this wholehearted and highly successful commitment to saving the lives of pregnant women. In the chapter concerning prenatal care in Eastman and Hellman's standard textbook, **Williams' Obstetrics** (fifth edition), the authors write:

> From a biologic point of view pregnancy and labor represent the highest function of the female reproductive system and *a priori* should be considered a normal process. But when we recall the manifold changes which occur in the maternal organism it is apparent that the borderline between health and disease is less distinctly marked during gestation than at other times, and derangement so slight as to be of little consequence under ordinary circumstances may readily be the precursor of pathologic conditions which may seriously threaten the life of the mother or the child or both. *It accordingly becomes necessary to keep pregnant patients under strict supervision and to be constantly on the alert for the appearance of untoward symptoms* [emphasis supplied]. . . It is in the prevention of such calamities [as eclampsia and dystocia] that care and supervision of the pregnant woman has been found to be of such value. *Indeed, antepartum care is an absolute necessity if a substantial number of women are to avoid disaster; and it is helpful to all* [emphasis supplied].[15]

The authors then describe in detail a very sound regimen of antepartum care.

The implications of this passage are clear: Pregnancy is normal—the "highest function" of a woman's reproductive system. Ergo, that highest function is not reached while a woman remains not pregnant. Yet the risks of serious morbidity and mortality are so much increased over the nonpregnant state that constant medical supervision is required when pregnancy occurs, particularly at the extreme ends of the reproductive spectrum.[16] If the risks were not so considerable, there would be no need for medical supervision.

There is a contradiction here: Pregnancy is a process in which the normal (nonpregnant) physiology is markedly altered for a time and a process that carries a significantly higher risk of morbidity and mortality than nonpregnancy. But if nonpregnancy is normal, how is it possible that pregnancy also is normal? Answer: If we say it is normal, it is normal.

Of course, Eastman and Hellman are seeking primarily to describe the difference between an uncomplicated (normal) pregnancy and a complicated (abnormal) pregnancy, a highly useful distinction in the context of obstetric practice. However, their highest function argument is extended by others to define a woman as most "normal" when she is pregnant or delivering a baby.

It would appear that part of the reason for the ambivalence about viewing pregnancy as normal and a state that requires constant supervision is that many physicians accept, implicitly or explicitly, the widely shared teleological definition of a woman as essentially a reproductive machine.

One physician suggested that woman be defined as "a uterus surrounded by a supporting organism and a directing personality."[17]

Adherence to this perspective clearly tends to inhibit critical examination of the corollary assumption that human pregnancy is not only normal but also an especially desirable event from the viewpoint of the woman's physiological, psychological, and social functioning and that failure (or, worse, refusal) to become or remain pregnant is, therefore, pathologic. In this context, it is not surprising that even the classical textbooks of obstetrics pay little or no attention to how a woman feels when she is pregnant, how she feels after an abortion, and whether she regarded her pregnancy as normal or desirable.

Suchman has pointed out that the way an individual perceives his or her health status may be more predictive of how he or she behaves in the face of illness than the actual medical diagnosis.[18] However, physicians trained in the Western tradition of medical practice tend to be much more disease oriented than patient oriented. Thus, their definitions of normality and abnormality tend to be stated in terms of the physician's perceptions and cognitive categories rather than those of the patient.[19]

The institutionalized view of pregnancy as a hypernormal state is perpetuated and enhanced by the linguistic categories of medical education and practice. The typical, routine pregnancy in a young and otherwise healthy woman is called a "normal pregnancy" unless it is complicated by various problems, such as preeclampsia, hydramnios, threatened abortion, abruptio placentae, hypofibrinogenemia, amniotic fluid embolism, or any one of the other numerous clinical syndromes associated with pregnancy.

"Normality" has always been subject to arbitrary social definition. In fact, anthropologist Ruth Benedict once proposed that normality is culturally defined.[20] She gave examples of behavior in Kwakiutl society that, while considered normal in that culture, would be considered unhealthy and delusional to the point of being psychotic in Western society. Anthropologist Margaret Mead later suggested that the question of health is whether it is regarded as an existing average or an ideal or goal to be attained.[21] In Western society, it tends to be the latter.

If "normal" health is defined as the existing average, however, it is likely to have a different connotation than if it is regarded as a goal to be attained. For example, if almost every child in the village has such a heavy roundworm burden that his stools look like spaghetti, and the existing average is taken as normal, it is normal for a child to have worms.

Using the same analysis, we can say that it was normal for the Cocos-Keeling Island women and it is normal for Shipibo Indian women to be pregnant for 25 percent to 30 percent or more of their reproductive years (and therefore relatively normal to be pregnant).[22] By comparison, the average suburban American woman may expect to be pregnant for only 5 percent of her fertile years. For the American woman, it is quite a bit less normal to be pregnant.

Medical sociologist David Mechanic points out that many diseases are not defined as illness states because they occur so frequently as to be regarded as the common state of humanity.[23] Perhaps pregnancy is such a condition, and its ubiquity previously had certain advantages for the human species.

Our culturally defined linguistic categories have accordingly come to shape our perceptions of biologic reality and thereby reinforce patterns with survival value.[24] There has been some cultural lag, however, with respect to our view of pregnancy. We cling to the outmoded view of pregnancy as women's highest, most normal function, even though Western medicine has begun treating pregnancy as a specialized kind of illness and various authors have called attention to the pathologic features of pregnancy.[25] In 1668 Mauriceau referred to it as "a disease of nine months' duration" (*maladie de neuf mois*) .[26] In any case, its resemblance to other illness states is no stranger to women, and it displays many nonspecific features of illness.

In terms of cultural function, Western society already defines pregnancy as an illness for which it has devised specific treatment programs ranging from medical management in the form of prenatal care to surgical intervention in the forms of abortion and cesarean delivery. These treatment programs have had positive results, which the patients themselves recognize and seek out whenever they can afford it.

When the specialty of obstetrics began developing in the early part of the twentieth century, for example, maternal mortality began a dramatic decline. In 1930 maternity directly or indirectly caused 11 percent of all deaths in women aged 15 to 45, whereas this proportion had declined to 3 percent by 1959.[27] Part of the decline was related to better living conditions and nutrition. However, a significant part of the decline arose from the increasingly effective medical management of pregnancy, including the prevention and treatment of eclampsia, post-partum hemorrhage, and post-partum infection.[28]

Successful surgical intervention, including cesarean delivery, in the cases of soft tissue and bony dystocia, also saved many lives. Studies regarding the disadvantages for both mother and offspring when there are short birth intervals have found that these improvements in mortality may also be the consequence of greater practice of fertility control, with resultant smaller completed family size and greater intervals between births.[29] Indeed, the greater normality of pregnancies in recent years (i.e., fewer complications and risks to the average mother) is certainly to some extent the result of a greater prevalence of normal nonpregnancy.

In the United States, the combination of factors, including longer birth intervals and fewer total pregnancies in the average fecund woman, has resulted in a lowering of the maternal mortality rate from 680 per 100,000 in the early 1920s to 11.1 per 100,000 live births in 1978.[30] The risks of serious morbidity and mortality have always been a part of pregnancy and may continue to be for some time, but some authors have contended that mortality rates can be brought still lower.[31]

Clearly, the view that pregnancy is a woman's most normal state has low survival value for the individual in terms of our growing understanding of the risks inherent in pregnancy, and it has a decreasing survival value for the species in the context of rapid population growth. Instead of being adaptive, the view of pregnancy as normal—or, rather, as a modified state of health—has become maladaptive both for individuals and for the species. Moreover, it does not explain the biologic and social realities that accompany pregnancy.

This analysis leaves us with the dilemma of having to cope with varying concepts of what is normal, what is health, what is illness, and what is disease.

In defining health and illness, anthropologist Steven Polgar uses the World Health Organization definition of health as the starting point; that is, not only the absence of disease and symptoms but also the presence of a sense of complete physical, mental, and social well-being.[32] He goes on to define illness as temporary or permanent impairment of functioning or appearance that need not be restricted to a decrease in the ability to function in ordinary ways. This definition is concerned with the person as a member of a group as well as with his or her biologic function.

Polgar also points out that explanations of illness serve, among other things, to indicate courses of preventive and curative action as well as to explain reality. Defining pregnancy as an illness would appear to be consistent with Polgar's definition.

There may be a difference between the disease entity as diagnosed by the physician, however, and illness as experienced by the person. As has been noted, health status as perceived by the patient may be more important in determining behavior in the context of illness than the correct medical diagnosis itself.

If the patient who is pregnant perceives herself as ill, for example, this may be much more important in terms of pregnancy outcome than the view of the physician that she is not.[33] Moreover, Engel points out that the presence of a complaint (i. e. , symptoms of pregnancy) must be regarded as presumptive evidence of disease.[34]

The symptomatic aspects of pregnancy, while based on certain physiological changes, are undoubtedly accentuated when the pregnancy is unwanted or when it occurs in the context of disturbed interpersonal relationships or other forms of stress. This has been demonstrated by Grimm, Rosengren, Davids, Poffenberger, and other investigators.[35] Sontag and others have suggested that this may also have adverse effects on the fetus.[36] There is clearly an interaction between physiological changes, cultural patterns, and psychological stress, and this is particularly true when the pregnancy does not occur under socially approved circumstances. Accordingly, it appears that "unwantedness" may be regarded as a major complication of pregnancy, with surgical intervention in the form of abortion as the indicated treatment rather than medical management, as would be the case with a wanted pregnancy.[37]

In spite of a woman's desire to terminate a pregnancy or a certain physiological basis for a sense of physical illness or discomfort, the behavior and statements of health professionals often summarize the predominant view that it is not the woman's physical condition or the fact of pregnancy that is the "illness," but her thinking that is "diseased."[38] Since in Western culture pregnancy has traditionally been defined as normal and the desire to terminate a pregnancy as pathologic, it follows that every woman who wants an abortion must need to have her head examined. That is exactly what happened in the late 1960s, when liberalized abortion laws required psychiatric consultation for women seeking legal abortion.

According to this logic, deviation from the accepted norm of pregnancy, especially once the pregnancy has begun, is *prima facie* evidence of abnormality. Thus, psychoanalyst May Romm once declared that intense conflict about a pregnancy or about giving birth to a child is "psychopathological.[39] The treatment suggested for women with these allegedly psychopathologic tendencies was, variously, psychotherapy, marriage, offering the baby for adoption, or some combination of these measures.

In fact, *a woman seeking an abortion is making a circumstantial self-definition of pregnancy as an illness for which she considers the appropriate treatment to be abortion.* In Mechanic's terminology, she is displaying "illness behavior."[40] Similarly, the woman who perceives the signs and symptoms of a *desired* pregnancy may also display illness behavior and seek medical attention in the form of prenatal care.

Newman has described certain kinds of ritualistic and symbolic communications with pregnant women by nonphysicians that imply urgency and danger while calling attention to the status of pregnancy.[41]

These communications, while tacitly or unconsciously recognizing the pregnancy itself as an illness, may be seen as magical attempts to ward off such unhealthy or dangerous patterns of thinking by ritual affirmation of the pregnant status.

In medical practice, *pregnancy is treated as a specialized form of illness even though physicians regard it as normal*. This may be seen as an example of *cognitive dissonance*.[42]

If illness is ordinarily viewed as a departure from the usual state of well-being, it is a priori, therefore, not normal.

The basis for these contradictions lies in the medical profession's failure to recognize the biosocial nature of illness and treatment and the role of the patient in their determination.[43] Recognition of the patient's role in the identification of illness and the choice of treatment invades the realm of professional exclusivity with its attendant prestige and status. This dilemma becomes particularly acute when a pregnant woman defines her own pregnancy as an illness for which she considers the appropriate treatment to be abortion.

Some studies have found that from 750,000 to more than 1 million births annually in the United States are unwanted by one or both parents.[44] Other studies indicate that reasons for a large proportion of unwanted births are primarily those that may be broadly defined as socioeconomic. Either the additional child results in increased economic hardship for the family unit or the birth occurs in the context of disturbed social relationships or there is some variation of thse reasons.[45] In addition to a large number of unwanted births, over 1.5 million abortions have occurred annually in the United States, with 300 abortions per 1000 known pregnancies.[46]

A study of motivations for abortion has found that the majority are sought for socioeconomic reasons.[47] Women seeking abortion seldom give the real reason for doing so to investigators studying this issue. The impression from clinical practice is that all but a few women seek abortions for reasons that can be broadly defined as socioeconomic, and many cite strictly economic reasons. Small-scale studies have supported this pattern, but national studies of this issue have not been done.[48]

It appears that *one-third of all pregnant American women each year define pregnancy as an illness for which they regard the appropriate treatment to be abortion*. The illness is not just biologic but is also social and economic; it is not just social but has a biologic basis in fact.

In view of these facts and analyses, it appears to be helpful to note those features, or parameters, of pregnancy that coincide with our traditional cognitive framework for illness, to see how well it fits. The test of the strength of the hypothesis lies in whether it explains reality and whether it predicts events.

The "null" hypothesis, then, in epidemiological terms (H°) is that pregnancy exhibits *none* of the identifying characteristics, or measurable parameters, of pregnancy.

Here's how that works out:

The illness parameters of pregnancy

The following illness parameters of the condition of pregnancy may be described:

1. *Etiology*

Fertilization and implantation of ovum

2. *Pathogenesis*

Host-parasite relationship

3. Pathophysiology

Displacement and compression of abdominal contents
Ureteral dilation[49]
Increased venous pressure[50]
Increased estrogen and progesterone levels[51]
Elevated basal metabolism rate[52] Glycosuria[53]
Increased aldosterone secretion[54]
Sodium and water retention[55] Decreased CO_2[56]
Hypercoagulability of blood[57]
Increased blood volume[58]
Bone marrow hyperplasia[59]
Increased renal blood flow[60]
Increased glomerular filtration rate[61]
Increased hepatic metabolic activity[62]

4. Clinical manifestations

Include a *subclinical* phase followed by distinct clinical *signs* and *symptoms*, which provide the basis for *clinical diagnosis*. Diagnosis may be also obtained through gross examination of the products of conception.

Positive signs of pregnancy[63]
Hearing and counting the fetal heartbeat
Perception of active fetal movements by the examiner
Radiologic recognition of the fetal skeleton
Sonographic recognition of the fetal parts

Probable signs of pregnancy[64]
Enlargement of the abdomen
Changes in the size, shape, and consistency of the uterus
Changes in the cervix
Braxton Hicks contractions
Ballottement
Outlining the fetus
Positive hormonal test for pregnancy

Presumptive signs and symptoms of pregnancy[65]
Cessation of menses
Changes in the breasts
Nausea and vomiting[66]
Discoloration of the mucous membranes of the vagina and vulva
Pigmentation of the skin and development of abdominal striae
Urinary disturbances
Fatigue
Perception of fetal movements

Other symptoms of pregnancy[67]
Pica[68]
Increased irritability[69]
Marked fluctuations in libido[70]

Leg cramps
Abdominal pain
Backache
Dyspnea

5. *Laboratory findings*

Chorionic gonadotropin present[71]
Hyperlipemia[72]
Decreased serum calcium[73]
Decreased serum iron[74]
Decreased hemoglobin[75]
Increased iron-binding capacity[76]
Decreased serum folic acid[77]
Increased serum copper[78]
Increased neutrophil alkaline phosphatase[79]
Alterations in serum protein pattern; decreased immunoglobulin G[80]
Increased fibrinogen level[81]
Positive C-reactive protein[82]
Bacteriuria[83]
Histologic study of the products of conception

6. *Complications*

Both acute and subacute exacerbations specifically associated with conception and pregnancy[84]
Diseases of the trophoblast: *benign*—hydatidiform mole; *malignant*—chorioadenoma destruens, choriocarcinoma[85]
Preeclampsia[86]
Eclampsia
Anemia
Placenta previa
Placenta accreta[87]
Abruptio placentae
Hypofibrinogenemia
Acute fatty liver[88]
Dystocia
Uterine rupture[89]
Amniotic fluid embolism[90]
Diabetes
Urinary tract infection
Multiple pregnancy
Ectopic pregnancy[91]
Hyperemesis gravidarum
Displacement of the uterus
Thromboembolic disease[92]
Puerperal psychosis
Hemorrhage
Puerperal infection

Retention of placenta
Placenta percreta[93]
Uterine dysfunction
Sickle cell crisis[94]
Right ovarian vein syndrome[95]

7.   *Differential diagnosis;*[96] Requires distinction between

Uncomplicated pregnancy
Hydatidiform mole
Pseudocyesis
Hematometra
Uterine sarcoma
Enlargement of uterus due to interstitial or submucous myomas
Extrauterine tumors

8.   *Treatment*

Medical management in the form of prenatal care
Medical management in the form of medication abortion
Surgical intervention in the form of abortion[97]
Hysterotomy
Hysterectomy
Late surgical intervention as in cesarean delivery
Late surgical intervention as in forceps delivery
Supportive psychotherapy

9.   *Prognosis*

Characteristic *duration*, which varies within certain limits; *recovery*, which may be spontaneous or induced; definable *recovery rate*; and risk of permanent or temporary
sequelae. The *case fatality rate* varies according to the patient's general health status
and the availability of effective medical care, and pregnancy can be listed as a *cause
of death*. Its recurrence is *episodic* among *survivors* not practicing effective preventive measures.

10.   *Epidemiology*

Universally occurring among females
Susceptibility highly variable and dependent on both biologic and nonbiologic factors. A
fecund woman engaging in coitus with a fertile man at the time of maximum susceptibility is said to be *exposed to the risk* of pregnancy.
Definable population at risk, an *incidence* of both conception and pregnancy among
the population at risk, a *point prevalence* and *period prevalence* of pregnancy, and
periodicity in the latter three characteristics[98]
Community *case-finding techniques*: urine *screening test* for the detection of pregnancy,
followed by *referral* of patients for appropriate *treatment*

11.   *Prevention*

A wide variety of methods of variable effectiveness, including abstinence and sterilization[99]

12. *Behavioral aspects*

Health behavior in anticipation or prevention of pregnancy
Illness behavior in seeking medical or surgical treatment
for an existing pregnancy
Participation in a *sick role*[100]
Other overlaid functions, such as *status affirmation*[101]

Other pathologic features of pregnancy

The relationship between the gravid female and the fetoplacental unit can be understood best as one of host and parasite. Local and systemic defense mechanisms on the part of the host may include increased uterine circulation, uterine contraction, increased blood volume, and a variety of other reactions, including isoimmunization. Billingham has suggested that parturition may represent an immunologic rejection similar to rejection of a homograft. [102] Aggressive mechanisms on the part of the fetoplacental unit include local invasion by the syncytial trophoblast, which is initially protected from maternal immunorejection; compression of the abdominal viscera and vessels; rupture of the uterus or establishment of ectopic pregnancy; elaboration of a luteotropic hormone; and nutritional competition with the host.[103] Kaplan and Grumbach hypothesize that the increased maternal resistance to insulin produced by the placental lactogen has the effect of sparing glucose for transfer to the fetus.[104] Page has speculated that the placenta elaborates a substance that results in an increased placental blood perfusion by producing maternal hypertension, leading, in turn, to the development of preeclampsia and eclampsia.[105]

Cameron enumerates several conditions on which the successful existence of a parasite depends: penetration into the host, adequate conditions of survival within the host, protective mechanisms of the parasite against the defenses of the host, and absence of effective reaction of the host.[106] Conditions of penetration into and persistence within the host are known as *invasiveness*. The capacity of parasites to produce disease is referred to as *pathogenicity*, while *virulence* is the measure of this capacity.[107] These features do not depend exclusively on the parasite but rather are determined by the interaction between parasite and host.

In this context, it may be seen that pregnancy, while exhibiting certain *neoplastic* characteristics, including actual *malignancy* at times, is most easily categorized as a *host—parasite* relationship. To this end, the effect of medical treatment, as in other parasitic conditions, is aimed at three fundamental goals: the blocking of the deleterious effects of the parasite or its destruction, the facilitation of the action of host systemic defense mechanisms, and the improvement of the general conditions of the host, which in itself results in an increase in defense mechanisms.[108]

The institutional arrangements and technology through which such goals are identified and accomplished may be regarded as *cultural adaptations* that augment *maternal biologic adaptations* (i.e., maternity hospitals or units; physicians and nurses with specialized training in obstetrics and gynecology).

The idea that pregnancy could be considered a pathologic process does not seem at first to be consistent with the continued survival of the human species for the past million or more years. However, any biologic event, and particularly disease process, can be considered in the light of adaptive responses that result in species survival and, secondarily, survival of the individual organism.[109] In this respect, *pregnancy is a highly successful biologic adaptation to the survival needs of the species*, although its survival value is changing under conditions of rapid population growth.[110] As is true of other adaptations, it may have disadvantages for all or a portion of the individuals in that species.

The best-known example of another biologic adaptation with *species survival advantages* and *individual disadvantages* is sickle cell trait and sickle cell disease of West Africa.[111] Heterozygous inheritance results in protection against lethal falciparum malaria, but homozygous inheritance is itself lethal for the small proportion of people who receive it. Pregnancy seems to be in the same general category: It has had outstanding survival advantages for the species but definite and often lethal disadvantages for individuals experiencing it. Our persistence in calling it normal in the face of these facts has been a *cultural adaptation* with a *high survival value for the species* – until recently.

The present situation is changed in three significant respects from previous human evolutionary experience:

1. A greater assurance of individual survival has reduced anxiety that the majority of a given couple's offspring will not survive to adulthood.
2. Technological developments, such as effective contraception and safe abortion techniques, now provide choices and offer perspectives about pregnancy that previously were unavailable or, at least, less obvious.
3. Under current conditions of phenomenal human population growth, *normal (i. e. , unlimited) reproduction, if anything, endangers survival of the human species and other species as well.*[112]

The preceding discussion allows us to view pregnancy in the context of both individual human illness and species adaptation.

Pregnancy is viewed, by Western society at least, as a normal phenomenon to be distinguished from illness states, even though *defining pregnancy as normal neither explains what we know about pregnancy nor predicts events surrounding pregnancy*. The strength of any hypothesis is its utility in dealing with reality. The hypothesis that pregnancy is merely an altered state of normal health does not meet this test, nor does the null hypothesis that pregnancy is not an illness.

The questions become these: Does the hypothesis that pregnancy is an illness explain the fact that people everywhere often seek its prevention, whatever the effectiveness of their methods, and have done so since the earliest historical and prehistoric times?[113]

Does it explain the fact that once pregnancy occurs, important physiological changes take place, subjective symptoms appear, and a significant excess risk of death is experienced?

Does it explain the fact that medical supervision will be sought whether the pregnancy is desired or not?

Does it explain the fact that this is true in nearly all human cultures and that the same cultures respond by the maintenance of rituals, procedures, and specialized persons or skills in order to meet the demand for supervision or assistance of some kind?[114]

Does it explain the fact that these activities continue in spite of countless and repeated assertions that pregnancy is normal?

Pregnancy may not be an illness. If it is not, though, one must ask: In what way is it not an illness? In fact, human pregnancy can be viewed as an episodic, moderately extended chronic condition with a definable mortality risk to which females are uniquely, although not uniformly, susceptible and to which the following obtain:

- It is almost entirely preventable through the use of effective contraception and is entirely so through sterilization or abstinence.
- When not prevented, it is the individual result of a set of species-specific biosocial adaptations with a changing significance for species survival.
- It is a neoplastic, endoparasitic (i. e., neoparasitic) autoinfection of relatively high pathogenicity and low average virulence, which is localized, self-limited, and nontransmissible.
- It may be defined as an illness requiring medical supervision through cultural traditions (functional or explicit) or individual illness behavior.
- It may be treated with a variety of surgical and medical procedures and with supportive psychotherapy, as indicated.
- It may be tolerated, sought, or valued for the purposes of reproduction, self-expression, or status affirmation.
- It has an excellent prognosis for spontaneous recovery if managed under careful medical supervision.

Notes

1 Garrow, D.J. *Liberty and Sexuality: The Right to Privacy and the Making of* Roe v. Wade. New York: Macmillan, 1994. p. 401.
2 Mauriceau, F. *Des maladies des femmes grosses et accouchées*. Paris, 1668.
3 Bodanis, D. *Passionate Minds: The Great Love Affair of the Enlightenment, Featuring the Scientist Emilie du Chatelet, the Poet Voltaire, Sword Fights Book bBrnings, Assorted Kings, Seditious Verse, and the Birth of the Modern World*. New York: Crown, 2006.
4 Lerner, M., and O.W. Anderson. (1963): *Health Progress in the United States:1900–1960*. Chicago: University of Chicago Press. Chapter 4, p. 34.
5 Hoyert D.L. Maternal mortality rates in the United States, 2021. *NCHS Health E-Stats*. 2023. DOI: https://dx.doi.org/10.15620/cdc:124678.
6 Hern, W.M. Pregnancy kills. Abortion saves lives. *New York Times*, May 21, 2019. https://www.nytimes.com/2019/05/21/opinion/alabama-law-abortion.html
7 Hurley, L. Supreme Court allows Idaho to enforce abortion law against emergency room doctors ahead of hearing case. *NBC News*, January 5, 2024.
8 Omran, A.R. Population epidemiology. *American Journal of Public Health* 64:674, 1974. https://ajph.aphapublications.org/doi/pdf/10.2105/AJPH.64.7.674
9 Hern, W.M. The illness parameters of pregnancy. *Social Science and Medicine* (England) 9:365, 1975. https://www.drhern.com/wp-content/uploads/2018/05/illness-param-pregnancy-1975.pdf
10 Benedict, B. Social regulation of fertility. In Harrison GA, and Boyce, A.J. (eds). *The Structure of Human Populations*. Oxford: Clarendon Press, 1972; Ford C.S.: *A Comparative Study of Human Reproduction*. New Haven, CT: Human Relations Area File Press, 1964; Nag, M. *Factors Affecting Human Fertility in Nonindustrial Societies: A Cross Cultural Study*. New Haven, CT: Human Relations Area File Press, 1976; Lorimer, F. *Culture and Human Fertility*. New York: UNESCO, 1954; Browner, C. The management of early pregnancy: Colombian folk concepts of fertility control. *Social Science and Medicine* (B) 14:25, 1980. PMID: 7394561 DOI: 10.1016/0160-7987(80)90037-x
11 Stout, D.B. *San Blas Cuna Acculturation: An Introduction*. New York, Viking Fund Publications in Anthropology, No. 9, 1957.; Mead, M., and Newton, N. Cultural patterning of perinatal behavior. In Richardson, S., and Guttmacher, A.F. (eds). *Childbearing: Its Social and Psychological Aspects*, p. 142. Baltimore:, Williams & Wilkins, 1967; Newton. N. The effect of psychological environment on childbirth: Combined cross-cultural and experimental

approach. *Journal of Cross Cultural Psychology* 1:85, 1970.; Firth, R. *We, the Tikopia*. Boston: Beacon Press, 1963; Firth, R. *Social Change in Tikopia*. New York: Macmillan, 1959; Lewis, O. *Tepoztlan: Village in Mexico*, chap 6, p. 69. New York: Holt, Rinehart & Winston, 1967; Hilger, I.: *Araucanian Child Life and Its Cultural Background*. Washington, DC: Smithsonian Institution Miscellaneous Collections, No. 113, 1957.

12 Foster. G.M., and Anderson, B.G: *Medical Anthropology*, p. 285. New York: John Wiley & Sons, 1978.

13 Devereux, G. A typological study of abortion in 350 primitive, ancient and preindustrial societies. In Rosen, H. (ed). *Abortion in America*, p. 97. Boston: Beacon Press, 1967; Devereux. G. *A Study of Abortion in Primitive Societies: A Typological, Distributional, and Dynamic Analysis of the Prevention of Birth In 400 Preindustrial Societies*. New York: Russell Sage Foundation, 1955.

14 Shain, R.N. Abortion practices and attitudes in cross-cultural perspective. *American Journal of Obstetrics and Gynecology* 142:245, 1982. https://doi.org/10.1016/0002-9378(82)90725-6.

15 Eastman, N.J., and Hellman L.M. *Williams' Obstetrics*, 12th ed, Chap 12, p. 337. New York: Appleton-Century-Crofts, 1961.

16 Eastman and Hellman, ibid.; Yerushalmy. J., Palmer, C.E., and Kramer, M. Studies in childbirth mortality: 2. Age and parity in childbirth fatality. *Public Health Reports* 55:1195, 1940; 29.; Perkin, G.W. Assessment of reproductive risk in nonpregnant women. *American Journal of Obstetrics and Gynecology* 101:709, 1968; 30.Menken, J. The health and social consequences of teenage childbearing. *Family Planning Perspectives* 4:45, 1972.

17 Calderone, M. (ed). *Abortion in the United States*, p. 118. New York: Harper Hoeber, 1958.

18 Suchman, E.A.: Social patterns of illness and medical care. *Journal of Health and Human Behavior* 6:2, 1965.

19 Lewis, A. Health as a social concept. *British Journal of Sociology* 4:109, 1953.

20 Benedict, R. Anthropology and the abnormal. *Journal of Genetic Psychology* 10:59, 1934.

21 Mead, M. *Cultural Patterns and Technological Change*. p. 229. New York: Mentor Books, 1963.

22 Smith, T.E. The Cocos-Keeling Islands: A demographic laboratory. *Population Studies* 16:94, 1960; Hern, W.M. High fertility in a Peruvian Amazon Indian village. *Human Ecology* 5:355, 1977. PMID: 12337376 DOI: 10.1007/BF00889176

23 Mechanic, D. *Medical Sociology*, p. 16. New York: Free Press, 1968.

24 Carroll, J.B. (ed.). *Language, Thought and Reality: Selected Writings of Benjamin Lee Whorf*. Cambridge, MA: MIT Press, 1964.; Frake, C.O. The diagnosis of disease among the Subanum of Mindanao. In Hymes, D. (ed). *Language in Culture and Society*, p. 142. New York: Harper & Row, 1964.

25 Hern, W.M. Is pregnancy really normal? *Family Planning Perspectives* 3:5, 1971, https://www.drhern.com/wp-content/uploads/2020/09/Is-Pregnancy-Really-Normal_.html; Delee, J.B., and Greenhill, J.P. *Principles and Practice of Obstetrics*, 8th ed, p. xiii. Philadelphia: W.B. Saunders, 1943; Freeman, M.G. Obstetric triage in indigent women. *Obstetrics and Gynecology* 36:919, 1970.

26 Mauriceau F: *Des Maladies des Femmes Grosses et Accouchées*, p 105. Paris: Charles Coignard, 1668. (English translation by Chamberlen H: *The Accomplished Midwife, Treating of the Diseases of Women with Child, and in Child-bed*. London, John Darby, 1673).

27 Lerner and Anderson, ibid., chapter 4, p. 34.

28 Willson, J.R. Health care for women: *Present Gynecology* 36:178, 1970; Marmol, J.G., Scriggens, A.L., and Vollman, R.F. History of maternal mortality study committees in the United States. *Obstetrics and Gynecology* 34:123, 1969.

29 Yerushalmy, J. On the interval between successive births and its effect on the survival of infants. *Human Biology* 17:65, 1945; 49.Yerushalmy, J. Neonatal mortality by order of birth and age of parents. *American Journal of Hygiene* 28:244, 1938; Westoff, C.F., Potter, R.G., and Sagi, P.C. *The Third Child*, chap 6. Princeton, NJ: Princeton University Press, 1963; Jaffe F.S., and Polgar, S. Epidemiological indications for fertility control. *Journal of the Christian Medical Association of India (Suppl)*, p. 12, 1967.; Eastman, N.J. The effect of the interval between births on a maternal and fetal outlook. *American Journal of Obstetrics*

and Gynecology 47:445, 1944; Morris, J.N., and Heady, J.A. Social and biological factors in infant mortality. *Lancet* 1:343, 1955; 54.Morris, J.N., and Heady, J.A. Social and biological factors in infant mortality: Variation in mortality with mother's age and parity. *Journal of Obstetrics and Gynaecology of the British Empire* 66:577, 1959; 55. Baird, D. The influence of social and economic factors on stillbirths and neonatal deaths. *Journal of Obstetrics and Gynaecology of the British Empire* 52:21, 1945; Wray, J.D. Population pressure on families: Family size and child spacing. In Revelle, R., Coale, A.J., and Freymann, M., et al. (eds): *Rapid Population Growth: Consequences and Policy Implications,* Vol. 2, p 403. Baltimore: Johns Hopkins University Press, 1971.

30 Lerner and Anderson, *op. cit.*, p 32; National Center for Health Statistics: Vital Statistics of the United States, Vol. 2, Mortality, 1940 through 1978. Washington, DC: U.S. Government Printing Office, 1980.

31 Phillips, O.C., and Hulka, J.F. Obstetric mortality. *Anesthesiology* 26:435, 1965.; Klein, M.D., and Karten, I. Maternal deaths: A health and socioeconomic challenge. *American Journal of Obstetrics and Gynecology* 110:298, 1971.; Benaron, H.B., and Tucker, B.E. The effect of obstetric management and factors beyond clinical control on maternal mortality rates at the Chicago Maternity Center from 1959 to 1963. *American Journal of Obstetrics and Gynecology* 110:1113, 1971.

32 Polgar, S. Health. In Sills, D.L. (ed). *International Encyclopedia of the Social Sciences*, pp. 330–36. Riverside, NJ: Macmillan, 1968.

33 Rosengren, W.R. Some social psychological aspects of delivery room difficulties. *Journal of Nervous and Mental Diseases* 132:515, 1961.

34 Engel, G. A unified concept of health and disease. *Perspectives in Biology and Medicine* 3:459, 1960.

35 Grimm, E.R. Psychological tension in pregnancy. *Psychosomatic Medicine* 23:520, 1961; Rosengren, W.R. Social sources of pregnancy as illness or normality. *Sociological Forum* 39:260, 1961; Rosengren, W.R. Social instability and attitudes toward pregnancy as a social role. *Social Problems* 9:371, 1952; Davids, A., and Rosengren. W.R. Social stability and psychological adjustment during pregnancy. *Psychosomatic Medicine* 24:579, 1962; Poffenberger, S., and Poffenberger, T. Intent toward conception and the pregnancy experience. *American Sociological Review* 17:616, 1952; Davids, A., and Devault, S. Maternal anxiety during pregnancy and childbirth abnormalities. *Psychosomatic Medicine* 24:464, 1962; Squier, R., and Dunbar, F. Emotional factors in the course of pregnancy. *Psychosomatic Medicine* 8:161, 1946; Weil, R.J., and Tupper, C. Personality, life situation, and communication: A study of habitual abortion. *Psychosomatic Medicine* 22:448, 1960; Benedek, T. The psychobiology of pregnancy. In Anthony, E.J. and Benedek, T. (eds). *Parenthood: Its Psychology and Psychopathology,* p. 137. Boston: Little, Brown & Co, 1970; Wortis, H., and Freedman, A.M. Maternal stress and premature delivery. *Bulletin of the World Health Organization* 26:285, 1962; Coppen, A.J. Psychosomatic aspects of pre-eclamptic toxaemia. *Journal of Psychosomatic Research* 2:241, 1958; Wiehl, D.G., Berry, K., and Tompkins, W.T. Complications of pregnancy among prenatal patients reporting nervous illness. In Passamanick, B. (ed). *Epidemiology of Mental Disorders.* Washington, DC: American Association for the Advancement of Science, 1959; Zemlick, M.J., and Watson, R.I. Maternal attitudes of acceptance and rejection during and after pregnancy. *American Journal of Orthopsychiatry* 23:570, 1953.

36 Sontag, L.W. Differences in modifiability of fetal behavior and physiology. *Psychosomatic Medicine* 6:151, 1944; Wile, I.S., and Davis, R. The relation of birth to behavior. *American Journal of Orthopsychiatry* 11:32, 1941; Spelt, B.K. The conditioning of the human fetus in utero. *Journal of Experimental Psychology* 38:338, 1948; Stott, D.H. Psychological and mental handicaps in the child following a disturbed pregnancy. *Lancet* 1:1006, 1957; Stott, D.H. Evidence for prenatal impairment of temperament in mentally retarded children. *Vita Humana* 2:125, 1959.; Newton, N., Teeler, B., and Newton, M. Effect of disturbance on labor. *American Journal of Obstetrics and Gynecology* 101:1096, 1968.

37 Cates, W., Grimes, D.A., and Smith, J.C. Abortion as a treatment for unwanted pregnancy: the number two sexually-transmitted condition. *Advances in Planned Parenthood* 12:115, 1978.

38 Benedek, *op. cit.*, p. 137.

39 Romm, M. In Rosen, H. (ed). *Abortion in America*, chap. 14, p. 210. Boston: Beacon Press, 1967.

40 Mechanic, D., and Volkart, E.H. Stress, illness behavior, and the sick role. *American Sociological Review* 26:51, 1961.

41 Newman, L.F. *Culture and Perinatal Environment in American Society*, p. 138. Doctoral thesis, Berkeley, California, 1967 ; Newman, L.F. Folklore of pregnancy: Wives' tales in Contra Costa County, California. *Western Folklore* 28:112, 1969.

42 Festinger, L. *A Theory of Cognitive Dissonance*, p. 263. Evanston, IL: Rowe & Paterson, 1957.

43 Saunders, L. *Cultural Difference and Medical Care*. New York:, Russell Sage Foundation, 1954; Polgar, S. Health action in cross-cultural perspective. In Freeman, H.E., Levine, S., and Reeder, L.G. (eds). *Handbook of Medical Sociology*, p. 397. Englewood Cliffs, NJ: Prentice Hall, 1963.; Cassel, J.: Social science theory as a source of hypothesis in epidemiological research. *American Journal of Public Health* 54:1482, 1964.; Cassel, J. Health consequences of population density and crowding. In Revelle, R., Coale, A.J., Freymann, M., et al. (eds), *Rapid Population Growth: Consequences and Policy Implications*, Vol. 2, p. 462. Baltimore: Johns Hopkins University Press, 1971; Nuckolls, K.B., Cassel, J., and Kaplan, B.H. Psychosocial assets, life crisis, and the prognosis of pregnancy. *American Journal of Epidemiology* 95:431, 1972.

44 Bumpass, L., and Westoff, C.F. The "perfect contraceptive" population. *Science* 169:1177, 1970.

45 Sloane, R.B. The unwanted pregnancy. *New England Journal of Medicine* 280:1206, 1969; Liben, F. Minority group clinic patients pregnant out of wedlock. *American Journal of Public Health* 59:1868, 1969.; Furstenberg, F. Jr., Gordis, L., and Markowitz, M. Birth control knowledge and attitudes among unmarried pregnant adolescents: A preliminary report. *Journal of Marriage and the Family* 31:34, 1969; Furstenberg, F. Jr. Premarital pregnancy among black teenagers. *Transaction*, p. 52, 1970; Pohlman, E. "Wanted" and "unwanted": Toward less ambiguous definition. *Eugenics Quarterly* 12:19, 1965; Steele, B.F., and Pollack, C.B. Psychiatric study of parents who abuse infants and small children. In Helfer, R.E., and Kempe, C.H. (eds). *The Battered Child*, p. 103. Chicago: University of Chicago Press, 1968; Armijo, R., and Monreal, T. The epidemiology of provoked abortion in Santiago, Chile. In Muramatsu, M., and Harper, P.A. (eds). *Population Dynamics*, p. 137. Baltimore: Johns Hopkins University Press, 1965; Requena, M. Social and economic correlates of induced abortion in Santiago, Chile. *Demography* 2:33, 1965.

46 Henshaw, S., Forrest, J.D., Sullivan, E. et al. Abortion services in the United States: 1979–1980. *Family Planning Perspectives* 14:5, 1982; Tietze, C. *Induced Abortion: A World Review*, 1983, 5th ed, p. 33. New York: The Population Council, 1983.

47 David, H.P. Induced abortion: Psychosocial aspects. In Sciarra, J.J, (ed). *Gynecology and Obstetrics*, Vol. 6, chap 53. Philadelphia: Harper & Row, 1982.

48 Armijo, R., and Monreal, T. The epidemiology of provoked abortion in Santiago, Chile. In Muramatsu, M., and Harper, P.A. (eds). *Population Dynamics*, p. 137. Baltimore: Johns Hopkins University Press, 1965.; Requena, M. Social and economic correlates of induced abortion in Santiago, Chile. *Demography* 2:33, 1965.

49 Fainstat, T. Ureteral dilatation in pregnancy: A review. *Obstetrical & Gynecological Survey* 18:845, 1963.

50 Reid, D.E. *A Textbook of Obstetrics*, pp. 160–217. Philadelphia: WB Saunders, 1962.; Douglas, B.H., Colemann. T.G., and Whittington-Coleman, P.J. Circulatory dynamics of pregnancy: IV. Fluid accumulation. *American Journal of Obstetrics and Gynecology* 108:999, 1970.

51 Hytten, F.E., and Leitch, I. *The Physiology of Human Pregnancy*, p. 148. Philadelphia: FA Davis, 1963.

52 Sandiford, I., and Wheeler, T. Basal metabolism before, during, and after pregnancy. *Journal of Biological Chemistry* 62:329, 1924.

53 Sims, E.A.H.: Renal function in normal pregnancy. *Clinical Obstetrics and Gynecology* 11:461, 1968.

54 Watanabe, M., Meeker, C,I., Gray, M.J. et al. Secretion rate of aldosterone in normal pregnancy. *Journal of Clinical Investigation* 42:1619, 1963.

55 Abitbol, M.M. Weight gain in pregnancy. American *Journal of Obstetrics and Gynecology* 104:140, 1969.; Reid, *op. cit.*, p. 269.; Douglas, Colemann, Whittington-Coleman, *op. cit.*

56 Hellman, L.M., and Pritchard, J.A. *Williams' Obstetrics*, 14th ed, p. 252. New York: Appleton-Century-Crofts, 1971.

57 Markarian, M., and Jackson, J. Comparison of the kinetics of clot formation, fibrinogen, fibrinolysis, and hematocrit in pregnant women and adults. *American Journal of Obstetrics and Gynecology* 101:593, 1968.; Ygge, J. Changes in blood coagulation and fibrinolysis during the puerperium. *American Journal of Obstetrics and Gynecology* 104:2, 1969.

58 Hytten, Leitch, *op. cit.,* p 24.; Douglas, Colemann, Whittington-Coleman, *op. cit.*

59 Rothman, D. Folic acid in pregnancy. *American Journal of Obstetrics and Gynecology* 108:149, 1970.

60 Rudolph, J.H., and Wax, S.H, The 1^{131} renogram in pregnancy: Normal pregnancy. *Obstetrics and Gynecology* 30:385, 1967.

61 Sims, E.A.H., and Krantz, K.E. Serial studies of renal function during pregnancy and the puerperium in normal women. *Journal of Clinical Investigation* 37:1764, 1958; Lindheimer, M.D., and Katz, A.l. : The kidney in pregnancy. *New England Journal of Medicine* 283:1095, 19

62 Hall, D.G., Fahim, M.S., Griffin, W.T. et al. Hepatic metabolic activity related to reproduction. *American Journal of Obstetrics and Gynecology* 109:744, 1971.

63 Hellman, L.M., and Pritchard, J.A. *Williams' Obstetrics*, 14th ed, p. 252. New York: Appleton-Century-Crofts, 1971.

64 Hellman, L.M., and Pritchard, J.A. *Williams' Obstetrics*, 14th ed, p. 252. New York: Appleton-Century-Crofts, 1971; Markarian, M., and Jackson, J. Comparison of the kinetics of clot formation, fibrinogen, fibrinolysis, and hematocrit in pregnant women and adults. *American Journal of Obstetrics and Gynecology* 101:593, 1968; Ygge, J. Changes in blood coagulation and fibrinolysis during the puerperium. *American Journal of Obstetrics and Gynecology* 104:2, 1969; Hytten, Leitch, *op cit*, p. 24; Douglas, Colemann, Whittington-Coleman, *op cit*; Rothman, D. Folic acid in pregnancy. *American Journal of Obstetrics and Gynecology* 108:149, 1970; Rudolph, J.H., and Wax, S.H. The 1^{131} renogram in pregnancy: Normal pregnancy. *Obstetrics and Gynecology* 30:385, 1967; Sims, E.A.H., and Krantz, K.E. Serial studies of renal function during pregnancy and the puerperium in normal women. *Journal of Clinical Investigation* 37:1764, 1958; Lindheimer, M.D., and Katz, A.l. : The kidney in pregnancy. *New England Journal of Medicine* 283:1095, 19; Hall, D.G., Fahim, M.S., Griffin, W.T. et al. Hepatic metabolic activity related to reproduction. *American Journal of Obstetrics and Gynecology* 109:744, 1971; Pritchard, J.A., and MacDonald, P.C. *Williams' Obstetrics*, 16th ed. New York, Appleton-Century-Crofts, 1980.

65 Hellman, L.M., and Pritchard, J.A. *Williams' Obstetrics*, 14th ed, p. 252. New York: Appleton-Century-Crofts, 1971.

66 Brandes, J.M.: First-trimester nausea and vomiting as related to outcome of pregnancy. *Obstetrics and Gynecology* 30:427, 1967; Benson, R.C. *Handbook of Obstetrics and Gynecology*. Los Altos, CA: Lange Medical Publications, 1964.

67 Hellman, L.M., and Pritchard, J.A. *Williams' Obstetrics*, 14th ed, p. 252. New York: Appleton-Century-Crofts, 1971.

68 Hytten, Leitch, *op. cit.,* p 129.; O'Rourke, D.E., Quinn, J.G., Nicholson, J.O. et al. Geophagia during pregnancy. *Obstetrics and Gynecology* 29:581, 1967.

69 Jessner, L., Weigart, E., and Foy, J.L. The development of parental attitudes during pregnancy. In Anthony, E.J. and Benedek, T. (eds): *Parenthood: Its Psychology and Psychopathology*, pp. 209–24. Boston: Little, Brown & Co., 1970.

70 Ibid.

71 Reid, *op cit,* p. 160; Mizejewski, G.J., Quinones, J. and Baron, J. Radioglobulin localization and immunospecificity in the transplanted human choriocarcinoma. *American Journal of Obstetrics and Gynecology* 111:413, 1971.

72 Hellman, Pritchard, *op. cit.*

73 Ibid.

74 Apte, S.V., and Iyengar, L. Absorption of dietary iron in pregnancy. *American Journal of Clinical Nutrition* 23:73, 1970.

75 Sturgeon, P. Studies of iron requirements in infants: III. Influence of supplemental iron during normal pregnancy on mother and infant. Pt. A. *The mother. British Journal of Haematology* 5:31, 1959.

76 Apte, Iyengar, *op. cit.*

77 Rothman, *op. cit.;* Kahn, S.B., Fein, S., Rigberg., S. et al. Correlation of folate metabolism and socio-economic status in pregnancy and in patients taking oral contraceptives. *American*

Journal of Obstetrics and Gynecology 108:931, 1970; Iyengar, L. Folic acid requirements of Indian pregnant women. *American Journal of Obstetrics and Gynecology* 111:13, 1971.

78 Burrows, S. and Pekal, B. Serum copper and ceruloplasmin in pregnancy. *American Journal of Obstetrics and Gynecology* 109:907, 1971.

79 Polishuk, W.Z., Diamant, Y.Z., Zuckerman, H. et al. Leukocyte alkaline phosphatase in pregnancy and the puerperium. *American Journal of Obstetrics and Gynecology* 107:604, 1970; Elder, M.G., Bonello, F., and Ellul, J. Neutrophil alkaline phosphatase in pregnancy and its relationship to urinary estrogen excretion and serum heat-stable alkaline phosphatase levels. *American Journal of Obstetrics and Gynecology* 111:319, 1971.

80 Maroulis, G.B., Buckley, R.H., and Younger, J.B. Serum immunoglobulin concentrations during normal pregnancy. *American Journal of Obstetrics and Gynecology* 109:971, 1971.; Mendenhall, H.W. Serum protein concentrations in pregnancy. *American Journal of Obstetrics and Gynecology* 106:388, 1970.

81 Markarian, Jackson, *op. cit.*; Ygge, *op. cit.*

82 Connel, E.B., and Connell, J.T. C-reactive protein in pregnancy and contraception. *American Journal of Obstetrics and Gynecology* 110:633, 1971.

83 Norden, C.W., and Kass, E.H. Bacteriuria in pregnancy: A critical appraisal. *Annual Review of Medicine* 19:431, 1968.

84 Hellman, L.M., and Pritchard, J.A. *Williams' Obstetrics*, 14th ed, p. 252. New York: Appleton-Century-Crofts, 1971; Markarian, M., and Jackson, J. Comparison of the kinetics of clot formation, fibrinogen, fibrinolysis, and hematocrit in pregnant women and adults. *American Journal of Obstetrics and Gynecology* 101:593, 1968; Ygge, J. Changes in blood coagulation and fibrinolysis during the puerperium. *American Journal of Obstetrics and Gynecology* 104:2, 1969; Hytten, Leitch, *op cit*, p 24; Douglas, Colemann, Whittington-Coleman, *op cit*; Rothman, D. Folic acid in pregnancy. *American Journal of Obstetrics and Gynecology* 108:149, 1970; Rudolph, J.H., and Wax, S.H. The 1^{131} renogram in pregnancy: Normal pregnancy. *Obstetrics and Gynecology* 30:385, 1967; Sims, E.A.H., and Krantz, K.E. Serial studies of renal function during pregnancy and the puerperium in normal women. *Journal of Clinical Investigation* 37:1764, 1958; Lindheimer, M.D. and Katz, A.l. : The kidney in pregnancy. *New England Journal of Medicine* 283:1095, 19; Hall, D.G., Fahim, M.S., Griffin, W.T. et al. Hepatic metabolic activity related to reproduction. *American Journal of Obstetrics and Gynecology* 109:744, 1971; Pritchard, J.A. and MacDonald, P.C. *Williams' Obstetrics*, 16th ed. New York, Appleton-Century-Crofts, 1980.

85 Teoh, E.S., Dawood, M.Y., and Ratnam, S.S. Epidemiology of hydatidiform mole in Singapore. *American Journal of Obstetrics and Gynecology* 110:415, 1971.; Hohe, P.T., Cochrane, C.R., Gmelich, J.T. et al. Coexistent trophoblastic tumor and viable pregnancy. *Obstetrics and Gynecology* 38:899, 1971.

86 Sims, E.A.H. Pre-eclampsia and related complications of pregnancy. *American Journal of Obstetrics and Gynecology* 107:154, 1970.

87 Weeks, L.R., and Grieg, L.B. Placenta accreta: A twenty-year review. *American Journal of Obstetrics and Gynecology* 113:76, 1972; Whitham, R.G., and Malberg, B.J. : Placenta accreta: A case report. *Rocky Mountain Medical Journal* 76:241, 1979.

88 Ober, W.B., and Lecompte, P.M. Acute fatty metamorphosis of the liver associated with pregnancy: A distinctive lesion. *American Journal of Medicine* 19:743, 1955; Holzbach, R.T. Acute fatty liver of pregnancy with disseminated intravascular coagulation. *Obstetrics and Gynecology* 43:740, 1974.

89 Schrinsky, D.C., and Benson, R.C. Rupture of the pregnant uterus: A review. *Obstetrical and Gynecological Survey* 33:217, 1978.; Dainer, M.J. Spontaneous uterine rupture. *Journal of Reproductive Medicine* 26:35, 1981.; DeWane, J.C. and McCubbin, J.H. Spontaneous rupture of an unscarred uterus at 19 weeks' gestation. *American Journal of Obstetrics and Gynecology* 141:222, 1981.

90 Grimes, D.A., Cates, W. Jr., Ziskin. L.Z. et al. Maternal death at term as a late sequela of failed attempted abortion. *Advances in Planned Parenthood* 14:77, 1979.; Roche, W.D., and Norris, H.J. Detection and significance of maternal pulmonary amniotic fluid embolism. *Obstetrics and Gynecology* 43:729, 1974; Resnik, R., Swartz, W.H., Plumer, M.H. et al. Amniotic fluid embolism with survival. *Obstetrics and Gynecology* 47:295, 1976.

91 Schneider, J., Berger, C.J., and Cattell, C. Maternal mortality due to ectopic pregnancy: A review of 102 deaths. *Obstetrics and Gynecology* 49:557, 1977; Rubin, G.L., Cates, W. Jr., Gold, J., et al: Fatal ectopic pregnancy after attempted legally induced abortion. *Journal of the American Medical Association* 244:1705, 1980.

92 Byrne, J.J. Thrombophlebitis in pregnancy. *Clinical Obstetrics and Gynecology* 13:305, 1970.

93 Teteris, N.J., Lina, A.A., and Holoday, W.J. Placenta percreta. *Obstetrics and Gynecology* 47 (Suppl):15, 1976.

94 Perkins, R.P. Inherited disorders of hemoglobin synthesis and pregnancy. *American Journal of Obstetrics and Gynecology* 111:120, 1971.

95 Reynolds, S.R.M. Right ovarian vein syndrome. *Obstetrics and Gynecology* 37:308, 1971; Brown, T.K., and Munsick, R.A. Puerperal ovarian vein thrombophlebitis: A syndrome. *American Journal of Obstetrics and Gynecology* 109:263, 1971.

96 Hellman, L.M., and Pritchard, J.A. *Williams' Obstetrics*, 14th ed, p. 252. New York: Appleton-Century-Crofts, 1971.; Markarian, M., and Jackson, J. Comparison of the kinetics of clot formation, fibrinogen, fibrinolysis, and hematocrit in pregnant women and adults. *American Journal of Obstetrics and Gynecology* 101:593, 1968; Ygge, J. Changes in blood coagulation and fibrinolysis during the puerperium. *American Journal of Obstetrics and Gynecology* 104:2, 1969; Hytten, Leitch, *op cit*, p. 24; Douglas, Colemann, Whittington-Coleman, *op cit*; Rothman, D. Folic acid in pregnancy. *American Journal of Obstetrics and Gynecology* 108:149, 1970; Rudolph, J.H., and Wax, S.H, The 1^{131} renogram in pregnancy: Normal pregnancy. *Obstetrics and Gynecology* 30:385, 1967; Sims, E.A.H., and Krantz, K.E. Serial studies of renal function during pregnancy and the puerperium in normal women. *Journal of Clinical Investigation* 37:1764, 1958; Lindheimer, M.D., and Katz, A.l. : The kidney in pregnancy. *New England Journal of Medicine* 283:1095, 19; Hall, D.G., Fahim, M.S., Griffin, W.T. et al. Hepatic metabolic activity related to reproduction. *American Journal of Obstetrics and Gynecology* 109:744, 1971; Pritchard, J.A., and MacDonald, P.C. *Williams' Obstetrics*, 16th ed. New York, Appleton-Century-Crofts, 1980; Benson, R.C. *Handbook of Obstetrics and Gynecology*. Los Altos, CA, Lange Medical Publications, 1964.

97 Hern, W.M. *Abortion Practice*. Philadelphia: J.B. Lippincott Company, 1984. Soft cover edition, Boulder: Alpenglo Graphics, 1990. Available from author; Hern, W.M. Laminaria in abortion: use in 1368 patients in first trimester. *Rocky Mountain Medical Journal* 72:390395, 1975. https://www.drhern.com/wp-content/uploads/2018/06/first-tri-laminaria-75.pdf; Hern, W.M. Fetal diagnostic indications for second and third trimester outpatient pregnancy termination. *Prenatal Diagnosis* 34(5):438-444, 2014. At https://obgyn.onlinelibrary.wiley.com/doi/10.1002/pd.4324; Hern, W.M. Second-trimester surgical abortion. In *Global Library of Women's Medicine*, 2nd edition. Hern, W., Glob.libr.women's med., (ISSN: 1756-2228) 2011; DOI 10.3843/GLOWM.10442 Revised August 2016 At https://www.glowm.com/section_view/item/441; Hern, W.M. Late abortion: Clinical and ethical issues. *In Whose Choice Is It? Abortion, Medicine and the Law*, 7th edition (David F. Walbert and J. Douglas Butler, Eds.). Chicago: American Bar Association, 2021. https://www.drhern.com/wp-content/uploads/2023/05/Late-abortion-clinical-ethical-issues-8-1-2021.pdf

98 Erhardt, C.L., Nelson, F.G., and Pakter, J. Seasonal patterns of conception in New York City. *American Journal of Public Health* 61:2246, 1971; Teoh, Dawood, Ratnam, *op. cit*.

99 Peel, J., and Potts, M. *Textbook of Contraceptive Practice*. London: Cambridge University Press, 1969.

100 Mechanic, Volkart, *op cit*; Kasl, S.V., and Cobb, S. Health behavior, illness behavior, and sick role behavior. *Archives of Environmental Health* 12:246, 1966; Suchman, *op cit*; Newman, *op cit*, doctoral thesis; Newman, *op cit, Folklore of Pregnancy*; Lewis *op cit*; McKinlay, J.B. The sick role: Illness and pregnancy. *Social Science and Medicine* 6:561, 1972.

101 Jessner, Weigart, Foy, *op cit*; Mead, Newton, *op. cit.*; Pohlman, E.H. Motivations in wanting conceptions. In Pohlman, E.H. (ed). *The Psychology of Birth Planning*, pp 48–81. Cambridge: Schenkman Publishing, 1969.; Himes, N.E. *Medical History of Contraception*, pp. 59–104. New York: Gamut Press, 1963.

102 Billingham, R.E. Transplantation immunity and the maternal-fetal relation. *New England Journal of Medicine* 270:667, 1964.

103 Simmons, R.L., and Russell, P.S. The immunologic problem of pregnancy. *American Journal of Obstetrics and Gynecology* 85:583, 1963.; Douthwaite. R.M., and Urbach. G.I. In vitro antigenicity of trophoblast. *American Journal of Obstetrics and Gynecology* 109:1023, 1971.
104 Kaplan, S.L., and Grumbach, M.M. Serum chorionic "growth hormone-prolactin" and serum pituitary growth hormone in mother and fetus at term. *Journal of Clinical Endocrinology* 25:1370, 1965.
105 Page, E.W. Some evolutionary concepts of human reproduction. *Obstetrics and Gynecology* 30:318, 1967.
106 Cameron, T.W.M. *Parasites and Parasitism*, pp. 226–36. New York: John Wiley & Sons, 1956.
107 Perez-Tamayo, R. *Mechanisms of Disease*, pp. 329–30. Philadelphia: W.B. Saunders, 1961.
108 Ibid., p. 338.
109 Dubos, R. *Man Adapting*, pp. 254–79. New Haven, CT: Yale University Press, 1965.; Cassel J, *op cit,* Social science theory; Engel, G. A unified concept of health and disease. *Perspectives in Biology and Medicine* 3:459, 1960.
110 Page, *op. cit.*; Torpin, R. Placentation and mammalian phylogeny. *Obstetrics and Gynecology* 37:942, 1971.
111 Medawar, P.B. *The Future of Man*, pp. 27–34; 95–103. New York: Basic Books, 1960.
112 Hern, W.M. *Homo Ecophagus: A Deep Diagnosis to Save the Earth*. London: Routledge, 2022.
113 Himes, *op. cit.*; Potts, D.M. History of contraception. In Sciarra, J.J. (ed). *Gynecology and Obstetrics*, Vol. 6, chap 8. Philadelphia: Harper & Row, 1982.; Newman, L.F. *Birth Control: An Anthropological View*, No. 27. Reading, MA: Addison-Wesley Modular Publications, 1972; Hern, W.M. Knowledge and use of herbal contraceptives in a Peruvian Amazon village. *Human Organization* 35:9, 1976; Dumond, D.E. The limitation of human population: A natural history. *Science* 187:713, 1975. PMID: 1090000 DOI: 10.1126/science.1090000; Hart, D.V., Rajadhon, P.A., and Couglin, R.J. *Southeast Asian Birth Customs: Three Studies in Human Reproduction*. New Haven, CT: Human Relations Area File Press, 1965.
114 Maccormack, C.P. (ed). *Ethnography of Fertility and Birth*. New York: Academic Press, 1982; Spencer, R.F. Embryology and obstetrics in preindustrial societies. In Landy, D. (ed). *Culture, Disease, and Healing: Studies in Medical Anthropology*. New York: Macmillan, 1977.

Plates

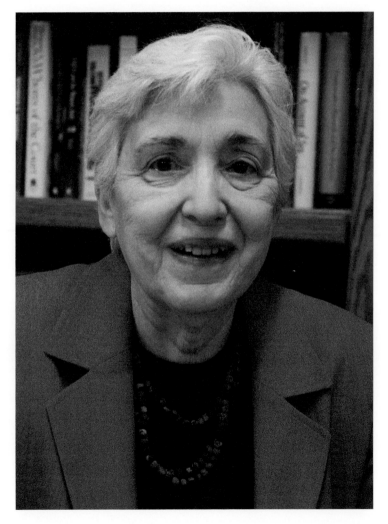

Figure P.1 Ellie Smeal, founder and president, Feminist Majority Foundation; president, National Organization for Women, 1977–82, 1985–87; organizer, 1986 Women's March on Washington. She has played an indispensable role as a leader in the women's movement. Photo © Warren Martin Hern.

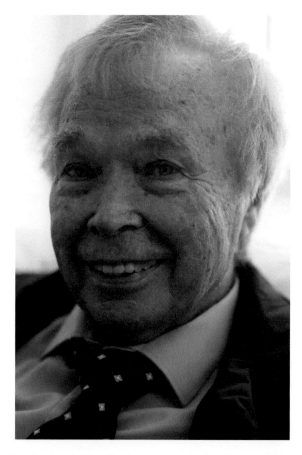

Figure P.2 Bill Baird. Early champion of birth control and reproductive rights, the only non-lawyer with three U.S. Supreme Court victories. Photo © Warren Martin Hern.

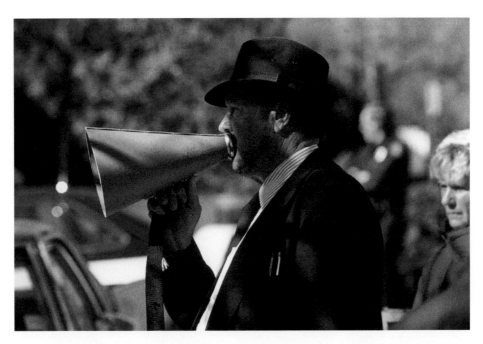

Figure P.3 Joe Scheidler with megaphone shouting obscenities at patients entering Boulder Abortion Clinic, October 1985.

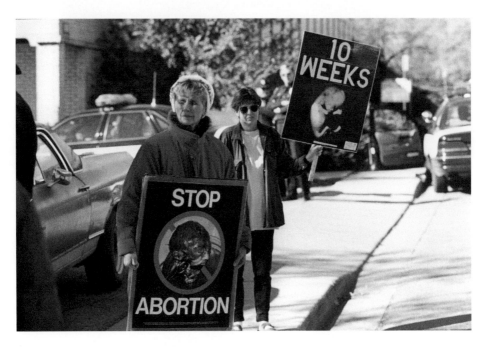

Figure P.4 Anti-abortion demonstrators with Joe Scheidler on sidewalk obstructing patients entering Boulder Abortion Clinic.

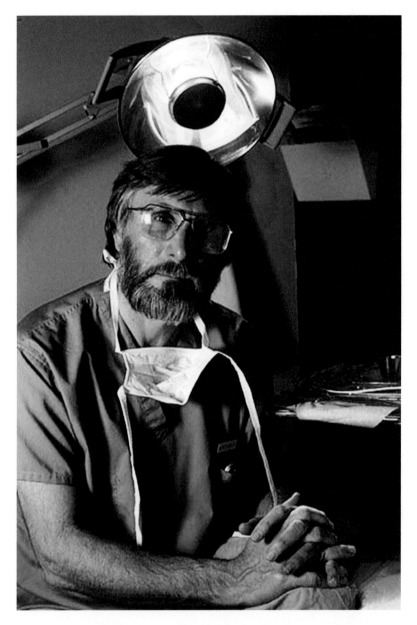

Figure P.5 Portrait of Dr. Warren Hern, director of the Boulder Abortion Clinic, by Eric Lars Bakke for the *New York Times* accompanying an article by Gina Kolata on late abortion, January 5, 1992, "In late abortion, decisions are painful and options are few."

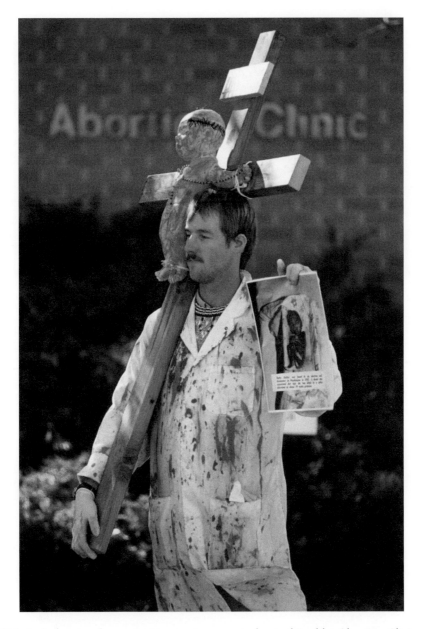

Figure P.6 Anti-abortion demonstrator carrying cross in front of Boulder Abortion Clinic.

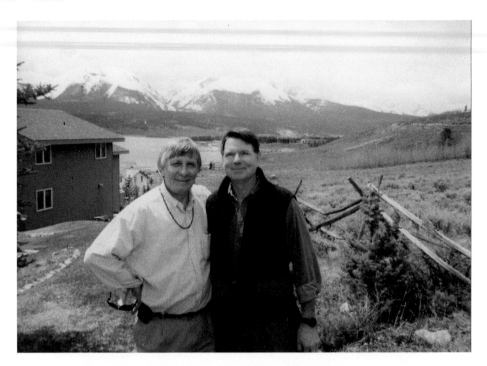

Figure P.7 Dr. Warren Hern together with Dr. George Tiller in Colorado.

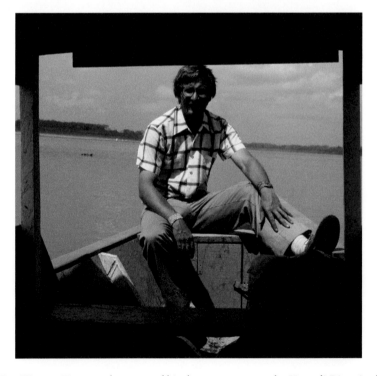

Figure P.8 Dr. Warren Hern on the prow of his dugout canoe on the Ucayali River in the Peruvian Amazon, 1983. Photo © Warren Martin Hern.

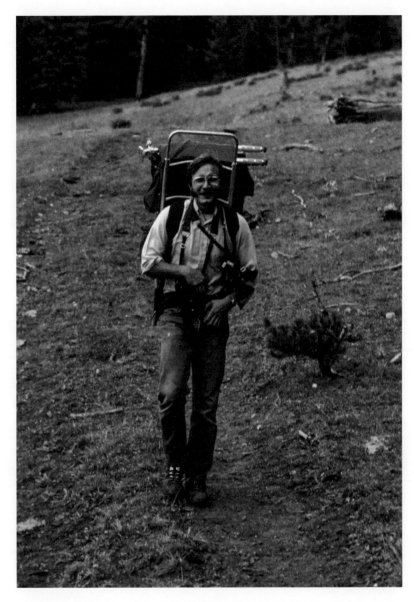

Figure P.9 Author/photographer Warren Martin Hern hiking to wilderness photography workshop in Wyoming, 1977. Photo © Boyd Norton.

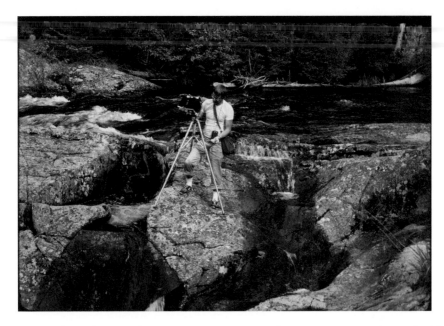

Figure P.10 Author / photographer Warren Martin Hern making a view camera photo of wilderness waterfall, Holy Cross Wilderness, 1985. Photo © Warren Martin Hern.

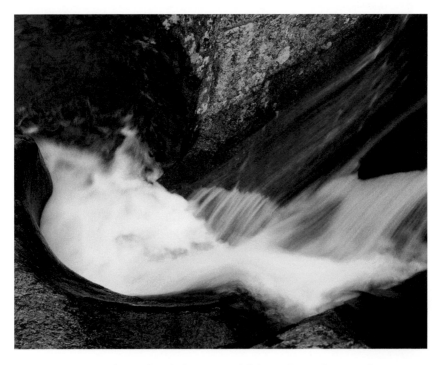

Figure P.11 View camera photo of pothole in waterfall by author / photographer Warren Martin Hern. Photo © Warren Martin Hern.

13 When is an egg not an egg?

THIS ... IS A PERSON.

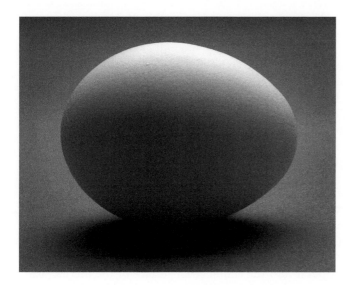

NO! IT'S A CHICKEN!!!
THIS...

1 Be it enacted by the people of the state of Colorado:
2 Article II of the constitution of the state of Colorado is amended BY THE ADDITION
3 OF A NEW SECTION to read:
4
5 **Section 31. Person defined**
6
7 AS USED IN ARTICLE II, SECTIONS 3, 6, AND 25 OF THE COLORADO
8 CONSTITUTION, THE WORDS "PERSON" AND "PERSONS" SHALL INCLUDE
9 ANY HUMAN BEING FROM THE MOMENT OF FERTILIZATION

IS A TURKEY.

DOI: 10.4324/9781003514961-14

On November 4, 2008, the people of Colorado were asked to approve or disapprove the above Ballot Initiative # 48 "Definition of a person."

The U.S. Constitution defines a person as existing from the moment of live birth. Initiative #48 was unconstitutional on its face. If adopted, it would have meant that live birth is not a significant legal event. This idea has many absurd and catastrophic consequences, but the principal purpose of its sponsors was to outlaw safe abortion. It failed.

An egg is a person. No, an egg is a chicken. A fertilized human egg is a person. An acorn is a tree. A seed is an apple. A set of plans is a house. A blastocyst is a "pre-born baby." An adult human being is a "pre-dead corpse." Up is down. Black is white. War is peace. Facts are not important. Belief is what matters. And people who know the truth will tell you what to believe. And they carry Guns. So you'd better Believe.

Anti-abortion fanatics have been saying for decades that a human embryo – or even a fertilized human ovum – is a person. The "Human Life Amendment" was introduced in Congress in 1975 by Senator Jesse Helms. It defined a fetus as a person. Colorado's anti-abortion fanatics wanted to define a fetus as a person existing "from the moment of fertilization." Their purpose, of course, was to outlaw all abortions.

The U.S. Constitution refers to "All persons born...," not "all persons conceived..." or "all fertilized eggs..." No live birth, no person. To be sure, this is an arbitrary judgment that is defined by our culture. In some cultures, a person does not exist until the first three or six months or first birthday has passed.

Among the Shipibo Indians of the Peruvian Amazon, with whom I have worked and studied for over 60 years, a baby is not given a name – and thereby personhood – until it is at least three months old. There is an important reason for this. In some Amazon villages, as many as 20–30 percent of the children die before they are a year old. A child's death hurts.

Stating that a person exists from the moment of live birth solves a practical problem. It is almost impossible to know when conception, however defined, occurs. Does conception mean the moment that the sperm penetrates the covering of the ovum or does it mean when the fertilized ovum (zygote) divides and forms a morula (clump of 16 cells)? Does conception occur when a blastula (hollow clump of cells) forms or does conception refer to implantation of the blastocyst into the endometrial surface of the uterine wall? What if the fertilized egg gets hung up in the Fallopian tube and forms an ectopic ("out of place") pregnancy that can easily kill the woman?

Does it matter that a woman may spontaneously abort ("miscarry") a pregnancy before she is even aware of it? Does it matter that this may happen in at least 75 percent of all conceptions? What about a spontaneous abortion (miscarriage) that happens when the woman is aware of the pregnancy? This happens in about 10–15 percent of all known pregnancies. Is the spontaneously aborted embryo a person? What if the woman smokes or drinks or takes drugs or rides the roller-coaster or hangs out with weird people like Republicans? Is she guilty of homicide if she has a miscarriage because some or all of these activities are known or thought by some to cause damage to the embryo or cause a miscarriage? Who will document this damaging behavior, and who decides what is damaging?

Does the census-taker count each known pregnancy as a person? What if there are twins or triplets? Who would know this, and how would they find out? Must each woman submit to a pregnancy test or a vaginal-probe ultrasound exam? How accurate are pregnancy tests? Which tests? There are various kinds with various levels of sensitivity. What if the positive pregnancy test is registering a hydatidiform mole (a kind of pregnancy that does not result in formation of an embryo), a choriocarcinoma (a kind of highly malignant cancer), or a chorioadenoma destruens (another kind of cancer)? Are these pregnancies counted as persons? They all resulted from fertilization of an ovum by at least one sperm.

How will the positive pregnancy test counts affect the census, and how will this affect political representation? Are districts in which women use less birth control likely to get more representatives because there are more fertilized eggs and embryos that count as persons? How will the people living in high birth control use (or low fertility) districts feel about having less representation than fetuses, embryos, and even hydatidiform moles? Senior citizens may not like this.

If women object to being forced to submit to regular pregnancy tests, we can just throw them in jail as they did during Romania's communist dictatorship under Nicolae Ceaușescu from 1965 to 1989. Women were required to produce children in order to have more workers and soldiers. After all, that's what women are *for*, right?

If a pregnant woman gets a passport, does she also get one for her six-week embryo? How will immigration authorities know if a legally registered woman is not sneaking an unregistered and undocumented embryo into the country? The border patrol will need a lot of pregnancy tests.

Anticipating the overturning of the *Roe v. Wade* by an increasingly conservative anti-abortion U.S. Supreme Court, and since the *Dobbs* decision overturning *Roe*, many states have passed into law "heartbeat" bills that prohibit abortion after an embryonic "heartbeat" (pulsation of a primordial cardiac tube) is observable with ultrasound. In mammals, primitive cardiac tissue develops very early. In humans, pulsations in cardiac tissue that will become the heart are visible when the woman is only about six weeks pregnant or earlier. She may not know that she is pregnant, and if she doesn't know it, the time when she could get an abortion legally in such a state would easily pass before she knew that. This effectively prohibits abortion even though the law would have clearly been unconstitutional under *Roe v. Wade*. Since the 2022 *Dobbs* decision overturning *Roe*, the "heartbeat" bills triggered by that decision prevent all women from getting abortions in states where that gun was loaded. It has the same effect on abortion as declaring the embryo a person with full legal status from the moment of conception.

The absurdity of this proposition that the fertilized egg is a person and the chaos that would ensue *should* make it unlikely that it will ever become the law of the land. The problem is, we are not dealing with rational people. The Alabama Supreme Court, in its theological *dictum, just made exactly that decision* on February 16, 2024.[1] It's the law of the land in Alabama.

Advocates of this insanity are Christian fanatics who have worked successfully for over 50 years to get us to this point. This idea is the syncretic product of blind religious fanaticism and blind lust for total power. This is a fatal combination for civilized society much less rational law. In the Age of Unreason, it is a mistake to dismiss it as impossible.

It's happening as we speak.

The Republican Party is now seeking a national ban on abortion, and the Republican Party now controls the U.S. Supreme Court. It is not unrealistic to imagine or even predict that the current Court, following the Alabama terminal stupidity, could rule that human life begins at conception and that the fertilized egg is a person. This would impose a view of human existence on our society which is appealing in its apparent simplicity: Human life begins at conception.

On examination, however, this question proves to be more complex. Does conception mean "fertilization" or "implantation?" Which conception? Could it have been the one (which one?) that occurred three million years ago near Olduvai Gorge in Africa?

The view of a theoretical instant in which each individual comes into being is in conflict with the view of life as a continuous stream reaching back into the origins of life itself billions of years ago. It is in conflict with the fact that each sperm and ovum is a human cell, that each diploid cell in the rest of the body has 46 chromosomes, and that, while the cells in each of our bodies are constantly dying and being replaced, our structures remain.

The idea that each fertilized ovum is a person amounts to the same thing as saying that each set of house plans is a house. Calling an ovum a person does not make it so. Calling a fetus an unborn person (and perhaps baptizing it) is as illogical as burying an undead body.

It is worthwhile to examine some of the health and social consequences that making abortion illegal by such an action would have.

In 1920 the maternal mortality rate in the United States was 680 per 100,000 live births. By 1960 maternal mortality had fallen to around 38 per 100,000 live births. This reduction was brought about by a number of things, including better prenatal care, better obstetrical care; the introduction of blood transfusion, antibiotics, and other drugs; longer birth intervals; postponed first births; fewer total pregnancies per woman; and better nutrition.

Nearly half of all maternal deaths in both 1920 and 1960, however, were due to induced abortion in some areas of the country. In New York City, as late as 1965, 55 percent and 65 percent of maternal mortality among Black and Puerto Rican women, respectively, was because of septic abortion.

Since 1970, however, abortion has become the safest surgical procedure – and the most heavily monitored – in the United States. The number of abortion deaths dropped from an average of 250 in the mid-1960s to less than 10 per year currently, while more than twice as many abortions are now being performed.

This improved safety is almost entirely because of the legalization of abortion, first in Colorado and in other states, then nationally, which permitted the introduction of improved techniques and the accumulation of skills and experience by physicians performing abortions. The risk of death from early abortion is now less than one per million procedures.

Overall, the risk of death due to abortion is currently less than two per 100,000 procedures, whereas the risk of death due to term birth is approximately 14 per 100,000 live births under the best circumstances. The risk of major complications in abortion is 1/200th the risk a woman experiences in term birth. Caesarean section is one major complication that occurs in one-third of all term deliveries, and, if this is necessary, her risks are magnified many times.

It is important to understand that these risks are experienced by women who are pregnant whether they wish to be pregnant or not and whether they are rich or poor.

From a medical point of view, abortion should be the indicated treatment of choice for pregnancy unless a woman has a desire to carry the pregnancy to term and reproduce. Safe abortion is a fundamental component of women's health care.

The effort to criminalize abortion through the mechanism of according the fetus the status of personhood, however, would have serious public health consequences not envisioned by its proponents. If interpreted literally by a zealous prosecutor, such a law would have the following consequences:

- It would proscribe all abortions, even if the woman's life is in immediate danger.
- It would criminalize the use of intrauterine devices.
- It would prevent the use of certain oral contraceptives and drugs, such as diethylstilbesterol, used in preventing pregnancy following unprotected intercourse, as in rape.
- It would prevent treatment, emergency or otherwise, of hydatidiform mole, chroioadenoma destruens, choriocarcinoma, and unruptured ectopic pregnancy. The first three, including the third, which is a cancer, arise from conception to become an undifferentiated mass of cells or water sacs. These products of conception would be classified as "persons" under the law.
- It would prevent the treatment of women for conditions unrelated to pregnancy without absolute proof of non-pregnancy, which is impossible under most circumstances.
- It would result in the prosecution of women experiencing spontaneous abortion (miscarriage) for negligent homicide if evidence could be found that the woman engaged in any physical activity or substance use that might lead to spontaneous abortion.
- It would prohibit the use of amniocentesis for the diagnosis of genetic defects.
- It would probably interrupt current research on in-vitro fertilization (test tube babies) for the benefit of infertile couples. This has already happened in Alabama and other states.
- It would prohibit evaluation of infertility in women since non-pregnancy would have to be proved before tests could be performed.
- It would prevent the use of x-rays on women who had suffered trauma and who were currently pregnant or might be.
- It would disrupt a confidential doctor-patient relationship in all cases of women in the reproductive age range.
- It would increase the number of unplanned pregnancies due to the criminalization of effective contraceptives.
- It would result in a catastrophic increase in the number of deaths and life-threatening complications due to improperly performed abortions.

As the result of criminalization, the number of abortions performed would probably drop to no less than half of the one million currently being performed nationally. An unknown number would be added to this fraction as the result of an increase in the number of unplanned pregnancies because of the criminalization of contraceptive methods. Women would seek and obtain the medications for "medication" abortion as they have already begun to do since the passage of oppressive state law throughout the United States following the *Dobbs* decision.

Women who experience "high risk" pregnancies – teenagers, older women, women who have recently delivered or who have had many pregnancies – would be forced to carry pregnancies to term whereas they are likely to choose abortion under the current circumstances for their own reasons. The result will be an increase in maternal mortality and complications due to pregnancy and increases in infant mortality, percentage of low birth weight infants, percentage of premature births as well as an increase in the proportion of developmental and functional abnormalities, an increase in the number of birth defects, and a higher neonatal mortality rate. The financial costs of these consequences will be met, in many cases, by the taxpayers.

One-third of all abortions currently are performed on teenagers. Most of these young women are unprepared for the emotional, intellectual, social, and economic responsibilities of parenthood in a complex society and are unprepared to form stable families with their partners. The argument that they should be forced to continue unplanned pregnancies in order to increase the supply of adoptable babies is both cruel and delusional. More than 90 percent of teenagers who continue unplanned pregnancies to term do not give up their babies for adoption.

What is the possible benefit to anyone of forcing a 12-year[old girl who has been sexually abused by a family member to carry a pregnancy to term? Her life is in danger from the pregnancy, she cannot care for herself much less a child, and there is no justification for what would be cruel and unusual punishment for being a victim of rape or incest.

The technology of abortion is so widely available among physicians and non-physicians alike that enforcement would be hopeless, so what is the point of this exercise? Are we willing to have a police state and keep all women under constant surveillance to ensure the law is observed? Or will we simply put doctors in jail for performing abortions, leaving transgressions to the untutored? In most societies throughout human existence, various fertility control measures have been used, including abortion. Laws have never prevented abortion, and they never will.

Anthropologist George Devereux studied 450 traditional tribal societies and found many ways of causing an abortion. Women have been having abortions for thousands of years.

The effort to outlaw abortion appears to be a response of a conservative minority to the relentless social change of the last 75 years. This social change has been fueled to a considerable degree by the introduction of highly effective, safe fertility control measures that are available on a wide scale for the first time in human history. From the point of view of cultural change, it is probably equivalent in importance to the domestication of fire at the human hearth.

An important consequence of this new availability of fertility control is the enhancement of the status and independence of women, which has been increasing over the past 100 years. The new role of women, however, collides head on with the view that the principal function of women is to bear children. This view is no longer shared by a great many people.

The view that women should confine their activities to reproduction, however, is held by a majority of Christians and Republicans. Their logic is that society must be protected against individuals (doctors who perform abortions; women who want them) to protect the embryos. Could it be that there is a scarce supply of human embryos? Could it be that we need a pronatalist public policy because of the shortage of people? Hardly. Could it be that some people think we have a shortage of white babies to counteract the increasing ethnic and racial diversity in the American population? Hmmm.

Anthropologist Virginia Abernethy, an expert on the cultural aspects of reproduction and population, concludes that certain populations exhibit "competitive reproduction."[2] The American population is becoming browner by the minute. People who regard themselves as white will become the minority in America soon. The white Nationalist "pro-life" movement is essentially a white supremacist movement. Could this be why white Christians are so opposed to abortion?

One important problem is that women are uppity: They vote, and they are now competing with men for jobs, money, and power. Fetuses, on the other hand, are apolitical, don't argue, present no economic threat, and may be defended along with the flag, apple pie, and motherhood before the voters at election time. They can be defended against sin and immorality, thereby throwing political opponents into disarray.

This conflict brings us clearly to an understanding of the struggle before us. The issue is not the protection of human life. We are already doing that by providing safe abortions for women. The real issue posed by anti-abortion legislation is the definition of power: who has it and who doesn't.

The issue is whether power in America will be wielded absolutely by those who cannot get pregnant or whether it will be shared with those who can. The issue is whether women are considered first-class citizens in the United States entitled to modern health care for a life-threatening condition that only women can have, namely pregnancy.

A more basic question before our society is not when life begins, but who is best prepared to decide when to transmit life to a new generation – the individual or the state? The right of the individual woman to make this choice should be supported. In this matter, she is more competent than any government. *

- An earlier version of this essay was published originally in the *Colorado Statesman*. It was then published as a full-page ad containing the photo of the egg in various Colorado newspapers during the campaign against Ballot Issue #48 in 2008. Colorado voters rejected the ballot issue, "Definition of a person," by a 3–1 margin (73.21 percent to 26.79 percent).

The idea that an egg is a person is so ridiculous, the only thing you can do is make fun of it. But tens of millions of people in this country believe things that are completely ridiculous, and they want the rest of us to believe them. They are ready to use lethal force to make this happen.

I have been looking down the barrel of that gun for a long time. So have my medical colleagues and everyone who helps me to do this work

Notes

1 Chandler, K. Warnings of the impact of fertility treatments in Alabama rush in after frozen embryo ruling. Associated Press, February 21, 2024. https://apnews.com/article/alabama -supreme-court-from-embryos-161390f0758b04a7638e2ddea20df7ca; Supreme Court of Alabama, October Term 2023-2024. SC-2022-0515; SC-2022-0579. https://publicportal -api.alappeals.gov/courts/68f021c4-6a44-4735-9a76-5360b2e8af13/cms/case/343D203A -B13D-463A-8176-C46E3AE4F695/docketentrydocuments/E3D95592-3CBE-4384-AFA6 -063D4595AA1D
2 Abernethy, V. *Born Abroad*. London: Arktos, 2023, p. 66.

14   Abortion and the Supreme Court

Roe v. Wade, 410 U.S. 113 (1973) and *Doe v. Bolton*, 410 U.S. 179 (1973)

Any discussion of the impact of legal decisions on the availability of abortion services in the United States must begin with an understanding of *Roe* and *Doe*, two companion cases, simultaneously argued and decoded by the U.S. Supreme Court on January 22, 1973. It has proven to be one of the most important and controversial decisions in the High Court's history. The decision has affected the lives of literally hundreds of millions of people.

Approximately 60 million abortions have been performed in the United States since those decisions were announced. Each abortion represents a woman whose life, as well as the lives of those around her, were changed in important and dramatic ways. These decisions changed American society in many ways, starting with the newly established freedom of women to end a pregnancy safely, in a clean, professional medical setting, instead of some unsterile back room or garage, by a non-medically trained operator. Aside from the medical safety that the legalization of abortion has provided, the new circumstances are healthier as well as less terrifying for women who seek the procedure. It allows health professionals who want to assist women to obtain abortion services in a humane, supportive, and dignified setting that helps women manage a most difficult decision and time in their lives.

On December 13, 1971, Sarah Weddington, a 26-year-old attorney from Texas with little trial experience, argued her first case before the U.S. Supreme Court in the case of *Roe*. Jane Roe was the pseudonym for the Texas plaintiff, a young pregnant woman who wished to terminate her pregnancy, and Henry Wade was the Dallas County district attorney. Ms. Weddington argued that the Texas law prohibiting abortion was unconstitutional because it deprived her client of the right to decide whether or not to have children and that her right to make this decision was protected under the Ninth Amendment. A Texas physician, James Hallford, joined Roe as a plaintiff, arguing that the law interfered with his right as a physician to determine what was in the best health interest of his patients. The law allowing him to protect the life of his patient by performing an abortion was vague, and he could not determine whether he would be prosecuted for performing an abortion.

Citing *Griswold* and the right of privacy established under that decision, the U.S. District Court decided for the plaintiffs, but it did not issue an injunction to prevent prosecution under the law. Ms. Weddington and her colleagues appealed directly to the U.S. Supreme Court in 1970.

DOI: 10.4324/9781003514961-15

At the same time, Margie Pitts Hames, an Atlanta attorney, filed *Doe* in the U.S. Northern District Court of Georgia on the behalf of her client, Mary Doe, pseudonym for Sandra Cano, who had a medical disorder requiring her to stop taking oral contraceptives and that could prove fatal if she became pregnant. Cano wanted to be able to preserve the right to obtain an abortion on medical grounds, if a future pregnancy occurred. The District Court refused her request for an injunction against prosecution under the Georgia law, and she appealed to the U.S. Supreme Court.

The Court decided to accept simultaneous review of the two similar cases, and they were argued on the same day, December 13, 1971.

Only seven of the justices were sitting. Ms. Weddington argued that a woman's right to privacy in reproductive matters was protected under the *Griswold* decision and that her rights to make decisions about whether to bear a pregnancy and have a child were protected under the Ninth and Fourteenth Amendments. She also argued that the Texas statute interfered with a physician's right to give the patient optimum medical care and was unconstitutionally vague.

Ms. Weddington further argued that the state of Texas must show a compelling interest in regulating a woman's reproductive behavior, but that the state had no compelling interest in regulating abortion. She stated that the fetus had no rights under either Texas state law or the Fourteenth Amendment since it was not a person until born alive. She cited evidence that properly performed abortions were safer than childbirth. Soon after the first oral argument, two justices, William Rehnquist and Lewis Powell, joined the Court, and Justice Harry Blackmun pressed to have the case reargued with the full Court. The case was reargued on October 11, 1972. In addition to her previous arguments, Weddington asserted that women have a fundamental right to abortion because of the impact of an unwanted pregnancy had on their lives.

On January 22, 1973, the Court handed down its *Roe* and *Doe* decisions, two of the most significant cases in American jurisprudence. By a 7–2 majority, the Court declared the Texas statute to be unconstitutional.

Justice Harry Blackmun wrote the majority opinions in *Roe* and *Doe*. It should be noted that prior to being appointed to the federal bench, Justice Blackmun had served as General Counsel to the Mayo Clinic in Rochester, Minnesota. The opinions in *Roe* and *Doe* can be read as protecting physicians' rights as well as those of women. He wrote a lengthy tour de force of legal scholarship that explored the ancient origins of abortion and current official policies of organizations, such as the American Bar Association and the American Public Health Association. His arguments and findings are briefly summarized here.

First, Justice Blackmun stated that concerns for the safety of abortion services and an interest in protecting lives were the only two reasons for applying state power to the abortion decision.

Second, Blackmun stated that the right to privacy extended beyond marriage to include reproduction, contraception, and decisions concerning childrearing. He stated that this right was protected under the First, Fourth, Fifth, Ninth, and Fourteenth Amendments. He asserted that the Texas law prohibiting abortion was unconstitutional under several of these amendments. He stated that states have the right to regulate abortion to protect the health of women and "potential life" of the fetus.

According to Justice Blackmun's information, he viewed abortion after the first trimester to have the same or more risks to the woman's life as childbirth, and therefore the state had a "compelling state interest" in regulating abortion in the second trimester to protect maternal health. After the second trimester, the viability of the fetus meant that the state had a compelling state interest in protecting the life of the fetus and could prohibit abortion except to save the woman's life.

Therefore, in Justice Blackmun's opinion, abortion in the first trimester of pregnancy was a constitutionally protected right for the woman in consultation with her physician; in the second trimester, the state may make reasonable regulations to protect maternal health; and in the third trimester, the state may prohibit abortion, unless it were necessary to save the woman's life. It is under this framework of the trimester system and constraints enunciated by Justice Blackmun that *Roe* and *Doe* have functioned as the principal guiding US Supreme Court decision since 1973.

In the *Doe* decision, the Supreme Court invalidated the Georgia law requiring approval for an abortion to be made by three physicians and a special committee of three other persons, following strict conditions for approval and prohibiting abortion for any woman who was not a resident of Georgia. The companion case of *Roe* invalidated the remaining portions of the Georgia abortion law.

Griswold v. Connecticut, 381 U.S. 479 (1965)

The *Roe* and *Doe*_decisions had important precedents. One of them was *Griswold*. Estelle Griswold was the director of the Planned Parenthood affiliate in New Haven, Connecticut. Dr. C. Lee Buxton from Yale Medical School was its medical director. They believed that they should be able to supply married women and married couples with contraceptives upon request, but Connecticut law since 1879 prohibited the distribution of contraceptives. They arranged to be arrested giving out contraceptives and then they challenged the law in court. The Court ruled that a married couple were entitled to privacy in this matter under the First, Third, Fourth, and Ninth Amendments of the Bill of Rights. The 7–2 majority opinion was written by Associate Justice William O. Douglas. Justice Arthur Goldberg in a concurring opinion found that this right of privacy was protected under the Ninth and Fourteenth Amendments. Justice Harlan found that privacy was protected under the Due Process Clause of the Fourteenth Amendment. Justice White concurred with Justice Harlan that privacy was protected under the Fourteenth Amendment. Two other Justices, Black and Stewart, dissented even though they found the law "uncommonly silly."

Griswold has become the seminal case for many later Supreme Court decisions. It came at a time when abortion laws were being changed and challenged throughout the United States. Colorado passed the first abortion reform law in the country in 1967, and this precedent was followed by changes in many other state laws, with New York completely repealing its abortion law in 1970.

Eisenstadt v. Baird, 405 U.S. 438 (1972)

Eisenstadt permitted the distribution of contraceptives to married couples, but a Massachusetts law forbade giving contraceptives to unmarried women. A nineteenth-century Massachusetts law under the heading of "Crimes against Chastity," made it a felony to distribute contraceptives. Bill Baird, who watched a woman die from an illegal abortion in 1963, set out to prevent such deaths by helping people secure access to birth control. He was giving a lecture at Boston University in 1967 when he invited audience members to come up to the stage and help themselves to contraceptive materials. He was arrested by the sheriff of Suffolk County, Thomas Eisenstadt, for the act of giving condoms and contraceptive foam to an unmarried 19-year-old woman. Baird was convicted and served three months in prison before his conviction was partially overturned. Baird carried his appeal to the Supreme Court, which ruled in his favor in 1972 citing the *Griswold* decision, holding that Baird's conviction violated the Due Process Clause of the U.S. Constitution. Justice Brennan's majority opinion was joined by Justices Douglas, Stewart, and Marshall, with Justice Douglas writing a concurring opinion, stating that Baird's arrest violated his right of free speech under the First Amendment.

Eisenstadt has been widely cited in other court decisions bearing on personal privacy.

United States v. Vuitch, 402 U.S. 62 (1971)

Dr. Milan Vuitch, a Yugoslavia-born physician specializing in outpatient abortion services in Washington, D.C., and Silver Spring, Maryland, was arrested on the grounds that he was violating the District of Columbia statute prohibiting abortion except to protect the woman's health. Judge Gerhard Gesell of the U.S. District Court for the District of Columbia, ruled in Dr. Vuitch's favor in 1969, saying that the D.C. statute was unconstitutionally vague and could not be enforced. Writing for the majority with Justices Burger, Blackmun, Harlan, and White, Justice Hugo Black reversed Judge Gesell's ruling. In the process, he changed the standard of enforcement by stating that the burden of proof was not on the physician to show that the abortion was medically necessary but on the prosecution to demonstrate why the abortion was *not* medically necessary and that the defendant's actions broke the law. Supporters of abortion rights saw this as a positive step forward because the decision included a "health" provision.

Planned Parenthood of Central Missouri v. Danforth, 428 U.S. 52 (1976)

The plaintiff, Planned Parenthood of Central Missouri, challenged the Missouri law restricting abortion, saying that it was unconstitutional and overly broad. The U.S. Supreme Court upheld the right of women to have an abortion and declared that the statute's requirements for parental and/or spousal consent were unconstitutional. The Supreme Court upheld the statute's requirement for recordkeeping and the provision that an abortion must be performed by a physician.

Bellotti v. Baird, 428 U.S. 132 (1976)

Bill Baird, founder of the Parents' Aid Society in New York and Massachusetts, filed suit on behalf of a minor seeking to have an abortion without her parents' consent. In this case, the Court upheld the Massachusetts law that required the consent of a parent, but it refused to lift the injunction against prosecution under the law. Bill Baird was known to walk the streets of Boston, dressed in a self-made condom suit, passing out literature and free contraceptives.

Maher v. Roe, 432 U.S. 464 (1977)

The Connecticut Welfare Department issued a ruling that it would use Medicaid funds only for first trimester abortions that were "medically necessary." Susan Roe, who was indigent, filed suit against Edward Maher, the Connecticut commissioner of social services.

In a 6–3 decision, the U.S. Supreme Court decided that the rule against the use of Medicaid funds did not violate the Equal Protection Clause of the Fourteenth Amendment and did not interfere with a woman's right to have an abortion.

Poelker v. Doe, 432 U.S. 519 (1997)

The City of Saint Louis chose to pay for public hospital services for childbirth but not to pay for "nontherapeutic" abortions. Citing *Maher*, the U.S. Supreme Court upheld the city's right to make this policy choice because it did not violate a woman's constitutional right to have an abortion. In addition and challenged was the city's assignment of all obstetrical and gynecological services to a single city public hospital that forbid the performance of abortion.

Bellotti v. Baird, 443 U.S. 622 (1979)

In an 8 to 1 majority ruling written by Justice Harry Blackmun, the U.S. Supreme Court ruled that teenagers do not have to secure parental consent to obtain an abortion.

Colautti v. Franklin, 439 U.S. 379 (1979)

John Franklin, M.D., was the medical director of the Planned Parenthood Association of Southeastern Pennsylvania. Colautti was the secretary of welfare of Pennsylvania. Franklin and his associates filed suit to invalidate the Pennsylvania Abortion Control Act, which held a physician to be criminally liable if "he or she performed an abortion and failed to use a technique prescribed by law when the fetus is viable or when there is sufficient reason to believe that the fetus may be viable." Writing for the 6–3 majority, Justice Blackmun held that this section of the Pennsylvania's 1974 Abortion Control Act was unconstitutionally vague and thus void.

Harris v. McRae, 448 U.S. 297 (1980)

In 1976 Congress passed the Hyde Amendment that prohibited the use of federal funds to pay for abortion services under Medicaid. That same year, Cora McRae, who was in her first trimester of pregnancy, filed a class action suit in the U.S. District Court for the Eastern District of New York requesting the court to enjoin the amendment's restrictions on the use of funds to pay for her abortion in a public hospital. The district court certified the class action and permitted U. S senators James Buckley and Jesse Helms and U.S. congressman Henry Hyde, sponsors of the amendment, to be defendants. The district court granted the injunction and found that the Hyde Amendment violated the Fifth Amendment's protection of Due Process and the Establishment Clause of the First Amendment prohibiting the establishment of religion.

In 1980 the Supreme Court found that the amendment did not interfere with a woman's right to have an abortion and that the state had no obligation to pay for her abortion. The court found that the fact that the restrictions happened to be consistent with Roman Catholic doctrine was purely coincidental.

Akron v. Akron Center for Reproductive Health, 462 U.S. 416 (1983)

The City of Akron, Ohio, passed a statute that imposed certain restrictions on abortion services that impacted the Akron Center for

Reproductive Health. These restrictions included the following:

- A first trimester abortion must be performed in a hospital.
- A physician may not perform an abortion on an unmarried minor under the age of 15 without obtaining the consent of one of her parents or a judicial bypass.
- The statute required that before performing an abortion, the physician must read to the patient from a prepared script containing a detailed description of the embryo or fetus, including the statement that the embryo is a "human life from the moment of conception," when it would be viable, the risks of abortion, and the availability of adoption resources.
- It required a 24-hour waiting period after the patient signs the consent form.
- It required that the fetal remains be disposed of in a "humane and sanitary manner."

Writing for the 6–3 majority, Justice Lewis Powell dismissed all of these provisions as unconstitutional for various reasons, including vagueness. This decision was later over-ruled in *Casey*.

Thornburgh v. American College of Obstetricians and Gynecologists, 476 U.S. 747 (1986)

The Pennsylvania law contested by the American College of Obstetricians and Gynecologists was similar to the Akron law, but the Reagan administration asked the Court to use *Thornburgh* to overturn *Roe*.

Justice Harry Blackmun, writing the opinion for a 6–3 majority, rejected the Reagan administration's request and reaffirmed *Roe*. Justice Sandra Day O'Connor dissented and disputed "not only the wisdom but also the legitimacy of the Court's attempt to discredit and pre-empt abortion regulation" by the states.

In his opinion, Justice Blackmun supported women's rights in the abortion decision over the rights of physicians, as he had in *Roe*. "Few decisions are more personal and intimate, more properly private, or more basic to individual dignity and autonomy, than a woman's decision – with the guidance of her physician and within the limits specified in *Roe* – whether to end her pregnancy. A woman's right to make that choice freely is fundamental."

Webster v. Reproductive Health Services, 492 U.S. 490 (1989)

William Webster was the Attorney General of Missouri. The Missouri law restricting abortion stated in its preamble that "the life of each human being begins at conception" and that "unborn children have protectable interests in life, health, and well-being." Attorney General Webster procured the services of former Solicitor General of the United States and then Harvard Law School professor Charles Fried to act as his co-counsel during Supreme Court arguments in this case. The law required:

- "Unborn children [are protected] with rights equal to those enjoyed by other persons."
- Before performing an abortion, the physician must determine the exact age of the fetus; if it were 20 or more weeks gestational age, the doctors had to determine whether it was viable, and had to test it for fetal lung maturity (difficult to determine in utero at that time and associated with significant risks).

- Government employed physicians may not abort a fetus they believe to be viable.
- State employees or facilities may not be used to perform or assist with abortions, except when the woman's life was in danger.
- Public funds, facilities, or employees may not "encourage or counsel" a woman to have an abortion, except when her life is in danger.
- Abortions performed after 16 weeks must be performed in a hospital.

The case was first heard in the U.S. District Court for the Western District of Missouri in Kansas City, Missouri. Frank Susman argued the case for the defendants before Judge Scott O. Wright, who wrote the opinion. I would note that Susman has over the years been counsel in nine abortion related maters before the U.S. Supreme Court and argued the majority of those cases, more than any other single attorney. (As a side note, Susman is the only lawyer to have argued two totally unrelated cases before the U.S. Supreme Court on the same day.)

During the trial of this case, I was an expert witness for the defendant, Reproductive Health Services, testifying that I had performed thousands of second trimester abortions on an outpatient basis in my private office with an extremely low complication rate. I testified that it was unnecessary to perform a second trimester abortion in a hospital using my surgical protocols and ordinary safety precautions.

The district court ruled that most of the Missouri law was unconstitutional on various grounds. The statements in the law that the fetus is an "unborn child" were thrown out on grounds of the Establishment Clause. The requirement that second trimester abortions be performed in a hospital was ruled to be unconstitutional. These elements of the law were not appealed in this case, which ultimately went to the Supreme Court.

The U.S. Supreme Court upheld most of the remaining Missouri law, affirming that states can regulate abortion care, and this decision became the basis for many new state laws regulating abortion. The arguments in the original district court hearing are fascinating and convoluted; and the Supreme Court justices had many opinions among them about various elements of the law. Their discussions, concurrences, and dissents are highly instructive.

In *Webster*, there were 78 *amicus curiae* briefs filed by non-parties, but purportedly interested parties, favoring one side or the other, more than in any other case in the history of the Supreme Court, up to that time.

The analysis prepared for *The Embryo Project Encyclopedia* is indispensable for any lay person who wishes to understand this Supreme Court decision.

Planned Parenthood v. Casey, 505 U.S. 833 (1992)

This is a critical decision in the history of U.S. Supreme Court decisions because it made fundamental changes in the interpretation and application of the *Roe* and *Doe* decisions.

Five odious provisions in the Pennsylvania Abortion Control Act of 1982 included:

- Requirements of a waiting period of 24 hours.
- Requirement that the doctor inform the woman about the dangers to her health by having an abortion and that the doctor give specific information about the development of the fetus.
- Requirement that the woman notify her husband in writing about her intention to have an abortion.

- Requirement of parental consent for minors seeking an abortion.
- Requirement of reporting certain data and keeping certain records.

The Supreme Court heard this case under strikingly different circumstances than with previous abortion cases. Two justices regarded as liberal and likely to support *Roe*, William Brennan and Thurgood Marshall, had been replaced by Justice David Souter and Justice Clarence Thomas, who were both regarded as conservative, since they were appointed by Republican president George H.W. Bush, and they were likely to be willing to overturn *Roe*. All but one of the justices had been appointed by Republican presidents opposed to *Roe*, Presidents Reagan and Bush, and the remaining Democratic appointee, Justice Byron White, had dissented from the *Roe* majority that legalized abortion. It was widely anticipated that this would be the case that would overturn *Roe*.

Kathryn Kolbert from the ACLU was the lead counsel for the plaintiff, Planned Parenthood of Pennsylvania. After the case reached the Supreme Court following split decisions by the district court and the Court of Appeals, Solicitor General,Ken Starr, argued on behalf of the defendants that the Court should overturn *Roe*.

To the amazement of many and the consternation of those opposed to *Roe*, Justices Souter and Kennedy joined a plurality opinion with Justice Sandra Day O'Connor, along with Justices Blackmun and Stevens, in upholding the "essential holdings" of *Roe* and *Doe* that a woman's right to choose to have an abortion was protected under the Due Process Clause of the Fourteenth Amendment as long as the abortion was to occur before the point of viability. In doing so, the justices substituted a viability criterium as the demarcation for protection of the abortion right and abandoned the trimester system devised by Justice Blackmun in *Roe*.

In addition, the Court, pressed by Justice Sandra Day O'Connor, substituted the "undue burden" standard for laws restricting abortion for the prior "compelling state interest" standard. With Justices Rehnquist and White, Justice O'Connor had advocated this change before in the *Akron* decision. This meant that instead of the state having to prove a "compelling state interest" in restricting access to abortion, the woman now had to prove that an enacted law gave her an "undue burden" in seeking an abortion. The "undue burden" standard also replaced the "strict scrutiny" standard of review that had been required under *Roe* to determine whether a law interfered with a woman's access to abortion services. The plurality also affirmed the right to privacy in the abortion decision as enunciated in *Eisenstadt*.

The abandonment of the trimester system specified under *Roe* allowed states to create laws restricting access to abortion during the first trimester of pregnancy, whereas a woman's right to have an abortion in the first trimester was totally protected under *Roe*. Under the "undue burden" standard, laws restricting abortion would only be unconstitutional if they were perceived as having the purpose of placing an unreasonable or "substantial obstacle" in the way of the woman seeking an abortion. Neither "undue burden" or "substantial obstacle" were defined, leaving the definition up to local, partisan interpretation.

Under these criteria, the only part of the Pennsylvania law that was deemed an "undue burden" was the provision requiring that the woman obtain the consent of her husband to get an abortion, previously held unconstitutional in *Planned Parenthood of Central Missouri*.

At the last minute, Justice Anthony Kennedy changed his mind about supporting all provisions of the Pennsylvania law and voted to uphold the "substantial holdings" of *Roe*. The "essential holdings" of Roe were considered to be:

1. A woman has the right to choose to have an abortion prior to viability, without undue interference from the State;
2. The State can restrict the abortion procedure after the point of viability, provided the law contains exceptions for pregnancies that endanger the woman's life or health;
3 The State has legitimate interests in protecting the health of the woman and the life of the fetus.

Four Justices, Rehnquist, Scalia, White, and Thomas, maintained that *Roe* should be struck down.

Stenberg v. Carhart, 530 U.S. 914 (2000)

In 1997, Nebraska's legislature passed a "Partial Birth Abortion" law (Nebraska Revised Statute 28-328) that prohibited any Nebraska physician from performing a "partial birth abortion." The statute presented an awkward problem in that there is no such thing as a "partial birth abortion" described in the medical literature. It is a political propaganda term coined by Douglas Johnson of the Right to Life Committee.

A Nebraska physician, Dr. Lee Carhart, used a procedure described in 1992 by a medical colleague for performing a late abortion (after 20 weeks gestation) in which the fetus is partially delivered feet first before its spinal cord is severed and cranial contents removed to permit easier and less traumatic delivery of the otherwise intact fetus. Carhart viewed this procedure as safer for women in several respects, including a diminished risk of fetal parts or other tissue remaining in the uterus at the end of the procedure. The term, "partial birth abortion," was applied by opponents of abortion as a pejorative reference to this procedure, merely for political purposes. It was not then or since considered a standard medical practice in late abortion. Carhart is a general surgeon who had been performing late abortions in Nebraska and Kansas for some time.

Under the Nebraska statute, there were no exceptions for the woman's health. It was not clear from the language of the statute whether the prohibition applied to other forms and protocols for second trimester abortion at any stage. The law had not been certified by the Nebraska Supreme Court.

Carhart sued Don Stenberg, the Attorney General of Nebraska, and both the federal district court and the Eighth Circuit Court of Appeals ruled that the law was unconstitutional. Both courts declared that the law placed an undue burden on a woman seeking an abortion.

Since there were several cases challenging this kind of medical procedure in lower courts, the U.S. Supreme Court decided to hear the case. In a 5–4 decision written by Justice Breyer and joined by Justices Ginsburg, Stevens, O'Connor, and Souter, the Court declared that the Nebraska law was unconstitutional since it had no medical exceptions. Justice Breyer also stated in his opinion that the law did not adequately distinguish between different types of abortion procedures and that it did not comply with precedents set in *Roe* and *Casey*.

Justices William Rehnquist, Clarence Thomas, Anthony Kennedy, and Antonin Scalia dissented in separate statements.

Hill vs. Colorado, 530 U.S. 703 (2002)

In 1986 anti-abortion demonstrations against two abortion facilities in Boulder, Colorado, were becoming increasingly disruptive. One of the clinics was Boulder Valley Women's Health Center, the first private, non-profit outpatient abortion clinic in Colorado, of which I was the founding medical director in 1973. The other facility was my private medical practice, Boulder Abortion Clinic, which I founded in 1975 after leaving Boulder Valley Clinic at the end of 1974.

Cynthia Pearson, the executive director of the Colorado chapter of the National Abortion Rights Action League, decided to request the Boulder City Council to enact a law that would protect patients coming to the two clinics as well as the physicians and staffs at these facilities.

During this time, extremely aggressive anti-abortion demonstrations were taking place at my office, Boulder Abortion Clinic, on a daily basis. There were several occasions when a massive police presence was necessary. On one occasion, there were two police command posts, the SWAT team, and more than 100 armed law enforcement officers from Boulder County were required. Demonstrators routinely cursed and screamed at patients walking along the sidewalk and into my office. Many patients found this to be the most stressful part of the abortion experience.

The result was the Boulder Buffer Zone Ordinance, which specified that any demonstrators who were within 100 feet of the entrance to either clinic must remain a minimum of eight feet from women and their companions entering the clinics. There was great controversy about the measure itself and the specific components of the statute. The American Civil Liberties Union demanded a modest distance for the demonstrators, and mediators arrived at the specified limits.

It was my opinion that the distance the demonstrators should be required to stay from the entrance to my office was the distance that a rifle bullet could travel since I assumed that the demonstrators were armed and ready to commit violence. As an alternative, I recommended that they be required to keep their demonstrations in New Jersey. There would be no restrictions on their freedom of speech at that distance.

The Boulder City Council passed the ordinance that was known as the Boulder Buffer Zone Ordinance. It was challenged in federal district court under the title *Buchanan v. Jourgensen.*

At a federal district court hearing presided over by Judge Zita Weinshienk, I testified that the proximity of the demonstrators had a traumatic effect on the emotional status as well as the physical well-being of my patients. Professor Edward T. Hall, a distinguished anthropologist and author of the proxemics theory of the social and cultural use of space, testified that the demonstrators were deliberately violating unwritten codes of social conduct by infringing on the patients' intimate distance and thereby causing them discomfort. Social psychologist Marianne LaFrance testified concerning the psychological stress caused by the proximity of the demonstrators.

Judge Weinshienk declined to order an injunction against implementation of the Buffer Zone Ordinance, and it remains in effect today.

In 1993 state representative Diana DeGette sponsored a law in the Colorado legislature, co-sponsored by state senator Mike Feeley, that codified components of the Boulder

Buffer Zone Ordinance as Colorado law. It was signed into law by Governor Roy Romer on April 19, 1993.

The law was immediately challenged in court by Jeannie Hill of the Colorado Right to Life Committee. The attorney for the Right to Life Committee, Jay Sekulow, who was chief counsel for the American Center for Law and Justice, was the lead counsel for the plaintiffs and deposed me in developing the legal attack on the state buffer zone law.

At the beginning of his deposition of me, Sekulow refused my request that he identify himself. I refused to proceed with the deposition and answer his questions until he did. After several exchanges, he gave me his name.

Sekulow has most recently served as personal attorney for former president Donald Trump during the time that he held office.

In lower court pleadings, the Colorado Buffer Zone Law was upheld. Oral arguments for the state of Colorado as defendant in the U.S. Supreme Court were made by Jean Dubofsky, an attorney who had been a justice of the Colorado Supreme Court. In a reversal of position, the American Civil Liberties Union argued for the plaintiff, Hill, against the Buffer Zone Ordinance on grounds that it limited free speech under the First Amendment.

On June 29, 2000, the U.S. Supreme Court upheld the constitutionality of the Colorado law. The 6–3 majority opinion was written by Justice Stevens, joined by Chief Justice Rehnquist and Justices O'Connor, Souter, Ginsburg, and Breyer in saying that the law prevents unwanted approaching, not speech. The Supreme Court held that the First Amendment right of free speech for the demonstrators was not violated by limiting their activities and requiring them to remain eight feet from patients entering a health-care facility.

Justices Kennedy, Scalia, and Thomas dissented. Justices Kennedy and Scalia issued strongly worded dissents, choosing to read their denunciations of the majority opinion aloud in Court.

Gonzalez v. Carhart, 550 U.S. 124 (2007)

In 2003 Congress passed the "Partial-Birth Abortion Ban Act," outlawing a procedure that is not described in the medical literature. In numerous hearings before the U.S. Senate and House of Representatives in 1994, 1995, and 1997, members of Congress heard not a word of testimony from any physician expert on late abortions. I was present at a hearing of the U.S. Senate Judiciary Committee on November 17, 1995, to which I was invited to testify by the Minority Counsel at the request of Senator Ted Kennedy, but I was not permitted by the chairman of the committee, Republican senator Orrin Hatch from Utah to testify, in spite of an appeal during the hearing by Republican senator Hank Brown from Colorado, who was sitting next to Senator Hatch. My prepared testimony was submitted for the record and was published in the *Congressional Record*.

The 2003 "Partial-Birth Abortion Ban Act" was signed into law by President George W. Bush on November 5, 2003, while surrounded by aging white men in blue suits who could not get pregnant. Previous versions passed in 1995 and 1997 had been vetoed by President Clinton.

During his campaign for reelection in 2004, President Bush proudly made reference to the fact that he had signed the "Partial-Birth Abortion Act" into law during one of his debates with the Democratic candidate, Senator John Kerry.

A previous version of this law passed by the Nebraska state legislature had been struck down by the U.S. Supreme Court in *Stenberg* because it had no health exception and because it interfered with the physician's judgment about the proper medical procedure for the patient. In the previous ruling, the Supreme Court also noted that the statute did not distinguish between different abortion procedure techniques and therefore could not be reliably interpreted as a guide to action.

In *Gonzalez*, the same physician, Dr. Leroy Carhart, challenged the federal partial-birth abortion ban in federal court. It was struck down in three federal district courts on the grounds that it had no health exception citing *Stenberg*. The district court decisions were all affirmed in the federal appeals courts.

Writing for the 5–4 majority, Justice Kennedy, joined by Justices Alito, Scalia, Thomas, and Chief Justice Roberts, stated that the Partial-Birth Abortion Ban Act did not violate the Constitution. Justice Ginsburg wrote a dissent, joined by Justices Breyer, Souter, and Stevens.

Kennedy's majority opinion stated that the Partial-Birth Abortion Ban Act was more clearly stated than the Nebraska law and therefore it was constitutional. The reversal of the Supreme Court's decision in *Stenberg* that the Nebraska law was unconstitutional and the Supreme Court's later decision in *Gonzalez* of constitutionality was due to the fact that Justice Sandra Day O'Connor had been replaced by Justice Alito.

Whole Women's Health v. Hellerstedt, 579 U.S.____ (2016) (The official page number has not yet been published.)

A Texas law passed in 2013 required physicians performing abortions to have admitting privileges to a hospital within 30 miles of the abortion facility. It also required abortion clinics to have the same standards of construction and design as ambulatory surgical centers. Whole Women's Health opposed these requirements as unnecessary and, with other plaintiffs, challenged the hospital admitting privileges requirement in the U.S. District Court for the Western District of Texas in Dallas. The Court granted the plaintiffs an injunction against enforcement of the law. Their case eventually reached the U.S. Supreme Court, which granted a stay in 2015.

On June 27, 2016, the U.S. Supreme Court ruled 5–3 that "Texas cannot place restrictions on the delivery of abortion services that create an undue burden for women seeking an abortion."

This decision is highly significant for many reasons, among which is the continuing proliferation of regulations at the local and state level hindering physicians seeking hospital privileges as a method of preventing access to abortion services outside of statutory limitations. A similar law passed in Louisiana was upheld, reversed, upheld, and finally enjoined by the U.S. Supreme Court (*June Medical Services LLC v. Russo*).

Dobbs v. Jackson Women's Health Organization (No. 19-1392, 597 U.S.____ 2022) (No. 2022)

The final straw that broke the legal camel's back was the *Dobbs* decision on June 24, 2022. A Mississippi law based on a model created by the Christian legal organization, Alliance Defending Freedom, was adopted with the specific intent of using it to overturn *Roe v. Wade*. Based on *Planned Parenthood v. Casey*, lower courts enjoined the execution of the Mississippi law prohibiting abortion after 15 weeks. The Jackson Women's Health Organization, the only clinic in that state where abortions were being performed, challenged the law. But instead of simply upholding the law, which would have meant that abortions up to 15 weeks could be performed, the U.S. Supreme Court used the occasion to overturn the *Roe v. Wade* decision issued in 1973 guaranteeing the right of women to have safe abortions.

A total of 49 years of precedent of a constitutional right to abortion were erased by this decision. The *Dobbs* decision marked the successful culmination of efforts over 50 years by Christian organizations and the Republican Party to overturn *Roe* and make abortion illegal in as many states as possible. It is now impossible or almost impossible to have a safe abortion in 19 states in America.

To date, the U.S. Supreme Court has accepted and ruled in 45 cases involving the issues of contraception and abortion.[1]

Note

1 https://en.wikipedia.org/wiki/Dobbs_v._Jackson_Women%27s_Health_Organization 19-1392, 597 U.S. ___

15 Partial truth abortion – or, political pornography for Republicans

Birth attendants have known for thousands of years that childbirth is a dangerous time for women, and the world literature is full of evidence of this. There are also many references to abortion sought by women and performed by birth attendants, midwives, and others in tribal societies. Physicians in classical times had sophisticated surgical instruments for helping women in these situations.

Remarkably sophisticated vaginal speculums were found in the ruins of Pompeii, and the Greek physician Soranus wrote eloquently about the challenges of keeping women safe in childbirth.[1] Soranus and other physicians had instruments that were specifically designed to remove a baby from a woman who could not deliver it in a spontaneous normal birth process. So did the great French physician François Mauriceau, who wrote the first obstetrics textbook, *Malades de femmes gGrosses et acouchée*, first published in 1668.[2] These instruments, some in the shape of a very large hook, required killing the fetus. Without this, the woman would die.

Two thousand years after Soranus and more than three hundred years after Mauriceau, American physicians are still seeking the best ways to help women end advanced pregnancies. These requests have become more common for many reasons, among them the fact that many modern women have postponed childbearing until late in their reproductive years in order to follow and realize their dreams of professional careers in law, medicine, business, teaching, the arts, and other opportunities. Beginning a pregnancy in the later reproductive years (over 30 or 35) increases the risk of fetal abnormalities, particularly certain genetic disorders.

There are many reasons why women find themselves trying to find ways to end a pregnancy that has advanced into the second or third trimester, especially those with desired pregnancies in which a catastrophic fetal anomaly or genetic disorder has been discovered, but there are other reasons discussed in other parts of this book.

One of the techniques for ending an advanced pregnancy has become a flash point in the harrowing and interminable political controversy surrounding late abortion in America in the twentieth and twenty-first centuries.

Techniques for late abortion in the late twentieth century included intra-amniotic injection of hyperosmolar (concentrated) salt solution, which had the effect of killing the fetus *in utero* and causing the woman to go into labor. Another was the intrauterine infusion of a synthetic prostaglandin, which could cause labor, but a large proportion of the fetuses in these cases (as many as 10–15 percent) were born alive or with agonal (reflexive) movements. The women who delivered the fetuses were frequently alone in a hospital bed or were attended by nursing staff that was unsympathetic to the woman's situation and/or horrified by the result.

DOI: 10.4324/9781003514961-16

Increasingly, physicians learned, through both clinical experience and published research reports, that removing the fetus with instruments (dilation and evacuation) appeared to have lower complication and death rates than the induction methods (causing labor) using saline and prostaglandin. But this method had its own challenges, especially in a more advanced pregnancy.[3]

In 1992 Dr Martin Haskell, a physician in Ohio who specialized in outpatient abortion services, reported that he had discovered or developed a new abortion technique that he called the "D & X" procedure (abbreviation for "dilation and extraction"). This technique consisted of gradual dilation of the cervix over several days using *Laminaria japonicum* (stalks of a seaweed found in the Sea of Japan), induction of labor, podalic version of the fetus (bringing the legs down to the lower uterus and into the vagina), pulling the fetus down until the occipital space was exposed between the top of the fetal shoulders and its head, then cutting into the posterior cranial cavity with scissors and removing the cerebral tissue with a vacuum aspiration cannula. This is a modern version of what has been practiced by birth attendants for at least two thousand years.

One of the main differences between what Dr. Haskell described and what was performed in classical or historical times is that, in most cases, Dr. Haskell was treating a woman who wanted to end a pregnancy at about half-way through the pregnancy and not one who was about to die because she could not deliver a baby at term (40 weeks) in an uncomplicated childbirth. The 20-week fetus was still alive when the abortion began as distinguished from historical situations in which the fetus was probably already dead when the physician or birth attendant removed the baby from a woman who could not deliver it on her own at term.

A most unfortunate context prevailed when Dr. Haskell made his presentation to his medical colleagues at a national meeting. First, a bitter political battle was already raging in which abortion of any kind was being opposed by highly conservative religious groups; second, the abortion issue was being exploited by one political party to acquire power; third, a campaign of psychological warfare was being conducted by the anti-abortion fanatics; and fourth, the unprincipled and fanatic opponents of abortion were able to obtain copies of Dr. Haskell's information sheet about his operation immediately.

Within days if not hours, what Dr. Haskell had presented to his medical colleagues as a way of ending the woman's pregnancy safely was converted to a powerful propaganda tool with the title, "partial-birth abortion." A gruesome description of the procedure was accompanied by drawings of a full-term, completely developed baby that was alive and kicking.

At the same time, Dr. James McMahon, a physician in California who specialized in outpatient abortion, began performing the same operation, which he called "Intact D & E" (intact dilation and evacuation). Dr. McMahon saw many patients with diagnosed fetal abnormalities in which both the referring physicians and the patients wanted the fetus to be delivered intact in order to facilitate diagnostic studies and also to help the grieving process for women who were ending desired pregnancies.

In 1992 abortion became a critical issue in the presidential campaign.[4] Bill Clinton's campaign devised the slogan that Clinton wanted abortion to be "safe, legal, and rare." At that time, about 1.5 million abortions were being performed in the United States each year. Militant anti-abortion fanatics were invading abortion clinics and waging violent attacks on clinics in other ways across the country. The anti-abortion movement was growing in strength in many ways.

By 1994 the Republican Party was increasingly using the abortion issue as an organizing principle and attracting conservative voters away from the Democratic Party. Newt Gingrich was the new congressional leader of the Republicans, who won the 1994 mid-term elections and took control of the U.S. House of Representatives in 1995. With that, Republicans in the House, in payback to the anti-abortion movement, offered 13 bills restricting abortions and access to reproductive health care. One of them made "partial-birth abortion" – a term not to be found in any medical publication – illegal.

Dr. Haskell was called upon to defend his operation in public forums and in legislative investigations. He did, and he revealed that 80 percent of such procedures were "elective" – they were not being performed for a particular medical indication.

Legislative attacks on Dr. Haskell in Ohio and the U.S. House of Representatives brought out testimony by a nurse who reported that she had witnessed one of these procedures while she was being considered for a job at Dr. Haskell's office. Her vivid and gut-wrenching testimony became an inflammatory propaganda point, but it did serve to focus on the emotional conflict between helping women and ending the potential life of a fetus.

Dr. Haskell's office stated that, as a temporary three-day assistant, the nurse was not permitted in the operating room and could not have seen this procedure. She stated several things that were simply not true. The conflicting reports made it difficult for the public to discern the truth, but the psychological effects and perception of an inhumane procedure in the glare of publicity and political hostage-taking resulted in a successful psychological warfare for the opponents of abortion.

A focus on the health and safety of women seeking abortion became impossible and obscured by the so-called partial-birth abortion trope and propaganda. In politics, perception becomes the reality, and this image overwhelmed all logic, reason, facts, and other considerations.

Canady's bill passed the U.S. House of Representatives in November 1995. It was the first time in American history that Congress had passed a bill making a specific medical or surgical procedure illegal although there was no description of the procedure in any medical publication.

Anticipating that Canady's bill would pass the House and be considered in the U.S. Senate, a member of Senator Ted Kennedy's office called me and asked me to prepare testimony concerning what was now SB 939, the Senate version of Canady's "Partial-Birth Abortion Ban Act."

Senator Kennedy was the ranking member of the Senate Judiciary Committee that would have a hearing on the bill. His request to me was joined by Senators Joe Biden (D-DE) and Arlen Specter (R-PA).

This committee was chaired by Senator Orrin Hatch (R-UT), who was a vociferous opponent of abortion.

My testimony was also requested by both U.S. senators from Colorado, Hank Brown (R-CO) and Ben Nighthorse Campbell (R-CO). Attorney Katherine Kolbert from the Center for Reproductive Rights called me to discuss what I needed for my testimony and reviewed my early draft of it.

The Senate Judiciary Committee hearing was scheduled for November 17, 1995. I had prepared my testimony, it had been reviewed with suggestions from attorney Kolbert, and I was ready to present my views to the committee.

At the same time that I was preparing for this testimony, I was organizing a symposium on the subject of anti-abortion rhetoric and anti-abortion violence for the 1995 annual meeting of the American Anthropological Association, which was going to be held at the same time in Washington, D.C., as the Senate Judiciary Committee hearing. The title of my symposium was *Abortion: The Language of Ideology and the Language of Violence.*

My invited symposium speakers included Professor Celest M Condit, author of *Decoding Abortion Rhetoric;*[5] Professor Suzanne Hanchet, "Fetal Personhood: an Unviable Concept"; and Professor Dallas Blanchard, author of *The Anti-abortion Movement and the Rise of the Religious Right.*[6] The title of my own paper was "Anti-abortion Rhetoric: The Fetus as Fetish Object, tthe Doctor as Demon." The discussants were Professor Marvin Harris from Columbia University, one of the most distinguished and widely published anthropologists in the world; Professor Faye Ginsburg from New York University, who was the author of *Contested Lives: The Abortion Debate in an American Community.*[7]

In my own paper, I discussed what it was like as a physician to be demonized by the anti-abortion fanatics and fear for my life as a result: three of my medical colleagues had already been assassinated for doing what I do, and several other people who worked in abortion clinics or alongside physicians had been killed. I described the fetus as a fetish object which was politically useful for winning elections.

We had an extraordinary faculty and symposium, but the minute it was over, I left the meeting and took a taxi to the Senate Judiciary Committee hearing where I was committed to giving my testimony against Senate Bill 939, the "Partial-Birth Abortion Ban Act."

The Senate hearing

On arriving at the Senate room where the hearing was to be held, I learned that the pro-choice leaders had decided that I would not be permitted to testify even though my testimony had been requested by the ranking member, Senator Kennedy, and several other senators who were members of the Judiciary Committee.

Kate Michelman, the president of the National Abortion Rights Action League, gave me a "shame on you!" look and wagged her finger at me as though I were a misbehaving grade school student. The new president of the National Abortion Federation, Vicki Saporta, gave me a similarly unfriendly look and would not speak to me.

Both moved away from me without speaking. I could only speculate that the reasons for this treatment lay in the fact that I had not conformed to the official pro-choice "party line" – that the so-called "partial-birth abortion" was the safest way to perform a late abortion. National reporters had been told this by pro-choice leaders, but when these reporters had called me (such as Diane Gianelli, the reporter from the *American Medical News,* the publication of the American Medical Association) and asked me whether this was true, I stated, "No. There is no evidence for that."

The pro-choice leaders had even gone to Pat Schroeder, U.S. Representative from Colorado, and persuaded her to state on the House floor that "partial-birth abortion" was the "safest way to perform late abortions." As I had known Pat for 20 years and knew her staff, I had called her legislative assistant, Andrea Camp, and recommended that she tell Pat not to say this because it wasn't true. So there was a possible explanation for the antipathy toward me by pro-choice leaders at the Senate hearing although I did not anticipate this.

I learned several years later from James Wagoner, who at that time was Kate Michelman's chief assistant on political and other matters, that he advised Kate not to allow me to testify because I wasn't "politically reliable." He knew that I would testify that the so-called partial-birth abortion was *not* the safest way to perform a late abortion. Wagoner calmly told me this over lunch one day and seemed satisfied with his own advice and the fact that I was not allowed to testify. I thought it was politically stupid advice.

Two pro-choice physicians (who I knew personally and respected), Dr. Mary Campbell and Dr. Courtland Peterson, were chosen by the pro-choice leaders to testify against the bill. Both had experience in abortion, but neither had experience in late abortion.

Dr. Campbell repeated a statement by the late Dr. Jim McMahon that the analgesia/anesthesia given to the pregnant woman would kill the fetus so it would have no pain, a statement that I did not believe or accept. Other than this, both physicians gave reasonable testimony, and they both made it clear that deciding which were the best methods of safe abortion must be determined by physicians, not legislators, to say nothing of the issue of who should be making the decision to have or to perform an abortion, and neither should involve legislators.

Following the testimony by Dr. Campbell, the anti-abortion sponsors of the legislation called physicians who were anesthesiologists, and one of these physicians ridiculed the notion that the amount of anesthesia or analgesia given to the woman having the abortion would kill the fetus.

Except for me, there were no physicians present at the hearing who had any expertise on the subject of late abortion or how such a procedure should be performed in a safe way. Dr. McMahon had recently died of a brain tumor; Dr. George Tiller from Kansas had been shot in both arms in an assassination attempt and was not willing to testify for security reasons; Dr. Haskell had received enormous harassment and many death threats resulting from his testimony and appearances in Ohio; and there was no one else in the nation with the relevant experience. I sat in the back of the room listening to the testimony and hearing while holding a copy of my prepared statement.

In his opening remarks, Chairman Hatch had quoted my statements from press reports that I did not think that the described procedure called "partial-birth abortion" was an acceptable way to terminate an advanced pregnancy and that I couldn't defend the practice.

My friend and former college classmate, Senator Hank Brown (R-CO), was seated next to Chairman Hatch. I found myself sitting next to one of Hank's Senate staff members. I said, "Please tell Hank that I am here in the audience and I am prepared to testify concerning this bill." I showed him my statement. A few minutes later, Hank said to Hatch, "Dr. Hern is here and would like to have an opportunity to testify."

It appeared to me that Hatch turned him down on the spot. The published *Congressional Record* does not record this and appears to show that Hatch was not opposed to my testifying. No matter, I was not called, and I did not have an opportunity to testify.

After the hearing, I went out into the hallway by the hearing room. A member of the staff of a national pro-choice organization was there, and I greeted her. Then I was approached by a reporter from the *New York Times* with whom I had had previous telephone conversations. He wanted to speak to me, but the pro-choice organization staff member attempted to intervene. The reporter and I had to retire to the men's room in order for him to interview me without interruption.

It was a frustrating experience. I knew several members of the Senate Judiciary Committee personally aside from Senator Brown, who I had known for several decades. I had enjoyed a dinner with Senator Alan Simpson (R-WY), a neighbor from Wyoming. I had presented the suppressed OEO Sterilization Guidelines to Senator Kennedy in 1973 when he was conducting an investigation into the unethical sterilization of the Relf sisters, and I had met him at various political events; I had met Senator Paul Simon (D-IL), and I had been on the speaker's platform in 1989 with Senator Diane Feinstein (D-CA). Senator Hatch certainly knew who I was. I had reason to believe that these senators (except for Hatch) would take me seriously and listen to my testimony regardless of their views on the subject. I was the only physician in the nation who was an expert on the subject of late abortion and who was also present at the hearing.

I felt that I was strapped to a chair with a sock in my mouth as I listened to something that vitally affected the lives and safety of my patients and millions of other women, not just my medical career, and with expert knowledge and experience, without being able to speak or do anything about it. The issue had vital consequences for the availability of safe abortions of any kind for American women. It was very frustrating, to say the least.

Since I was not permitted to testify at the hearing, I submitted the following written testimony to the committee:

STATEMENT

of

Warren M. Hern, M.D., M.P.H., Ph.D.

Director, Boulder Abortion Clinic

1130 Alpine

Boulder, Colorado 80304

Assistant Clinical Professor

Department of Obstetrics & Gynecology

University of Colorado Health Sciences Center

Denver, Colorado 80220

Before the Judiciary Committee

of the

United States Senate

Concerning S. 939

17 November 1995

Thank you, Mr. Chairman, for the opportunity to submit a statement to this body concerning S. 939, the so-called "Partial Birth Abortion Ban Act" of 1995. I appreciate the invitation to prepare a statement that came to me from Senators Kennedy, Biden, and Specter as members of the Judiciary Committee. I also deeply appreciate the joint request by Senators Hank Brown and Ben Nighthorse Campbell of Colorado that I be given an opportunity to testify in person and that my remarks be inserted in the record. Since I was not permitted to testify in person, I request that this written statement be entered into the record as per the requests by Senators Brown and Campbell.

My name is Warren Martin Hern. I am a physician engaged in private medical practice in Boulder, Colorado, where I specialize in outpatient abortion services. My formal medical training includes graduation from the University of Colorado School of Medicine in 1965 followed by a one-year rotating internship at Gorgas Hospital in the Panama Canal Zone. I subsequently served for two years as a commissioned officer in the United States Public Health Service assigned as a Peace Corps physician in Brazil. Following that, I studied public health and epidemiology at the University of North Carolina School of Public Health in Chapel Hill, receiving my Master of Public Health degree in 1971. In March, 1970, I began service as Chief, Program Development and Evaluation Branch, Family Planning Division, Office of Health Affairs in the Office of Economic Opportunity, Executive Office of the President in Washington, D.C. I served in this capacity as a federal official until June, 1972.

Since 1973, I have provided abortion services in Boulder, Colorado. I have provided these services in my private practice, Boulder Abortion Clinic, since 1975.

In 1980, while continuing my medical practice, I resumed my graduate work in Chapel Hill, and in 1988, I received my Ph.D. in Epidemiology from the University of North Carolina School of Public Health. My dissertation research studied the health effects of cultural change among the Shipibo Indians of the Peruvian Amazon.

My publications since 1975 include three books and some 40 professional papers concerning abortion and other aspects of fertility.[1] My medical textbook, **Abortion Practice**, was published by J.B. Lippincott Company of Philadelphia in 1984. It remains in print as the principal textbook concerning abortion and is used internationally.

In addition to my private medical practice, I hold several academic appointments. I am Assistant Clinical Professor of Obstetrics and Gynecology at the University of Colorado Health Sciences Center and Professor Adjunct in the Department of Anthropology, University of Colorado at Boulder.

Senate Bill 939

The bill under consideration, S. 939, is called the "Partial Birth Abortion Ban Act," but there is no such thing as a "partial birth abortion." This is an operation which has never been described in the medical literature, and as far as I know, it does not exist. The bill's sponsors describe some procedures which have been performed for many generations in the case of obstetrical emergency. The operation mentioned in the Senate bill contains some elements of a procedure called an "Intact D & E," or "Intact Dilation and Evacuation" by some physicians during the course of scientific discussions of late abortions, but I have never heard the term, "partial birth abortion" in these discussions. As written, the bill describes aspects of an operation which is performed routinely by some physicians currently, but they are procedures with a long history and wide application by other physicians on a sporadic and unpredictable basis. The bill's language could be interpreted to refer to virtually any second trimester or later abortion. If made more specific, it has the potential to single out and discriminate against specific doctors, some of whose procedures may be alleged to be consistent with the language of the bill. Doctors are poor judges of these subtleties when presented with the exigencies of patient needs. These circumstances mean that the bill can produce a "witch hunt" atmosphere that chills medical practice and interferes with good patient care by conscientious doctors.

History of Intact D & E

Evidence from the ancient city of Pompeii indicates that an operation like this may have been performed by physicians and surgeons during that era, approximately 1,950 years or more before the present time. Breech extraction followed by perforation of the fetal skull by surgical instruments to allow delivery of the aftercoming head in an obstetrical emergency has been practiced by physicians and midwives for hundreds if not thousands of years. It has been practiced in the South American Amazon for a similar period. This is not a new idea.

The specific operation described by the bill's sponsors involves routine version of a 20-week or later fetus into a breech (feet first) position, followed by extraction of the fetus up to the neck, when the base of the fetal skull is perforated with surgical instruments. At that point, the contents of the fetal skull are removed by vacuum aspiration using a hollow cannula. Since the fetus is usually dead by this point, whether due to an induced abortion or miscarriage, and since the head is under great pressure, the cerebral contents are often extruded without any intervention by the surgeon. The head collapses, permitting delivery of the more or less intact fetus.

A variation of this procedure, which is usually preceded by several days of treatment to open the uterus so as to permit passage of the fetus, is decompression of the fetal skull as it presents first in the sequence of expulsion or delivery of the fetus. Again, the fetus is usually dead at the point at which this occurs. I think fetal death is often brought about by infarction (death) of the placenta as the result of other kinds of treatment such as those that cause uterine irritability.

A common approach to abortion by some obstetricians who have discovered a severe fetal anomaly in an advanced pregnancy is to place prostaglandin suppositories in the vagina followed by induction of labor and expulsion of the fetus. It is my understanding that the maneuvers described by the sponsors of S. 939 are followed by attending physicians throughout the nation when the safety of the woman having the abortion is at issue.

Another approach, which I favor and which is followed by some other physicians, is to induce fetal death on the first or second day of treatment of the cervix. This requires an injection of a medication into the fetus under (usually) ultrasound guidance. This is the procedure which I and one or two other physicians follow. It is accompanied by other forms of treatment, but these vary according to the physician. In the case of a breech presentation of a dead fetus, the procedure described by sponsors of S. 939 is routinely followed.

Advantages of Intact D & E

The principal purpose of an abortion is to end a pregnancy which threatens a woman's life or which she wants terminated. The manner of ending the pregnancy must be determined by safety factors for the woman and acceptability of the methods used. The considerations for the fetus are secondary to the safety and welfare of the woman seeking the abortion.

The possible advantages of Intact D & E procedure include a reduction of the risk of perforation of the uterus. Since most women seeking abortions are young women who hope to reproduce in the future, having a safe abortion technique for late abortion is of paramount importance, aside from the prevention of complications. Another advantage of the Intact D & E is that it eliminates the risk of embolism of cerebral tissue into the woman's blood stream. This catastrophe can be almost immediately fatal.

I support the right of my medical colleagues to use whatever methods they deem appropriate to protect the woman's safety during this difficult procedure. It is simply not possible for others to second guess the surgeon's judgment in the operating room. That would be dangerous and unacceptable.

Fetal Considerations

According to biologist Clifford Grobstein and others, fetal neurological development well into the early part of the third trimester is insufficient for the fetus to experience what we regard as "pain." In Professor Grobstein's book, Science and the Unborn (1988, Basic Books, New York), "...an adequate neural substrate for experienced pain does not exist until about the seventh month of pregnancy (30 weeks), well into the period when prematurely born fetuses are viable with intensive life support."[8] Like any other mammalian organism, fetuses have enough neurological development to permit certain reflexes, but this is not the same as pain. Interpretation of these reflexes as "pain" is highly misleading.

Duration of pregnancy and reasons for late abortion

While about 1% of all abortions are performed after about 20 weeks of pregnancy, only about .03%, or fewer than 500, are performed after 26 weeks. The majority of these are now performed by me or one of my medical colleagues. These abortions are almost always performed for the most tragic reasons of severe fetal anomaly, genetic disorder, or immediate risk to the woman's life. They are not performed for frivolous reasons, contrary to statements by those opposed to abortion.

For example, one woman was recently brought to me by air ambulance from Rapid City, South Dakota for an abortion because she was about to die from her pregnancy, which was desired. She was a diabetic and had developed hyperemesis gravidarum (uncontrollable vomiting from pregnancy). She was starving to death. Her doctors were having difficulty keeping her alive. Her blood chemical balance was severely altered to the point that her heart could stop at any time. She was profoundly dehydrated. She was critically ill and could barely speak. Since she and her husband wanted the pregnancy, they tried everything to get her through it, but she was finally advised that she must have the abortion. While being flown to Boulder so that I could see her, she almost died in the airplane. I began her treatment immediately and performed the abortion by one the techniques I have described here two days later. She recovered completely and felt healthy again the next day. Without this operation, she would have died.

Another woman with an advanced pregnancy was referred to me by a colleague in northern Colorado because her fetus had been found to have a severe genetic disorder. She and her husband both wanted the pregnancy to continue. The fetal disorder also caused a serious disease of the placenta, which, in turn, caused the woman's blood pressure to go up. When she arrived at my office, her blood pressure was starting to go up at an alarming rate. I put her in the hospital as I continued my treatment. Her urine output diminished. She became edematous. Her electrolytes (blood chemicals) were out of balance because she was not excreting urine. She developed pulmonary edema (water on the lungs) and began having difficulty breathing. Meanwhile, I was trying to prepare her for the abortion, which promised to be extremely dangerous because of a large placenta that obstructed the opening of the uterus and threatened to cause catastrophic bleeding. We crossmatched blood for her. At 2 AM on the second night, before her cervix was completely prepared for the abortion I needed to perform, I had to act. She was deteriorating rapidly and it was clear that she would die before morning if I did not perform the abortion. This operation took every bit of my skill and experience as a surgeon and everything I have learned in 22 years of performing abortions. Although she was ill for some days from the effects of the pregnancy, the patient recovered fully.

On another occasion, a woman had been referred to me from Michigan for a late abortion because the fetus had a severe anomaly. The pregnancy was complicated by polyhydramnios (too much amniotic fluid surrounding the fetus), which was the result of one of the fetal anomalies. She was resting in my recovery room in preparation for her abortion, accompanied by her husband, when suddenly, without warning, the woman developed signs of shock, and I made a diagnosis of placental abruption. The placenta had torn away from the wall of the uterus and she was bleeding to death into the uterus. I carried her into my operating room without waiting for assistance, placed her on the operating table, and assembled my surgical team. My nurse held her fist on the patient's aorta to keep her from bleeding to death while I did the abortion. As I began the procedure, two units of blood (about a quart) spurted out of her uterus, and she lost another unit during the operation. Without our preparations and my skill and experience, that woman would have died within minutes.

Mr. Chairman, I did not have time with any of these cases to consult the United States Senate on the proper method of performing the abortions.

Comparative risk of abortion and term birth

Without medical treatment, the risk of death due to pregnancy and childbirth is in the range of 1%. This is measured by the maternal mortality ratio, which is the proportion of women dying from pregnancy or its effects to the number of live births. For example, in 1920, the maternal mortality ratio was 680 per 100,000 live births. 680 women died for each 100,000 live births. In the Peruvian Amazon, where I conduct medical research from time to time, the maternal mortality ratio is about 1000 deaths of women per 100,000 live births, or about 1%.

By 1960, the U.S. maternal mortality ratio had dropped to about 38 per 100,000 live births. It is now about 8 per 100,000 live births for term pregnancy.

By contrast, the death rate in abortion is about 2 or 3 per 1,000,000 procedures, or about .2-.3 per 100,000 abortions. For early abortion, the abortion mortality rate is less than 1 per million procedures.

This means that a woman is ten or more times likely to die if she carries a pregnancy to term than if she has an abortion. For women at high risk of pregnancy complications, the risk of death may be 100 times greater for carrying the pregnancy to term.

Late abortion is a more dangerous procedure than early abortion, but the evidence is that it is still much safer in terms of mortality risk than carrying a pregnancy to term. The risk of a major complication is about 25-30% with term pregnancy, but it is much lower in late abortion. In a recent medical article of mine published in the journal *Obstetrics and Gynecology* in February 1993, I described the experience of 124 patients for whom I performed abortions in pregnancies complicated by severe fetal anomaly, diagnosed genetic disorder, or fetal death. The average length of pregnancy was 23 weeks with a few over 30 weeks. The major complication rate was less than 1% (one patient). In another comparative study of mine published one year ago in the *American Journal of Obstetrics and Gynecology*, 1001 patients whose pregnancies ranged from 13 to 25 weeks in duration experienced a major complication rate of 0.3%. Only 3 of these patients experienced a major complication.

Implications of S. 939 for medical practice

Late abortion as currently practiced in the United States is a safe procedure that saves women's lives. The medical community has not determined the very best way to perform these procedures, and that cannot be determined by any legislature. That is a matter for scientific study and medical judgment.

If S. 939 is passed into law, any physician performing any second trimester or later abortion could be prosecuted by an aggressive public prosecutor. It would cause each physician to have to make a legal and political judgment with each patient as to whether prosecution would follow the exercise of the physician's judgment. It is an unwarranted and unacceptable intrusion into the practice of medicine.

The women who seek late abortion always do so for serious reasons. My experience has been that the women who seek my services are experiencing great pain and anguish, along with their family members, as the result of a very difficult decision. Even those who have all the information in a particular case have difficulty in determining the best thing to do. As a practicing physician, I do not see how any governmental body can effectively or rationally control these decisions.

S. 939 is an irretrievably bad piece of legislation that cannot be made acceptable by any means, and I urge the Senate to defeat it at the first opportunity.

References [to written statement]

Hern, W.M.: Laminaria in abortion: use in 1368 patients in first trimester. *Rocky Mountain Medical Journal* 72:390–395, 1975.

Hern, W.M. and A. Oakes: Multiple laminaria treatment in early midtrimester outpatient suction abortion. *Advances in Planned Parenthood* 12:93–97, 1977.

Hern, W.M.: The concept of quality care in abortion services. *Advances in Planned Parenthood* 13:63–74, 1978.

Hern, W.M., W.A. Miller, L. Paine, and K.D. Moorhead: Correlation of sonographic cephalometry with clinical assessment of fetal age following early midtrimester D & E abortion. *Advances in Planned Parenthood* 13:14–20, 1978.

Hern, W.M. and B. Corrigan: What about us? Staff reactions to D & E. *Advances in Planned Parenthood* 15:3–8, 1980.

Hern, W.M.: Outpatient second-trimester D & E abortion through 24 menstrual weeks' gestation. *Advances in Planned Parenthood* 16:7–13, 1981.

Hern, W.M.: Correlation of fetal age and measurements between 10 and 26 weeks of gestation. *Obstetrics and Gynecology* 63:26–32, 1984.

Hern, W.M.: Serial multiple laminaria and adjunctive urea in late out patient dilatation and evacuation abortion. *Obstetrics and Gynecology* 63:543–549, 1984.

Hern, W.M.: *Abortion Practice.* J.B. Lippincott Company, Philadelphia, 1984. Reviewed in Family Planning Perspectives, New England Journal of Medicine, Journal of the American Medical Association.

Hern, W.M.: Evolution of second trimester abortion techniques. *In Prevention and Treatment of Contraceptive Failure*, U. Landy and S.S. Ratnam, eds. New York: Plenum Press, 1986.

Hern, W.M.: Use of prostaglandins as abortifacients. In Gynecology and Obstetrics, chapter 58, J.W. Sciarra, Ed., Philadelphia, J.B. Lippincott Co, 1982. Published in 1988.

Hern, W.M.: *Abortion Practice.* Softcover reprint. Alpenglo Graphics, 1990, 368 pages, 59 illustrations, 3 color plates, 16 tables. Available from Alpenglo Graphics, 1130 Alpine, Boulder, CO 80304.

Hern, W.M., C. Zen, K.A. Ferguson, V. Hart, and M.V. Haseman: Outpatient abortion for fetal anomaly and fetal death from 15–34 menstrual weeks' gestation: Techniques and clinical management. *Obstetrics and Gynecology* 81:301–306, 1993.

Hern, W.M.: Cervical treatment with DilapanTM prior to second trimester dilation and evacuation abortion: A pilot study of 64 patients. *American Journal of Gynecologic Health* 7(1):15–18, 1993.

Hern, W.M: Laminaria versus Dilapan osmotic cervical dilators for outpatient dilation and evacuation abortion: Randomized cohort comparison of 1001 patients. *American Journal of Obstetrics and Gynecology* 171:1324–1328, 1994.

Hern, W.M.: Abortion: Medical and Social Aspects. In *Encyclopedia of Marriage and the Family*, David Levinson, Ed. New York: Simon & Schuster MacMillan, 1995. pp. 1–7.

[end of submitted testimony]

---

* * *

Several weeks after I attended this hearing and submitted my testimony, on December 4, the Senate once again took up the "Partial-birth abortion" controversy and proposed legislation and spent another whole day on it in spite of other pending matters such as the national budget, a threatened government shut down, and other emergencies identified by Senator Barbara Boxer (D-CA). The hearing resumed:

The Presiding Officer:	The Senator from Utah is now recognized.
Mr. Hatch:	Mr. President, I rise today to speak in support of H.R.

1833, the Partial-Birth Abortion Ban Act of 1995. [Senator Hatch then spoke of several "misrepresentations" offered by opponents of the bill.]

This ties in closely to what I consider the next misrepresentation made about the partial-birth abortion procedure: the claim that in some circumstances a partial-birth abortion will be the safest option available for a late-term abortion. Testimony and other evidence adduced at the Judiciary Committee hearing amply demonstrate that this is not the case.

An article published in the November 20, 1995, issue of the *American Medical News* quoted Dr. Warren Hern as stating, "I would dispute any statement that this is the safest procedure to use." Dr. Hern is the author of *Abortion Practice*, the Nation's most widely used textbook on abortion standards and procedures. He also stated in that interview that he "has very strong reservations" about the partial-birth abortion procedure banned by this bill. Indeed, referring to the procedure, he stated, "You really can't defend it. I'm not going to tell somebody else that they should not do this procedure. But I'm not going to do it."

In fairness to Dr. Hern, I note that he does not support this bill in part because he feels this is the beginning of legislative efforts to chip away at abortion rights. We have included a statement from him in the Record. His opinion on the procedure, however, is highly instructive.

At this time, Senators Simon (D-IL), Boxer, and others submitted dozens of letters opposing the legislation from women who had been helped by Doctors Haskell and McMahon and from a wide variety of obstetrics and gynecology department chairs at university teaching hospitals from around the country. None of these communications deterred the opponents of abortion.

Soon after this, Representative Canady's bill passed the U.S. Senate in December, 1995 under the sponsorship of Senator Bob Smith (R-NH). President Clinton vetoed the bill on April 6, 1996, but the Republican-controlled House of Representatives overrode the veto on September 19, 1996. There were not sufficient votes in the US Senate to override the veto.

A focus on the health and safety of women seeking abortion became impossible and obscured by the so-called "Partial Birth Abortion" trope as part of the anti-abortion propaganda campaign. In politics, perception becomes the reality, and this image overwhelmed all logic, reason, facts, and other considerations. It became widely accepted in the public that all later abortions were done by the infamous "partial-birth abortion" method, and I had people coming up to me for years asking me how I could do that.

The hysteria over "partial-birth abortion" continued and spread the impression that all abortions had something to do with this. The trope was clearly useful and effective for helping Republicans win elections.

In 1997 the same bill was introduced in the U.S. Senate and was approved in May. But this was after endless debate, more hearings, more testimony, and the startling invocation of my name on both sides of the "debate."

This time, several women who had experienced late abortions by Dr. Jim McMahon using what was essentially the "intact D & E" procedure gave eloquent testimony in person about how important this procedure was to their lives, their health, and their families. There were witnesses on both sides.

Senator Rick Santorum (R-PA), who was newly elected, was the principal sponsor of the bill, and it was supported by Senator Orrin Hatch (R-UT). Amendments to protect the health and safety of women were introduced by Senators Diane Feinstein (D-CA) and Barbara Boxer (D-CA). An amendment introduced by Senate Minority Leader Tom Daschle (D-SD) attempted to assure that the procedure could be performed only if there would be otherwise a "grave risk to health" for the woman if she didn't have the procedure. What follows are excerpts and exact quotes from the *Congressional Record*:

On May 15, 1997, Santorum, quoting me, said that Daschle's restriction would not be a barrier to my performing the abortion because I had asserted in interviews and publications that every pregnancy is a threat to that woman's life and health.

Santorum: It lets there be abortion on demand, anytime, anywhere, on anybody. That is what this [Daschle's] amendment does. It has no restrictions. It is an exception that is not an exception. It is an exception that says that, while we cannot have post-viability abortions except for the health of the mother – let me tell you what Dr. Warren Hern, who wrote the definitive textbook on abortion, called *Abortion Practice*, said. Here it is: *Abortion Practice*, Warren M. Hern, from Colorado. My understanding is this is sort of the definitive textbook on teaching abortions. He does second- and third-trimester abortions and is very outspoken on this subject. He does not use partial-birth abortion, I might add; does not see it as a recognized procedure. But this is what an abortionist who does late-term abortions – in fact, has people come from all over the world to have abortions done by him – this is what he said about, not the Boxer-Feinstein amendment but the Daschle amendment, which we are going to debate next: "I will certify that any pregnancy is a threat to a woman's life and could cause grievous injury to her physical health."

In other words, abortion on demand, anytime during pregnancy. And he believes this. Some would say you are relying on the doctor's bad faith--no. He believes this. And he has a right to believe it. If you look at the statistics, I mean, you know, unfortunately some women do die as a result of pregnancy and, therefore, he could say legitimately there is a risk. Any pregnancy is a risk. It may be a small risk, but it is a risk. And all these bills require, that we are going to hear today, is just a risk. Not a big risk, a risk.

So what we have are limitations without limits. What we have is a farce, to try to fool all of you, to try to fool the press. It has done a very good job fooling the press. We have wonderful headlines about how we are trying to step forward and do something dramatic on limiting late-term abortions. *Phooey*, we have a step forward into the realm of political chicanery, of sham, of obfuscation, illusion, that does nothing but protect the politician at the risk of the baby.

Let me tell you what Dr. Warren Hern said – again, Dr. Warren M. Hern, author of *Abortion Practice*, what I am told is the definitive textbook on abortions who does second- and third-trimester abortions, said it yesterday in the Bergen County Record, and I will repeat it: "I will certify that any pregnancy is a threat to a woman's life and could cause grievous injury to her physical health."

The Boxer-Feinstein amendment does not say anything about physical health. This is the Daschle amendment he is referring to, which also does not do anything. But there is never a case, according to Dr. Hern, where he cannot do an abortion and claim physical health. He says it again, just in case he was misquoted, in today's USA Today: "I say every pregnancy carries a risk of death."

I will talk first about the health exception. I showed the quote today from Dr. Warren Hern. Again, Dr. Hern is an authority on abortion procedures and techniques. He has written *Abortion Practice*, Warren M. Hern. This is the definitive textbook on teaching abortion. He does second- and third-trimester abortions. He does them from all over the world. He instructs doctors through his book and directly on abortion practice. This is what Dr. Hern said yesterday to the Bergen County Record: "I will certify that any pregnancy is a threat to a woman's life and could cause grievous injury to her physical health."

Dr. Hern, who does second- and third-trimester abortions, was commenting on the Daschle amendment. This is one of the leading people in this field. I just suggest that Dr. Hern, while I could not disagree more with what Dr. Hern says, the fact of the matter is that he can stand there and, in good conscience, say that to not only the Bergen County Record, but to *USA Today* – he repeated the statement in case there is no validity to the original statement, a different quote, similar in nature – that any pregnancy could be a threat and could cause grievous injury – I know this is the language the press keeps honing in on, "grievous injury" to physical health. Here it is.

"I have a lot of other things I am going to say about health and why the health exception, as drafted in this amendment, is a very broad loophole and will not restrict abortions. The fact that the doctor is the one to certify, what does that mean? That is pretty much current law. The doctor certifies when there is a health reason to do an abortion, and we say we are going to ban these, but the doctors determine when there is an exception."

Senator Daschle responded: The Senator from Pennsylvania has offered legislation that will clearly not stop one abortion because every other abortion procedure is available. He recognizes that. So I don't know how anyone could argue that his ban of a procedure is a ban of abortion, because it doesn't stop all of the other procedures. So how does it stop abortion?

As to Dr. Hern, *that man is going to jail,* and I will just tell him on the record in public right now, *Dr. Hern, you're going to jail for perjury if this legislation passes and you lie about the need for unnecessary abortions you perform.* If you don't go to jail, there is something wrong with our legal system, not with the law as it is written.

With regard to making the determination, that it is up to the doctor, let me just say one last thing. I don't know what the Senator or any other Senator who supports H.R. 1122 would say if a doctor said, "Well, I'm going to take Dr. Hern's approach 'to save the life of a mother,'" which is a clause in their bill, "I'm going to use dilation and extraction to save the life of the mother. I can do that. It's legal." Dr. Hern should love that language. That is still available.

So if we distrust the veracity of a doctor in my circumstances, I would think we would be reciprocal in distrusting the veracity of any doctor who could use any out and, indeed, they allow an out, not to mention all the other alternative abortion procedures. So there are differences between us in spite of the good intentions we have, in spite of the fact I know we both want to come to the same conclusion.

My colleague from Pennsylvania, Senator Santorum, has already read the quote from Dr. Warren Hern, but it is appropriate to hear it again because it is directly on point to this issue. Dr. Warren Hern, a Colorado abortionist who has performed hundreds of late-term abortions, has already stated that he will certify that any pregnant woman can meet the standard of the Daschle amendment. "I will certify that any pregnancy is a threat to a woman's life and could cause grievous injury to her physical health." Any pregnant woman.

The Presiding Officer: The Democratic leader is recognized.

Mr. Daschle: I listened with great interest to the distinguished Senator from Ohio. He mentioned Dr. Hern's remark that he would use life or grievous injury. That was his term, life or grievous injury as a reason to continue an abortion practice. I cite his remark because, of course, H.R. 1122 uses life as a reason, justifiably, to allow the late-term abortion, the dilation and extraction method that the bill otherwise prohibits from being used. So, if Dr. Hern would use health, he would use life, as he indicated, making meaningless the language in H.R. 1122, as well. I just hope we apply the same standards to both bills in our debate as to what the efficacy of language will be. Indeed, if people are going to find loopholes, they will find them in H.R. 1122, as in our bill. But, again, *I reiterate that Dr. Hern, with our language, will go to jail, will go to jail.*

Keep Government out of this. Leave it with the physician. *But we will throw that physician in jail.* The Daschle abortion ban spares viable fetuses, proposals stricter than the GOP measure. *They will throw him in jail, and then, keep Government out.*[9]

This threat toward me was repeated various times, and Senator Mary Landrieu (D-LA) emphasized it by saying that "Dr. Hern" would "lose his medical license. He will not be able to practice." This went on and on. The Senate debate, citing my name various times, what quoted at length in newspaper columns including Robert Novack in the *Washington Post* and Frank Murray in the *Washington Times*.

Eventually, the Senate bill passed by an overwhelming 2–1 majority in the Senate in May 1997, was passed by the House with a 295–136 majority on October 8 and sent to the White House for approval by the president. Clinton vetoed the Partial-Birth Abortion Ban for the second time on October 10, 1997.

Here's my reaction to listening to and reading about the continuing debate on the floor of the United States Senate in which my name, comments to the news media, and published works were cited by the senators (published as an op-ed article in the *New York Times* on May 24, 1997):[10]

> As I watched the Senate debate on late-term abortions this week, I was struck by the surreal quality of the remarks. The oratory from both sides had nothing to do with the anguish faced by my patients and their families, yet the results will profoundly affect their lives.
>
> Families sometimes ask me to do things that might be illegal if the bill the Senate passed on Wednesday or anything like it ever becomes law. The bill's sponsors say it would only ban a procedure that abortion foes call "partial birth" abortion, in which a living fetus is partially delivered and its skull collapsed so it can be delivered intact. But the legislation is so vaguely worded that doctors have little idea of what would really be banned under it.
>
> It is true that the Senate does not have the votes to override a likely Presidential veto. But the foes of abortion will keep sponsoring legislation that keeps doctors guessing about what they are allowed to do.
>
> Many families that come to me for late-term abortions – after 24 to 26 weeks of pregnancy or later – want the fetus to be delivered intact. I never make a guarantee; my first objective is to make the procedure as safe as possible for the woman. But having the fetus delivered intact is safer at some stages of pregnancy than performing an abortion with forceps and dismembering the fetus in the womb. And sometimes there are other reasons to keep the fetus intact.
>
> A couple came to me recently in despair. The woman's fetus was missing both arms and most of one leg and had other deformities indicating that if it were born alive at term it would be severely impaired, physically and mentally, and would likely never gain consciousness. The woman and her husband wanted the fetus to be delivered intact. I was able to do so.
>
> After the abortion, my staff and I wrapped the fetus in a baby blanket and presented it to the couple. It was now their stillborn baby. The woman gently and lovingly stroked it with her fingers. She wept a little. Her husband held his head in his hands and was silent. After five or 10 minutes, she folded the blanket and covered her baby, and I took it away.
>
> If the bill to ban "partial birth" abortion were to become law, could I be prosecuted in a case like this? Absolutely. Could I be convicted? I don't think so, but I don't know. One reason is that the term "partial birth" abortion does not

occur anywhere in medical literature – the Senate wants to ban a procedure that doctors don't think exists.

One might also think I would be safe because the fetus was already dead when I delivered it. But the legislation is so vague that there is no way to find out except to see if the sheriff arrested me. If I were nervous about being arrested, I would be better off not performing any late-term abortions at all.

That, of course, is the intent of the bill: to keep doctors from performing any abortion. All the various Congressional proposals to ban "partial birth" abortion have shared this unconstitutional vagueness. "This legislation leaves doctors unable to determine whether the medical care they are providing is a criminal act," says Janet Benshoof, president of the Center for Reproductive Law and Policy. "Moreover, it prohibits second trimester abortion in violation of the Supreme Court's guarantee that women can make these private choices free of governmental interference."

But one part of the bill is not vague: It makes no distinction between second trimester abortions and those performed after the fetus is viable. "Partial birth" abortions would be banned even when the woman's health is jeopardized and when there is a serious fetal abnormality.

The American Medical Association's support of the bill – after the sponsors made a few "compromises" in language intended to better protect doctors from criminal prosecution – was misguided and cynical. The bill, as amended, protects only doctors who are performing complicated term deliveries; the A.M.A.'s sham protections would leave doctors who perform abortions vulnerable to prosecution. That's why the American College of Obstetricians and Gynecologists still opposes it.

President Clinton is right to object to this dangerous measure. And he would do well to be suspicious of all such attempts to limit late-term abortion – even those "compromise" proposals from legislators who claim to support abortion rights."

[*end of article*]

* * *

The following year, an extensive article reviewing the complex legal and medical arguments for and against the proposed ban was published in the *University of Pittsburgh Law Review* by Professor Ann MacLean Massie: So-Called "So-Called "Partial-Birth Abortion" Bans: Bad Medicine? Maybe. Bad Law? Definitely!" Citing my textbook, *Abortion Practice*, and my submitted testimony before the Senate Judiciary Committee, she states, "Dr. Hern's approach [of causing fetal demise by intrafetal injection prior to the abortion procedure as part of the operative protocol for late abortion] may turn out to be the better norm for defining the medical standard of care, whatever surgical technique the physician plans for the actual abortion. However, only the medical community can decide this."[11]

But it wasn't over. In 2002, the Republican-controlled House and Senate passed the "Partial-Birth Abortion Ban Act" again, and this time, President George W. Bush signed the bill into law on November 5, 2003 – one year before he was up for reelection.

At the signing ceremony, Bush was surrounded by aging white men in dark suits who could not get pregnant. There were no women present at the signing and no physicians.

Just before the signing of this bill, *Slate* magazine published my article, "Did I violate the partial-birth abortion ban?" on October 27, 2003.[12] In my article, I raised a number of questions that had not been answered prior to the passage of this bill and as it made its way to the president's desk:

> Exactly which procedures will be banned, and which doctors prosecuted? Will the anti-abortion lobby be happier with the alternative methods to which doctors will resort? If not, which methods and doctors will be targeted next? Will this ban have a chilling effect on related procedures? If so, will it prevent abortions—or births?

> I don't know the answers to the questions I've posed above, and neither does Congress. No physician expert on late abortion has ever testified in person before a congressional committee. No peer-reviewed articles or case reports have ever been published describing anything such as "partial-birth" abortion, "Intact D&E" (for "dilation and extraction"), or any of its synonyms. There have been no descriptions of its complication rates and no published studies comparing its complication rates with those of any other method of late abortion. What I do know is that the political exploitation of this issue is confusing and frightening my patients.

> Recently, I received a call from a woman whose physician had discovered catastrophic genetic and developmental defects in the fetus she is carrying. The pregnancy was profoundly desired, and the diagnosis was devastating for her and her husband. She called me with great anxiety to find out whether passage of the "partial-birth" ban by the Senate would mean that she could not come to my office for help because my work would be illegal. She was also horrified by the images that she had seen and the terminology she had heard in the congressional debates. I reassured her that I do not perform the "partial-birth" procedure and that there is no likelihood that the ban's passage would close my office and keep me from seeing her. The fetus cannot be delivered "alive" in my procedure—as the ban stipulates in defining prohibited procedures— because I begin by giving the fetus an injection that stops its heart immediately. I treat the woman's cervix to cause it to open during the next two days. On the third day, under anesthesia, the membranes are ruptured, allowing the amniotic fluid to escape. Medicine is given to make the uterus contract, and the dead fetus is delivered or removed with forceps. Many variations of this sequence are possible, depending on the woman's medical condition and surgical indications.

> On the same day I got that call, I received a call from another woman who hoped to become pregnant but wanted to be reassured that, in spite of passage of the "partial-birth" ban, she would still be able to terminate the pregnancy if a serious genetic defect were discovered at, say, 20 weeks of pregnancy. Because of her history, she has an especially high risk of such a scenario. Without reassurance, she would avoid pregnancy entirely. Again, I reassured her that I would be here for her if she needs me.

> But what if the people enforcing the "partial-birth" ban decide for some reason—because they doubt that my injection worked, for example—that it covers

what I do? Or what if other doctors decide to follow the same procedure of causing fetal death by injection some time—even a day or two—before the extraction is performed? If the intact delivery of the living fetus (the "birth" imagery) is what bothers lawmakers, will they ban this method as well? Depending on the doctor, the alternative to intact extraction could be dismemberment of the fetus in the uterus, which may be more dangerous for the woman and no less troubling to look at. Is that what Congress wants? Who gets to decide what is safer for the woman: the expert physician or Congress?

Earlier this year, I began an abortion on a young woman who was 17 weeks pregnant. Because of the two days of prior treatment, the amniotic membranes were visible and bulging. I ruptured the membranes and released the fluid to reduce the risk of amniotic fluid embolism. Then I inserted my forceps into the uterus and applied them to the head of the fetus, which was still alive, since fetal injection is not done at that stage of pregnancy. I closed the forceps, crushing the skull of the fetus, and withdrew the forceps. The fetus, now dead, slid out more or less intact. With the next pass of the forceps, I grasped the placenta, and it came out in one piece. Within a few seconds, I had completed my routine exploration of the uterus and sharp curettage. The blood loss would just fill a tablespoon. The patient, who was awake, hardly felt the operation. She was relieved, grateful, and safe. She wants to have children in the future.

Did I do a "partial-birth" abortion? Will John Ashcroft prosecute me? Stay tuned."

[*end of article in* Slate]

---

* * *

In his October 8, 2004, debate with John Kerry, Bush bragged that he had signed the ban on "partial-birth abortion" into law.

Dr. Lee Carhart, who was using the "intact D & E" method for late abortions, challenged Nebraska's prohibition against this procedure. He carried the day all the way to the U.S. Supreme Court, which ruled, in *Stenberg v. Carhart* (2000), that the law had no provision for saving the woman's life, and the law prohibited other forms of abortion that were safe for women. The law was declared to be unconstitutional. The principal lengthy dissenting opinion was written by Justice Anthony Kennedy, a Catholic. It could have been prepared in the offices of the anti-abortion National Right to Life Committee, and it probably was.

But once more, this was not the end of the story. Justice Sandra Day O'Connor, who had nominally supported abortion choice in *Casey*, was replaced by Samuel Alito, a conservative opponent of abortion, in 2006. When the Nebraska ban on "partial-birth abortion" came before the Court again in late 2006 in the form of *Gonzalez v. Carhart*, in which Dr. Carhart challenged the congressional Partial-Birth Abortion Ban of 2003, O'Connor's pro-choice vote had been replaced by Justice Alito, also a practicing Catholic opposed to abortion. In *Gonzalez v. Carhart*, because of a change in personnel, the Court decided that the Congressional "Partial-Birth Abortion Ban" was, in fact, constitutional, and they upheld the law. Lower courts had struck it down since, as with the Nebraska law, it had no health exception. But now the Court had another anti-abortion justice and an anti-abortion president who happily and proudly signed it into law.

So much for a "government of laws." A new justice gave the Court a new conservative majority, and they won the day.

The decision of the U.S. Supreme Court on *Gonzalez vs. Carhart* reversing the previous *Stenberg v. Carhart* decision of 2006 striking down the Nebraska law as unconstitutional, thereby upholding the constitutionality of the Nebraska law against "partial-birth abortion" because of this change of personnel in the Court, came down on April 18, 2007. Two weeks later, the *Colorado Statesman* published my editorial comment on this decision under the headline "The doctor's dilemma—truly delusional decisions from the Supreme Court":[13]

Many years ago, a young woman with a desired pregnancy was referred to me by her physician in northern Colorado because tests had shown a dangerous genetic disorder in the fetus. The chromosomal abnormality was not only lethal for the fetus; it posed a risk to the woman's health. She was in danger of developing severe high blood pressure due to changes in the placenta that accompanied this condition. She was about 22 weeks pregnant.

When the woman arrived at my office, she didn't feel well. Her blood pressure was normal. By the time I got her to the operating room for the first steps of a three-day abortion procedure, her blood pressure was elevated. By the time we had finished this first step, it was higher. After watching her for a short time, I decided that she needed to be in the hospital. Her blood pressure continued to go up dangerously in spite of medications now being administered by medical colleagues and nurses who were experts in the management of these problems.

By midnight, her kidneys started to shut down. She stopped producing urine. We were worried about her having seizures or a stroke. Meantime, the preparations that were necessary to perform an abortion safely at this stage of pregnancy had hardly begun. It soon became apparent that we could not wait for those measures to have their effect. By 3 a.m., I concluded that my patient would not survive until dawn if I didn't do the abortion right then, so I did. The chief of obstetrics, who had no experience with this kind of abortion, stood behind me as I operated. Without the abortion to empty the woman's uterus, she would die. Difficult as it was, it was safer for her than an abdominal operation to cut open her uterus or remove the uterus along with the fetus.

The woman survived without complications, but it took a long time to bring down her blood pressure and get other systems back to normal.

I couldn't stop at 3 a.m. to find out from a lawyer whether the operation I was about to perform was exactly as prescribed and not prohibited in any way by Congress. That is the kind of problem created by the law that was upheld by the Supreme Court on Wednesday, April 18.

There are innumerable problems with the "Partial Birth Abortion Ban Act of 2003" that was upheld by the Supreme Court in *Gonzales v. Carhart*, starting with the fact that no committee in either the House or the Senate has ever heard spoken testimony from or questioned a physician expert in late abortion before it was passed by Congress and signed into law by the President.

I was present at the only hearing before the U.S. Senate Judiciary Committee on November 17, 1995 with prepared testimony at the request of the minority counsel who worked for Senator Kennedy. Pro-choice leaders did not want me to testify because I disagreed with their statements that the "partial-birth abortion" technique was the "safest way to do late abortions." There has never been any evidence for this assertion, which was repeated in court by those opposing this absurd law.

There is no way for a physician to read this law and know whether he or she would be prosecuted for exercising their medical judgment for a patient. Justice Kennedy's opinion upholding the law does not help. It is an obscene and convoluted mass of contradictions that brings judicial micromanagement into difficult medical decisions that must be made in minutes or seconds. It is delusional to assert that this law, and worse, this decision, does not keep doctors from practicing good medicine for their patients. It is surreal.

The only certain way to avoid prosecution under this law is not to perform abortions.

Even though Congress passed the 'Partial Birth Abortion Ban Act of 2003' without reference to any facts or expert testimony, and even though Justice Kennedy stated that Congress had made assertions contrary to fact, he and his four male Catholic brethren, all appointed by Republican presidents, voted to uphold the law. It is the first time that Congress has passed a law prohibiting a specific medical or surgical procedure. There are no exceptions to protect a woman's health, even in an emergency.

In this case, it is a procedure reported by one physician at a private medical conference in 1992 and which has never been described in the medical literature. Although I specialize in late abortion, I do not personally know anyone who does this procedure including the physician who made the report in 1992. No one knows who performs it or how many are done.

What we do know now as the result of this decision is that the radical religious right has won the struggle for power in this country. It is a triumph of ideology and politics over facts and reason.

[end of article]

***

These facts and arguments obviously have had zero effect on the political hysteria and exploitation of the abortion issue.

In current abortion practice, this controversy was moot before it began because the standard of care in late abortion includes the induction of fetal demise before the surgical procedure of abortion begins. This has been the case for decades as shown by my own clinical reports beginning in 1980.[14]

The foregoing U.S. Senate debates and bills were meaningless political pornography for the sole purpose of electing Republicans although it also succeeded for the senators as lascivious entertainment. It was public voyeurism.

More fun than the issue of the national debt ceiling.

It is bizarre that the U.S. Senate, the "greatest deliberative body in the world," with issues before it such as war and peace; poverty; racial and ethnic equality in American society; economic and social injustice; the consideration and choice of federal judges and U.S. Supreme Court justices; the regulation of commerce, science, and industry; the necessity of understanding climate changes on our society; the inexorable growth of world population; the complex issues surrounding foreign affairs and defense of the country; should spend hours and days of its time considering the private decisions of unknown women and private parts of women's anatomy of which they have no understanding or knowledge much less medical expertise, is utterly baffling.

It was all pointless as well as inappropriate.

The foregoing debate and discussions among the male members of the U.S. Senate amounted to mutual masturbation – a U.S. Senate "circle jerk." What a way for the senators to spend their time. Children should not be allowed to watch. Even at that, it wasn't even very good as X-rated material.

Turn off the C-SPAN, please.

Notes

1 Temkin, O. *Soranus' Gynecology*. Baltimore: Johns Hopkins University Press, 1991.
2 Mauriceau, *op. cit.*
3 Hern, W.M. Second-trimester surgical abortion. In Global Library of Women's Medicine, 2nd edition. Hern, W, *Glob libr.women's med. (ISSN: 1756-2228)* 2011; DOI 10.3843/GLOWM.10442 Revised August, 2016 At https://www.glowm.com/section_view/item/441; Hern, W.M. Late abortion: Clinical and ethical issues. *In Whose Choice Is It? Abortion, Medicine and the Law*, 7th edition (David F. Walbert and J. Douglas Butler, Eds.). Chicago: American Bar Association. https://www.drhern.com/wp-content/uploads/2023/05/Late-abortion-clinical-ethical-issues-8-1-2021.pdf
4 Gregg, R.B. Rhetorical strategies for a culture war: Abortion in the 1992 campaign. *Communication Quarterly*, 42(3):229–43, 1994. https://doi.org/10.1080/01463379409369931; Dionne, E.J. Abortion rights supporters claim election gains. *Washington Post*, November 9, 1992. https://www.washingtonpost.com/archive/politics/1992/11/09/abortion-rights-supporters-claim-election-gains/962212a9-1c1f-44a3-9b08-51e01f471058/
5 Condit, C.M. *Decoding Abortion Rhetoric: Communicating Social Change*. Urbana: University of Illinois Press, 1990.
6 Blanchard, D.A., and Prewitt, T.J. *Religious Violence and Abortion: The Gideon Project*. Gainesville: the University Press of Florida, 1993.; Blanchard, D.A. *The Anti-abortion Movement and the Rise of the Religious Right: From Polite to Fiery Protest*. Woodridge: Twayne Publishers, 1994.
7 Ginsburg, F.D. *Contested Lives: The Abortion Debate in an American Community*. Berkeley: University of California Press, 1989.
8 Grobstein, C. *Science and the Unborn: Choosing Human Futures*. New York: Basic Books, 1988.
9 U.S. Senate debate on "Partial-birth abortion," May 15, 1997. Congressional Record pp 8328, 8347, 8348, 8351, 8354, 8358, 8363, 8366, 8379. https://www.govinfo.gov/content/pkg/GPO-CRECB-1997-pt6/pdf/GPO-CRECB-1997-pt6-6-1.pdf;C-SPANhttps://www.c-span.org/video/?81254-1/late-term-abortion-debate#!
10 Hern, W.M. Abortion bill skips the fine print. Op-Ed Page, *New York Times*, May 24, 1997. https://www.nytimes.com/1997/05/24/opinion/abortion-bill-skips-the-fine print.html ; https://www.drhern.com/wp-content/uploads/2019/05/Abortion-Bill-Skips-the-Fine-Print.pdf
11 Massie, A.M. So-Called "So-Called "Partial-Birth Abortion" Bans: Bad Medicine? Maybe. Bad Law? Definitely!" *University of Pittsburgh Law Review* 59(2): 301–80, 1998. https://heinonline.org/HOL/LandingPage?handle=hein.journals/upitt59&div=4&id=&page=https://scholarlycommons.law.wlu.edu/cgi/viewcontent.cgi?article=1098amp;context=wlufac
12 Hern, W.M. Did I violate the Partial-Birth Abortion Ban? *Slate*, October 22, 2003. At https://slate.com/technology/2003/10/did-i-violate-the-partial-birth-abortion-ban.html
13 Hern, W.M. The doctor's dilemma: Truly delusional decisions from the Supreme Court. Guest opinion, *Colorado Statesman* 108(18):6. May 4, 2007. https://www.drhern.com/wp-content/uploads/2018/05/doctors-dilemma.pdf.
14 Hern, W.M. *Late Abortion Clinical Reports, Book Chapters*. www.drhern.com/publication-category/late-abortion-clinical-reports-book-chapters/

16 The language of abortion – words matter

In the 1970s, Channel 7 in Denver ran a series of programs concerning abortion, and I was invited to participate in several of them. One program was designed as a sort of town hall, and people got to take turns expressing their views. On this occasion, I was in line with everyone else, including, of course, people who were sincerely opposed to abortion, and they knew that this was my clinical specialty as a physician.

A man who was standing next to me struck up a pleasant conversation and began expressing his anguish about the subject. He was a blue-collar worker from a Catholic family, and we began discussing his concerns. "When my wife is pregnant, she doesn't say, 'I'm going to have a fetus,' she says, 'I'm going to have a baby.' That seems normal to me. The other way doesn't." "Well," I said, "It is normal to say that she's going to have a baby, because that's what happens usually unless you decide to end the pregnancy. In medical terms, it's a 'fetus' until it's born, and then it's a 'baby,' but there's nothing wrong with calling it a 'baby' if that's how you feel about it. The issue is really who's going to make the decision to carry the pregnancy to term and have a 'baby' or decide to end the pregnancy with an abortion. The woman needs to make that decision," I said. "Well, that's not right," he said. "Nobody should be able to end that baby's life." "It depends on your point of view, but the law needs to let women make that decision themselves since they are the ones who are pregnant," I said. "I don't like this," he said. "It's a change in how we think about women and pregnancy," I said, "and many people don't like it. That's why we are having this discussion."

The man's anguish and discomfort was genuine and sincere. There was no rancor. He didn't threaten me or say anything nasty to me. It was a civilized conversation.

That kind of conversation no longer seems possible. A large part of that is because of the inflammatory language used by opponents of abortion. They call those of us who perform abortions and help women "baby killers," "child killers," "murderers," and many other epithets. Doctors are demonized and cast as subhuman animals. The fetus is fetishized and imbued with powers it does not have.

The human embryo has a specialized tube in the early weeks of growth that begins contracting rhythmically and pushing blood through primitive arteries, and that is called a "heartbeat" by enemies of abortion even though there is no "heart."

The language around abortion has become a weapon in the psychological warfare against abortion by enemies who take no prisoners. "Don't kill your baby," anti-abortion protesters scream at my patients, many of whom have desired pregnancies they are heartbroken to end for important medical reasons.

DOI: 10.4324/9781003514961-17

"Pro-life"

All of the physicians and others who are assassinated by "peaceful" anti-abortion demonstrators have been killed by people who call themselves "pro-life." This vicious, vile propaganda term is not only a lie, it is a slander against those of us who help women because it casts us as "pro-death" or "anti-life" even though we save many women's lives in our work. It is an Orwellian concealment of the consignment by anti-abortion fanatics of women to the unwanted risks of pregnancy and sometimes, too often, death. It shows that the anti-abortion fanatics care nothing about either the truth or the welfare and life of the woman. To them, she is an inanimate hollow vessel whose only purpose is as a reproductive machine. It is the fulfillment of one physician's inhumane description of women: "Think of a woman as a uterus surrounded by a supporting organism and a directing personality."

This insulting slander is perpetuated by some mainstream journalists and broadcasters, such as Chris Matthews and Ellen Goodman, writers like Willam Saletan, who poses as a pro-choice intellectual, and Mary Ziegler, a legal historian who writes loving odes to anti-abortion "pro-life" fanatics presented as "history."[1] Jennifer Holland has written a superb book, *Tiny You*, about the history of the Western anti-abortion movement, but her otherwise extremely important book is flawed by the disturbing use of this profoundly vicious propaganda term.

It is an unforgivable oxymoron.[2]

In these contexts, the propaganda term "pro-life" used as a neutral, objective adjective is a deadly weapon against those of us who help women. It is an enabling tool for those who think of themselves as "pro-life" that justifies killing those of us who are, by contrast in this fevered hall of mirrors, "pro-death." The woman whose life is at stake in many ways is an ignored non-entity. The focus is on the fetus, a small demigod to be protected at all costs, including killing doctors who perform abortions. It is a deeply pathological and dangerous delusion. It is called *Killing for Life,* which also happens to be the title of an indispensable book by Carol Mason.[3]

"The idea that the fetus has rights is preposterous: it poses a threat to the woman's life and health" (from *Tiny You*, by Jennifer Holland).[4]

The total, overwhelming success of the anti-abortion fanatics in this deadly psychological warfare is illustrated by the thoughtless and pervasive use of the term "pro-life" by all kinds of journalists and public intellectuals as though it were really a neutral, objective adjective.

"Pro-life" is a rally cry and slogan for a totalitarian white supremacist movement that forces white women to have babies and forces other women with fewer resources to face the higher death risks of pregnancy and childbirth without adequate care. Black women in the United States have a maternal mortality ratio three times as high as white women; in Alabama, it is five times higher for Black women.

For those of us who help women and understand that safe abortion is a fundamental part of women's health care, the use of this phrase is like using a racial epithet or a kick in the vital parts. It is inexcusable. It is worse coming from those who pose as neutral or "pro-choice" because it means that the speaker is thoughtless, careless, and indifferent to the real meaning of this cruel slogan.

"It's what they want to be called"

Writers like William Saletan and others who pose as "pro-choice" intellectuals insist on calling anti-abortion fanatics "pro-life" because – *"that's what they want to be called."*

This is an absurd and obscene reason for calling the anti-abortion terrorists the opposite of what they are, and it is a hideous lie and insult to those of us who help women. It is pure sophistry.

A thought experiment: What if the Nazis decided that they wanted to be called *"The Bringers of Mother's Milk, Love, and Honey?"*

Over a period of two days, on September 29 and 30, 1941, Nazi military units murdered 33,771 Jews at Babyn Yar in Ukraine.[5]

Did the Reuters headline on October 1 state *"The Bringers of Mothers' Milk, Love and Honey massacred 33,771 Jews at Babyn Yar earlier this week?"* No. They were murdered by the Nazis. And the Nazis were ruthless. So are the Christian anti-abortion fanatics.

"Providers" – the commodification of abortion

The commodification of abortion is seen in the classification of women who come to clinics for help as "clients." They are not seen as people receiving "medical care," and this enables the enemies of safe abortion to deny the fact that safe abortion services constitute an important kind of "medical care."

In a normal physician's office of any kind, and in a hospital, the people coming there for help are called "patients." This is distinguished from those who are going to insurance agents, who have "clients"; lawyers, who have "clients"; car salesmen, who have "customers"; and grocers, who have "customers." Physicians have "patients." But the pro-choice community, going along with the rest of the health-care community, no longer calls physicians "physicians" or nurses "nurses." They are "providers." This is a way of disinfecting the transaction from the stigma of abortion. There are "providers" of screwdrivers to the Pentagon, there are those who are "providers" of tires to the trucking industry, and there are the "providers" of Meals on Wheels. There are no "providers" of brain tumor surgery, no "providers" of heart transplants or "appendectomy providers," but there are "abortion providers."

It's absurd and dehumanizing.

I don't "provide" abortions. I am a physician. I "perform" abortions as a part of my personal service and care for a "patient" who is not a "client." She is a "person," not a "consumer." I am not selling bananas, candy bars, or toys.

Calling me a "provider" strips away my humanity, my identity, my long experience and training as a physician and surgeon, my practice of medicine in the long tradition of medical care, and my commitment to helping other people who, in this case, happen to be "women," not "clients." I am, therefore, not part of an economic machine that consists of "providers" and "consumers." How do you "consume" an abortion? Is it simply an economic act to be included with the Gross National Product? To economists, maybe. Economists don't see "patients." Economists see "numbers." I see people who are "patients."

Performing an abortion is a complex set of procedures beginning with my greeting my patient in a friendly and considerate manner and showing her that I am a compassionate and skilled medical practitioner who is there to help her solve a problem with her body, which, in this case, is a pregnancy that may be threatening her life or a process over which she herself has no control and wishes to end in the safest manner possible. She is not just a uterus on two legs. She is a "person" who is my "patient," and I am also a person who is a "physician." I am not a "provider." I went to "medical school," not "provider school."

"Abortionist"

"Abortionist" is an ugly term used to describe incompetent and unscrupulous criminals performing unsafe abortions in back-alley places like garages and workshops. It was commonly used in the past also to refer to non-medical practitioners performing abortions who may have been quite competent. It remains as a stigmatizing epithet the anti-abortion fanatics use to vilify and damage skilled, conscientious, and highly professional doctors and nurses who are performing safe abortions for women who need them. Its use is part of the psychological warfare against safe abortion by unscrupulous opponents of abortion. Its use is acutely pejorative and highly effective in continuing this stigma. It has no use in expressions that purport to support safe, legal abortion services.

Do you know any "appendectomists?"

"Baby" – or "fetus"?

When I am speaking to the patient, I do not refer to the fetus as a "baby" even though she may wish to do so. I use neutral language while respecting her feelings and her right to think about her pregnancy and developing embryo or fetus in any way she wishes. If she has a pregnancy with a serious fetal anomaly, I don't say, "I'm sorry your baby has.... (condition)…" I say, "I'm sorry about what has happened to your pregnancy." I try in this way to avoid adding to her emotional anguish. Women who have been brutally raped and who are horrified by a resulting pregnancy do not want to talk about their "baby."

After the abortion in the case of an advanced pregnancy with a serious fetal anomaly or genetic disorder, many patients want to have a viewing and hold their fetus. My staff prepares the fetus and dresses it in baby clothes that we provide for current patients, and one of us brings it into the patient's recovery room for viewing. Sometimes, patients want a family photo, including the husband or partner. I also take a photo of the clothed fetus in a blanket-covered basin as prepared by my staff. We do not refer to the fetus as a "baby," but sometimes the patients do, and they may give their baby a name.

These are tender and vulnerable moments in people's lives, and they need to be left alone and respected in their pain of a pregnancy loss. This fact is incomprehensible to those who oppose abortion, shout at women coming into my office or any other clinic, and whose policy is to kill doctors who help women. They have no pity.

We who help women through this crisis and difficult experience need to be left alone to help them.

Our most vicious adversaries against this human need at this time are self-righteous Christians and the Christians who control the Republican Party. As a woman enters my office to end a desired pregnancy that she desperately wants because of the prospect of endless pain and suffering for the child she would have after birth and the endless anguish of her family, the Christians shout "Don't kill your *baby*." So much for Christian love and compassion.

"*Projecting unearned guilt onto women is politically useful and effective for getting power.*" (Holland, ibid.)[6]

"Abortion on demand"

"Abortion on demand" is a term that was coined by a non-physician, Garrett Hardin, a brilliant scientist who was concerned about uncontrolled growth of the human population and the unjust limits women experienced in controlling their own fertility. This slogan commodifies abortion, which is a medical and surgical treatment of pregnancy; it is not a consumer product. "Abortion on demand" dehumanizes and trivializes the dedication, work, and risks and commitment of physicians, nurses, counselors, and others who risk their lives to help women. "Abortion on demand" was a cry taken up by the supporters of women's rights to "control their own bodies" (make decisions about their own bodies). In this context, the attack on anti-abortion laws wielded the weapons of "rights" and social justice, with an occasional nod to the risks faced by women in pregnancy.

Any woman who walks into my office and "demands" an abortion will not get one in my office. I am a physician, a person, and not an abortion-dispensing machine. Such a "demand" is disrespectful and denies my humanity. It is disrespectful of my skilled, experienced, dedicated staff of nurses, counselors, laboratory technicians, and patient coordinators who answer the phone, my medical record assistants, and everyone else on my staff who are dedicated to give women and their families the support they need for a crisis in their lives. Everybody in my office risks their lives every day to help women.

The woman has a right to "request" an abortion, which I, as a physician, am prepared to perform for her subject to many factors of medical judgment, among other things. But "demanding" an abortion ignores and discards the humanity and care that we offer the person in need.

As a political slogan, "abortion on demand" is not useful, is absurd, and is not politically helpful. Used by opponents of abortion, it is mindless. "Abortion is health care" is more to the point because it is, and it is critical to the health and safety of women. "Abortion on demand" obliterates that fact.

"Rights of the fetus" – or rights of the woman?

The emphasis on women's "rights," which is totally reasonable and correct, devolved into a struggle for power instead of an effort to help women have rational, safe, medical care for the condition of pregnancy. Most of the lawsuits reaching the courts exemplify this struggle for power, and this has contributed to the long-term successful political effort to control the coercive power of the state by appointment of anti-abortion judges as well as justices of the U.S. Supreme Court. This has taken the struggle for abortion rights and the basic rights of women to make decisions about their own lives and bodies directly into the voting booth and placed that power in the hands of people like Mitch McConnell who are indifferent to women's suffering. Unfortunately, the enemies of women, women's health care, and women's rights have understood this much better over the past 50 years than the people who regard themselves as "pro-choice" – with some exceptions. Some of those who are on the side of women in this matter understand the political stakes, but some of them are pushed aside by those who don't.

One national leader whose organization was dedicated to using votes and political power to defend women's rights to safe abortion was relieved of her job by those who thought this political effort was undignified. The respectable and correct alternative was considered to be lobbying anti-abortion legislators and trying to get them to vote the right way. Good luck with that. She was fired from her job of organizing pro-choice voters in the late 1970s.

How many elections have been lost since then to politicians who would enslave women by sponsoring anti-abortion legislation and confirming federal judges and Supreme Court justices who are against abortion?

"The idea that the fetus has rights is preposterous: it poses a threat to the woman's life and health." (Holland, ibid.)[7]

Exceptions in anti-abortion legislation

Speaking of exceptions, how do you have a law that outlaws abortion "except" for certain circumstances? How do you decide what the "exceptions" are, who makes that decision, and what is the justification for "exceptions" or "no exceptions?" Once the focus is off the real threat to each woman's life and health with each abortion, the argument about "exceptions" and "rights" and "abortion on demand" doesn't make any sense. It's absurd except to those who use these fraudulent phrases to keep women from having safe abortions by dominating the voting booths and electing Republican candidates.

The blatant fraudulence of the anti-abortion laws with "exceptions" for rape, fetal anomalies, or "life of the mother" was exposed in Texas with the case of Kate Cox, a mother of two and with a history of two cesarean deliveries with a desired pregnancy in which the fetus was fatally afflicted with Trisomy 18. Her life was threatened by complications in her pregnancy and the fact that she would have to have a third cesarean delivery if she was forced to give birth to a fetus that was hopelessly impaired and doomed. After going through the legal nightmare of successfully appealing to a court for an "exception" so she could end the pregnancy, the court was overruled by Ken Paxton, the anti-abortion Attorney General of Texas, and Ms. Cox had to leave the state to have an abortion. It was cruel and unusual punishment for having a life-threatening and complicated pregnancy. The "exceptions" in anti-abortion laws are dishonest and solely cosmetic. They are not meaningful.

Many women who seek abortions are not "mothers" because they haven't had children. They are "women." The anti-abortion legislation that calls for exceptions for "life of the mother" define the "woman" as a "mother," not a "woman" because, of course being a "mother" is what "women" are *for*. She is a "mother" after she has had a "baby," but she is primarily and first a "woman." The anti-abortion legislation erases this distinction and trivializes the survival and needs of the "woman" by using this terminology.

Anti-abortion legislation declares that a woman may have an abortion only if the pregnancy endangers a "major bodily function." What about "survival?" What's a "major bodily function," and how is it different from a "minor bodily function?" Who decides what's a "major bodily function?" How about a legislator who is a pest exterminator (think of Tom DeLay[8] as your medical advisor) or a corrupt real estate executive (think of Donald Trump)?

What if women take over the legislature and decide that men's penises are a "minor bodily function" compared to, say, the heart or lungs? After all, they're only good for having sex (especially rape) and being an extension of the urethra. Women have gotten by just fine for a long time without having penises.

Legislators without (or even with) a medical education deciding what kind of health care women can have according to whether or not it affects a "major bodily function" is obscenely ignorant, preposterous, delusional, and funny if it didn't have such deadly effects for women. It is grotesque. But it wins elections for Republicans. Time to stop that.

"Perf rate"

In 1986 I was asked by the Florida Abortion Council to be the principal speaker at their special Risk Management Seminar so I could help physicians and other abortion health practitioners learn how to improve safety and prevent complications in abortion services.

In one session, a physician at the back of the room (an old friend and colleague) asked me, "What's your perf rate?" "My *perf* rate? What are you talking about? What's a '*perf*?'" "When you perforate the uterus," he replied. "Oh, you mean my *perforation* rate. Do you want to know how many times I have made a hole in (perforated) the uterus in performing an abortion?" I asked. "Is that what you mean?" "Yes," he said. "None. Zero. It hasn't happened in over 5,000 abortions," I said. "A *perf* sounds cute and cuddly, like something you would hold on your lap and pet like a puppy or kitten, not something dangerous," I said. "A *perforation* of the uterus is a serious and potentially lethal injury to the uterus which is to be avoided at all costs. Calling it a 'perf' trivializes it and makes it sound innocuous."

"How did you manage to have zero perforations?" my friend asked. "I use laminaria for overnight dilation of the cervix so I don't have to force and tear the cervix open with steel dilators," I said. "And I do abortions very carefully." I explained the many advantages of using laminaria for this purpose. But it did require two visits for the patient.

"We can't do that," my friend replied. "Why not?" I asked. "Because it costs too much." He replied. "Well, raise your fee enough to meet the expense," I said. "We can't," he said. "Why not?" I said. "We would lose patients to the competition," he said. "Well, first things first," I said.

Here is an example of a philosophical point and a choice of values: Safety for the patient or profit first? It also illustrates the power of words. "*Perf*" trivializes an important, serious, and potentially fatal complication that is almost always completely preventable. Trivializing it with this word permits the user of the word to dismiss the steps necessary to protect the patient from injury. Those steps are expensive.

So are principles.

"Unborn child" "child"

On January 5, 2024, the Fifth Circuit Court of Appeals ruled that doctors may not perform emergency abortions even though such an emergency operation is required by the federal Emergency Medical Treatment and Labor Act (EMTALA). In the decision, judges of the Fifth Circuit, the most conservative in the country, all appointed by Republican presidents, referred throughout the decision to the "*mother*" and the "*unborn child*," reflecting a bias against abortion even if this would save the woman's life. The woman is not a "mother" until she has had a "baby," and the "fetus" is not an "unborn child." This framing places the focus on the "innocent victim" of the abortion instead of the "woman" whose life is in immediate danger. She's "guilty" because she's a "woman" who also happens to be a "person." *Who's got the guilt?* The Christians know.

This language and framing continues the psychological warfare of abortion opponents at the highest judicial level in the American legal system and codifies sectarian language that damages women.

Do you know anybody who is an "undead corpse?" Are you?

Notes

1 Ziegler, M. *After Roe: The Lost History of the Abortion Debate*. Cambridge, MA: Harvard University Press, 2015; Ziegler, M. *Abortion and the Law in America: Roe v. Wade to the Present*. Cambridge, UK: Cambridge University Press, 2020.
2 Holland, *Tiny You*. Ibid.
3 Mason, C. *Killing for Life: The Apocalyptic Narrative of Pro-life Politics*. Ithaca, NY: Cornell University Press, 2002.
4 Holland, *Tiny You*. Ibid.
5 Holocaust Encyclopedia: *Mass Shootings of Jews during the Holocaust*. Large scale massacres in 1941: Babyn Yar. https://encyclopedia.ushmm.org/content/en/article/mass-shootings-of-jews -during-the-holocaust
6 Holland, *Tiny You*. Ibid.
7 Holland, *Tiny You*. Ibid.
8 Tom DeLay, Republican House Majority Leader (2003–2005), came to Congress from a career in Texas as a pest exterminator. He was an opponent of abortion rights and also opposed the teaching of evolution in schools

17 "First, kill all the doctors"

In 1992, as chair-elect of the Population, Family Planning and Reproductive Health Section of the American Public Health Association (APHA), I responded to general concern in the pro-choice community about the apparently impending shortage of physicians who were willing to perform abortions. This followed an interview with me by *New York Times* reporter Gina Kolata on the stresses experienced by physicians doing this work. At the 1992 APHA meeting, I proposed organizing a symposium on this subject composed of physicians actually involved in performing abortions, academic leaders who were training physicians in these procedures, and other clinic personnel such as nurses and clinic administrators.

By the time we reached the 1993 annual APHA meeting, the decision had been made that this symposium was too important to be left to the doctors who were actually doing abortions. The panel should include only one physician (me) and seven other clinic workers from non-profit clinics. With the limited time, there was just enough time for each person to stand up and say, "Things are bad and they're getting worse" and then sit down: A bumper sticker symposium

At one point, one of the panelists said, "Nobody should be able to make a living doing abortions." So much for conducting professional medical service on a continuing basis.

This came at a time of turmoil in the pro-choice community and rising hostility toward doctors in clinics. There was a general desire to replace doctors with nurses, physician assistants, and the new "abortion pill," mifepristone ("'RU-648"), which caused a medically induced abortion without the care of a physician. The message to physicians, including many of those who had performed tens of thousands (overall, millions) of abortions over decades, was "Go Away!"

The following paper, which I was given only a few minutes to present in a summary form, and which was not published, follows:

Strategies for addressing the shortage of abortion providers
"First, kill all the doctors"
Warren M. Hern, M.D., M.P.H., Ph.D.
Director
Boulder Abortion Clinic
Assistant Clinical Professor
Department of Obstetrics & Gynecology
University of Colorado Health Sciences Center

DOI: 10.4324/9781003514961-18

Presented at the 121st meeting of the American Public Health Association, San Francisco, October 26, 1993, at a symposium, The Shortage of Abortion Providers: A Crisis in the Making.

Abstract

Recent news reports, studies, and editorials have raised questions about whether there are enough physicians to provide the 1.6 million abortions that are sought by American women each year. Is there a shortage? Is it real? What are its causes? What can be done, what is being done to train physicians in abortion care? What are the obstacles for training programs? What will be the effect of changing government policies after 12 years of anti-abortion harassment under Ronald Reagan and George Bush? What are the effects of assassination attempts against physicians who provide abortions, at least one political assassination of a physician, and open invitations by anti-abortion leaders to their followers to assassinate doctors? What is the national response to these threats and violent acts? How are doctors responding?

An attempt is made in this paper to answer some of these questions, although, in most cases, no definitive answer can be given.

> The first thing we do, let's kill all the lawyers."
> **King Henry VI, Part II; Act II, Scene IV.**

In Shakespeare's play, the characters who are plotting to take over the country decide that the best way to do it is to create anarchy and sow confusion by disrupting the legal system. The best way to do that, they conclude, is to kill the lawyers. The American anti-abortion movement has made a chilling decision to apply this reasoning to the doctors who perform abortions in this country.

But are the anti-abortion fanatics the only ones who think that getting rid of the doctors will solve the problem?

It is somewhat ironic that I have been asked to present my recommendations for strategies to deal with the "physician shortage" in abortion services even though I proposed such a session for this year's APHA meeting. It is ironic partly because, to some extent, the controversy and public concern can be traced to an informal conversation about other abortion-related matters I had with a reporter at the New York Times in December 1989. At the time, I had proposed a session dealing with anti-abortion harassment and violence at the 1990 APHA meeting. In the process of the conversation with the reporter, I casually mentioned to her some of the difficulties that we face as physicians who provide abortion services. She was shocked at some of the anecdotes I related to her. She resolved to write a story about it. In a few days, she called me and asked for the names of other physicians who had experienced these problems and for the names of physicians who had stopped providing abortions. The article appeared on the front page of the New York Times on January 3, 1990.[1] The article contained a few quotes from me, but principally, it concentrated on the problems of other physicians who had experienced far more difficulties, including my friend and colleague, Dr. Curtis Boyd. In the article, the Executive Director of the American College of Obstetricians and Gynecologists characterized those of us who specialize in abortion services as "extremists." Some of my pro-choice colleagues who were not providing abortion services criticized my willingness to divulge the problems of harassment of physicians. They said it would only prove the effectiveness of harassment and encourage it. The harassment is effective, I said. We may as well acknowledge it. Terrorism works.

Subsequently, Congressional hearings were held concerning harassment of physicians and attacks on abortion clinics. At the 1990 APHA meeting held in New York that fall, we held the symposium that I had organized on the subject. Several valuable papers were presented, the symposium was well attended, but there was no press interest of any kind. One of the papers presented at the 1990 APHA symposium, "An epidemic of anti-abortion violence in the United States," was published in 1991 in the American Journal of Obstetrics and Gynecology under the authorship of Dr. David Grimes, Dr. Jaqueline Forrest of the Alan Guttmacher Institute, and two staff members of the National Abortion Federation[2]. At about the same time as the APHA symposium, a national pro-choice organization sponsored a private blue-ribbon symposium on the question of the availability of abortion providers. Its report, "Who Will Provide Abortions?" was released 1991.[3] The 26-member symposium included only one physician in private specialty practice who provides abortions on a full-time basis, Dr. Boyd. As pointed out by Dr. Boyd at the conference, the question is not: "Why don't physicians do abortions?"; the question is, "Why do physicians do abortions?" The report is unfortunately marred by plagiarism: A statement falsely attributed to one of the conference participants was reproduced, word for word, from a statement made by Dr. William Rashbaum at the 1976 Western Regional Conference On Abortion, and published in 1977 in a book, *Abortion in the Seventies*, which I co-edited.[4]

The chair of the symposium, Dr. David Grimes, was later the author of a paper, "Clinicians who provide abortions: The thinning ranks," published in *Obstetrics and Gynecology* in 1992.[5] Several papers in addition to Dr. Grimes' 1992 paper have appeared in *Family Planning Perspectives* and other journals dealing with the shortage of physicians and the lack of residency training in abortion services, the most recent of which was by Dr. Westhoff in the February, 1993 issue of *Obstetrics and Gynecology*.[6] Numerous newspaper columnists, including Ellen Goodman of the *Boston Globe* and Anna Quindlen of the New York Times have written columns concerning the problem. There has been, in short, considerable commentary on the lack of availability of physicians to perform abortions and concern about who will do them. Authors of these reports and commentaries have noted anti-abortion harassment and declining pay as examples of factors that have discouraged doctors from performing abortions.

Is there really a lack of physicians to perform abortions? How meaningful, for example, is the Alan Guttmacher Institute's statistic that 83% of all counties in the U.S., where 31% of the women of reproductive age live, has no abortion provider?[7] If this is a crisis, and in some places it surely is, what are its origins?

In order to answer this question, it is necessary to go back in history a little to put the issue in a proper perspective.

When the movement to make abortion services legal gained momentum in the United States in the 1950s and 1960s, physicians were prominent advocates of that change.[8] The "charismatic" role of physicians in society as agents of legitimacy was critical in this process[9]. Medical data gathered by physicians were crucial in formulating both the New York law of 1970 and the subsequent U.S. Supreme Court decisions of 1973. When abortion became legal throughout the U.S. that year, physicians across the country were active in establishing abortion services and in defending their existence. The passive as well as active support of the medical community was an important component of public acceptance.

Subsequent to that time, notwithstanding the contributions of physicians to the increasing availability of abortion services, and notwithstanding the fact that physicians have performed nearly all of the 30 million abortions performed since 1970 in the United States, a strong movement developed which rejected both physicians and the role of men in the provision of abortion services. The fact that most 20th century American physicians have been men is not coincidental, but it has little to do with the attitudes of male physicians who have provided the bulk of abortion services during the past two decades. Many of those physicians performing abortions have consciously and openly rejected the attitudes that previously led to discrimination against women in the medical profession, and many of these physicians have been prominent in defending the right of women to make their own reproductive decisions. Yet the contributions of physicians, both males and females, have been progressively and consistently relegated to inferior status by leaders of the American pro-choice movement since 1973. That may be changing now, but it has been a clear pattern, and sometimes, official policy, for pro-choice organizations to disassociate themselves from physicians who specialize in providing abortion services. Doctors have been taken for granted. In feminist clinics, in particular, reports and observations consistently have indicated that the role of the physician is that of a technician to be seen and not heard. The classical role and status of the physician as an independent and educated professional whose good will is assumed and valued has been turned on its head: the physician, in many cases, came to be seen as the adversary, the enemy, the necessary evil to be tolerated in a setting exclusively devoted to the concerns of the woman receiving the service and the women involved in providing care. The physician's professional concerns were seen as unimportant, even offensive, and irrelevant at best. Terms such as "menstrual extraction" were invented to conceal the medical and surgical nature of pregnancy and the abortion operation, and other elaborate processes of denial of the risks of both pregnancy and abortion were established[10]. Strenuous efforts were mounted to demonstrate that physicians were unnecessary to the abortion procedure, and the difficulties of consistently performing safe abortions were minimized by everyone from clinic staff members to academic analysts.

Women coming for abortion services ceased to be called "patients," a term which implies a certain kind of relationship between the person with a medical condition seeking treatment and the physician providing the treatment. They were to be called "clients," implying the kind of commercial relationship one finds between a financial customer and a stockbroker, for example. Physicians found themselves relegated to the position of cogs in a machine called an "abortion service." Reports concerning the availability of abortion services constantly referred to the number of hospitals that "perform" abortions, ignoring the clear fact that hospitals do not perform abortions or any other surgical operations, for that matter; physicians perform abortions. Some hospitals permit physicians to do so, and some do not.

Unfortunately, most physicians providing abortion services have passively accepted this progressive diminution and deprecation of their contributions to women's health.

At critical moments in the legal and political history of abortion during the past 20 years, some pro-choice leaders have come together to have press conferences to make statements about public issues such as impending legislation, court cases, anti-abortion violence, and the like. Physicians who specialize in providing abortion services have virtually never been invited to participate in these events. The National Abortion Rights Action League, in particular, has consciously chosen on most occasions to avoid public associations with physicians who specialize in providing abortion services or to involve them in policy issues for the ostensible reason that such physicians have a pecuniary interest in the result. This begs the question that many of these physicians are committed to performing abortions for philosophical and ideological reasons; that is why they have that specialty. Also, performing abortions is still considered a disreputable activity among some prominent members of the "pro-choice" community.

Physicians rarely, if ever, have been asked to represent the views of pro-choice organizations in national forums, even though some of these organizations were founded to represent abortion service providers including physicians.

At an important national political event concerning abortion rights in the fall of 1989, nearly a hundred speakers were invited to participate in a day-long speak-out before the Lincoln Memorial. The speakers included rock stars, daytime soap opera stars, politicians of all kinds including members of Congress, feminist leaders, political candidates, labor union leaders, and leaders of political groups from as far away as Australia and South Africa. The speakers' list included a biochemist and three physicians, only one of whom was currently involved in performing abortions as a specialty. Dr. Etiene-Emile Baulieu, the biochemist discoverer of RU-486, was lionized and given a prominent first place on the program. Dr. Baulieu has earned and deserves all the recognition he gains from his contribution, but only a few thousand women in this country have received abortions with RU-486. Two other physicians not engaged in abortion services were asked to speak. By contrast, the physician specializing in surgical abortion services, who *defacto* represented the thousands of physicians in this country who have done so, was not originally invited but requested an opportunity to come to Washington to participate and speak. He was given a time in the later part of the program, but this was postponed several times. He was only permitted to speak after pleading with the organizers and then not until the event was closing and most of the 100,000 people attending and all of the press had left.

The symbolic treatment of the biochemist and first two physicians compared with the that of the third physician who was actually performing abortions, had performed thousands of them, and who left his operating room to speak at the event, spoke volumes about the very different ways their contributions were valued by the organizers, the National Organization for Women and other pro-choice organizations.

The discovery of RU-486, which is a welcome and extremely important scientific advance and as well as contribution to medical knowledge, and which offers great hope for the treatment of breast cancer, among other things, has been hailed as the "magic bullet" that will eliminate both the need for doctors and the abortion controversy. Feminist leaders and columnists have been prominent in holding out this false hope, but the message to the physicians who have been dedicated to performing abortions has been clear: we don't want to need you, and pretty soon, we won't need you.

The breathless and fantastic depictions of RU - 486 are wrong in many respects. The early complication rates of RU-486 were uncomfortably high, with a significant number of women requiring blood transfusions, whereas the rate in early surgical abortion is minuscule - in the range of 0.001%.[11] RU-486 must be used with adjunctive drugs such as prostaglandins that sometimes result in serious and uncomfortable side effects, and some women, after taking the drugs require completion of the abortion with a vacuum aspiration procedure. If taken improperly or too late in the pregnancy, the pregnancy continues. RU-486 is doubtless effective in most cases in the selected women for whom it is likely to be effective: those who are very early in their pregnancies. It should by all means be available for abortion, and it has great promise as either a contraceptive or "morning after" medication. But it will not replace doctors who perform abortions. It certainly will not eliminate the abortion controversy.

The rural "deficit" in abortion services

The Alan Guttmacher Institute concluded that over 80% of U.S. counties have no one who provides abortion services, and there is no reason to dispute this conclusion. But what does it mean? Physicians who do abortions are not found in rural areas for the same reason that other physicians are not found in rural areas. There has been a steadily diminishing availability of all medical specialties in rural counties as physicians have remained in larger cities after training for the availability of important amenities not found in small towns. Even where abortion services are available in small towns, women frequently do not wish to have their abortions in these locations because of the lack of privacy. They go to the big city where their decision and treatment can remain private instead of being known to other members of the community within minutes. The discrimination against physicians who perform abortions is often intense in rural areas. Physicians in rural communities who are willing to provide abortion services do so few that their complication rates are sometimes extremely and unnecessarily high. There is generally an inverse relationship between the number of abortions performed by an operator and the complication rates. The answer to this observation is not to put a physician or other practitioner on every street corner in small towns in order to increase local availability of abortion services.

The AGI conclusion also conceals some important facts.

In Gilpin County, Colorado, for example, not only is there no abortion provider, there are no resident practicing physicians of any kind. There are also no grocery stores or gas stations. But it takes less than 45 minutes to get from any part of Gilpin County to several Front Range cities, including Boulder and Denver, where most people buy their groceries and, as I can testify, have their abortions. How do the Gilpin Counties of America influence the AGI results?

Urban concentration of abortion services

The large number of physicians who perform abortions tend to be concentrated in the urban areas, particularly in states that do not have legislatures rabidly attacking them. In fact, there are so many abortion services and physicians to perform them in most metropolitan areas, the competition between clinics and physicians is fierce, even cutthroat. Abortion services are often organized in the urban areas around non-profit services dedicated to lowering fees as much as possible with the help of tax exemptions, deductible contributions, and economies of scale. In particular, Planned Parenthood services provide the bulk of abortion services in many communities. Planned Parenthood and other collective or non-profit clinic services frequently use physicians-in-training to perform abortions, meaning that these physicians, who sometimes perform abortions in violation of their residency program contracts, can be paid at lower levels.[12]

In order to pay the physicians even a token amount for performing the abortions, the clinics must then organize high-volume activities which shrinks physician contact with patients. This arrangement accentuates the "technician" role of the physician and reduction in status identified by the [previous] report as a source of dissatisfaction for the physicians. The declining income for physicians performing abortions is aggravated and overcome only by increasingly higher volumes, which means more competition among an increased number of providers trying to see the same or declining number of patients. These are not optimum working conditions for physicians. Private practitioners, when faced with this competitive situation, are inclined to turn to other more interesting, remunerative, or professionally rewarding activities not excoriated by everyone from the President on down, as was the case for 12 years. The competition is too keen to permit concentration on the professional goals of quality care and patient satisfaction. The physicians skilled at performing abortions and dedicated to doing so either have to organize their services to compete with the non-profits and feminist clinics or turn to other activities. The economic pressure means that quality care has suffered and shortcuts have been made in the provision of services. One of the consequences is increased complications and collapse of some services.

The economics of abortion services

One of the only ways we have of measuring value in this society is money. The fee for a first trimester abortion at Preterm Clinic in 1970 in Washington, D.C. was $185, which was reduced later to $165; the fees were less in New York City. Calculations by the Economics Institute at the University of Colorado indicate that cost-of-living increases alone would raise that to over $600 in today's economy. That does not reflect catastrophic increases in malpractice insurance costs and extreme increases in the costs of property damage insurance costs, security costs, and property replacement costs resulting from anti-abortion violence since 1981. However, the average cost for a first trimester abortion is little over $250 today, which means that the real cost of this operation is less than half or one-third of its cost in 1970, and it means that the amount paid physicians is a fraction of what it was in 1970 in real dollars[13].

Abortion has become a commodity, like soap. It is a retail product. The providers of abortion services have made it so. The professional organizations, which could educate the public to demand quality services instead of choosing services by the lowest fee, have not fulfilled this task, even when it is the organization's founding mandate. The paradoxical result is that while abortion services have become increasingly expensive to provide, sometimes requiring around-the-clock private armed security guards and military fortress security, while insurance and property costs have skyrocketed, and while physicians willing to be publicly associated with abortion services have become scarcer, the price of the service, or commodity, as it has become, has gone down. This is the opposite effect that would be expected in a market economy.

The explanation of the paradox are the cost externalities and the response externalities.[14] The cost externality has been the political pressure from, most visibly, the national Republican party as it has used the abortion issue to gain power, meanwhile encouraging antiabortion fanatics. One of the results has been the social devaluation of abortion services (and those who provide them, especially physicians) and devaluation in the marketplace. The response externality has been the willingness of the abortion service providers to absorb the excess costs by two means: reduction in the quality of services or personal sacrifice motivated by ideology or altruism; sometimes both. Efforts at removing the causative externality by the pro-choice community have been, until recently, minimal except for local aberrations. In the fall of 1989, after Candidate George Bush had advocated the imprisonment of doctors who do abortions and after President Bush had vetoed local Washington, D.C. funding for abortion services for poor women who had been raped, Americans who consider themselves pro-choice supported Bush in the polls by a margin of 2 to 1.

There are two ways to deal with the economic competition. If the objective is quality care, and if that is a priority, it means that the difference comes out of the lives of those providing the services. Incomes are lower, hours are longer, outside interests are sacrificed, family and personal activities are sacrificed, teaching and research activities are sacrificed, professional education is sacrificed, marriages disintegrate, debts accumulate, and mortgages mature. The second way is to cut corners on patient care, and that has been the choice of many abortion providers, especially those whose interest is commercial rather than altruistic. Those who make these decisions are candid about their choices.

Recommendations of the [previous] report

Among other things, the [previous] report recommended sending out invitations to physicians no longer in practice. It is absurd to think that sending out public relations packages to encourage retired old physicians to dodder down to the local abortion clinic will really do anything to solve the problem. The last thing most retired physicians want is to get shot at for doing something the Operation Rescue mob doesn't want them to do. Ben Munson entered a merciful retirement after more than 30 years of heroic and courageous service to women in Rapid City, South Dakota, the victim of a predatory State Attorney General who exploited Ben's abortion practice to gain the Governor's office, nearly costing Ben his practice and his life savings. Ben is now enjoying his life without the daily cares of being picketed and harassed every waking hour. Who needs it? The women go to Sioux Falls, Minneapolis, Denver, or Boulder, and get their abortions safely done by experts. Nobody would buy his practice.

The [previous] report makes several recommendations to deal with the lowered income and loss of status for physicians providing abortions. The first is to train many more physicians to do abortions and to patronize those who do them, and the second is to train "mid-level" clinicians to do abortions, some of whom are on record as having a professional commitment not to do abortions (the nurse-midwives). There are two examples of non-physicians performing abortions in the nation as the basis for this recommendation.

The obvious result of training many more physicians to perform abortions when we currently have so many who do them that the ones doing them cannot be adequately paid for doing them, of course, is to lower the amount paid for each abortion being performed. How lowering the amount available to pay physicians for performing abortions will rectify the low pay currently being experienced is a mystery that the report does not solve.

Since many physicians specializing in providing abortion services already feel that they are the lowest possible grade of clinician available, it is not clear who the "middle-level" clinicians would be, unless it means that nurses and physicians assistants are a higher level of clinician, the only obvious alternative conclusion. That will do little to raise the status of physicians who perform abortions. If we are so concerned about enticing physicians to perform abortions, how can we do so by telling them that they can be replaced by someone with far less medical education?

The logical consequence of the ambivalence about physicians performing abortions is the suicidal fantasy of women performing their own abortions on themselves and on each other, as advocated by some feminist groups. Aside from the ghastly medical consequences that are likely to ensue from this misguided idea, it short-circuits the big question of how we shall run our society and what shall be the status of women. If women can do this themselves and it is not necessary to have a political and legal climate where it can be done by skilled physicians in a modern and properly equipped setting where women are treated with care and dignity, then what are we fighting for? The public is likely to say that the heavy rhetoric about abortion rights is so much posturing. Let's move on to issues we can really do something about such as the budget deficit and Iranian dictators. The women will take care of themselves. Not to worry. And the doctors will go back to being respectable gentlemen in three-piece suits who show up for church or temple with the family in squeaky shoes every week at the right time, earn the unanimous love of their communities for curing every sore throat in sight, and get elected to Presidencies of grateful Rotary Clubs throughout the nation. It will certainly be easier on the doctors and their families.

All this sends another message to physicians who specialize in providing abortion services: We can get along without you, and we are going to see that you get even less for doing what you are doing. To me, this seems to confound two important questions: relative availability of services and issues of social/economic justice. Making services available is one objective; dealing with inequities in economic power for those who have limited income is another matter.

The [previous] report correctly notes that the fees charged for abortion have fallen by a factor of four since 1969 rather than keeping up with the cost of living index. The average national fee is approximately one-third what it was in 1971. It is simply not possible to provide quality services under these conditions. It is certainly impossible to provide quality services, to pay for the astronomically increased security costs, and to build long-term institutional stability. At this point, the [previous] report crosses over into sheer fantasy. Clinics are encouraged to offer attractive financial packages and other benefits to physicians. But who pays? Not the patients. If you raise the fee by $25 on a first trimester procedure to pay for a new, up-to-date ultrasound machine, to equip a new exam room, to hire a more qualified nurse, or to hire another physician, the patients go to the next clinic down the street or even to another clinic dozens, even a hundred miles away. This illustrates the fallacy of the report. There is no deficiency of physicians to provide abortions. There are hundreds if not thousands of physicians who perform abortions. They are, however, not distributed in a way that the report writers would like for them to be distributed.

The report deplores the "isolation" of free-standing outpatient abortion services and worries that they are more vulnerable to political pressure. In fact, the free-standing clinics, while plagued with certain problems, can be seen in another way: They are a positive and highly adaptive response to institutional hospital hostility to abortion services and to the cumbersome nature of those inpatient services. The "isolation" the report criticizes is sometimes consciously self-inflicted and is avoided by some physicians and clinics. On the contrary, outpatient abortion clinics have, in fact, provided a new model for efficient and highly competent health care that permits concentration on the specific needs of a specific group of patients. The counseling service included in many clinics, for example, is something that could be incorporated in other surgical programs at great benefit to patients as well as reducing both complication rates and lawsuits, as they have in abortion services.

Causes of declining availability

The single most important influence driving physicians from the abortion field during the past 20 years, however, has been the aggressive and absolutely cynical use of the abortion by right-wing groups, especially the Republican Party, to gain political power.[15] Ronald Reagan was the first American President to use opposition to abortion as an important part of his political appeal, but the extreme right wing of the Republican Party took over its platform in 1976, and that faction expelled the most moderate elements of the party in 1980. From that point until the present, fanatic opposition to abortion has been a mainstay of Republican political ideology.

The very first thing that Ronald Reagan said at his first press conference on the day after he was elected in 1980 was: "I am going to make abortion illegal." Two days later, Senator Strom Thurmond, on an interview on the Today Show, made it plain that he would seek the death penalty for those who perform abortions.

On his inaugural day, Ronald Reagan brought the main anti-abortion leaders into the White House and welcomed them in the Oval Office. His Secretary of Health and Human Services, Richard Schweiker, spoke at an anti-abortion rally and announced, "We are going to give you a pro-life [sic] administration." From that point until 1993, every person appointed to important responsibilities for public health in the Reagan and Bush Administrations was chosen on the sole basis of his or her fanatic opposition to abortion as distinguished from other qualifications. An unpredictable result was Dr. Everett Koop, who had no public health credentials prior to being appointed Surgeon General, and whose nomination was opposed by the American Public Health Association for the first time in its history, but who subsequently showed his independence of thought and action by rejecting a White House demand that he issue a report claiming a pattern of damaging long-term effects from abortion.

At every turn during his time as President, Ronald Reagan condemned abortion and those who perform them. He invited anti-abortion leaders into the White House every January 22, and he never failed to address anti-abortion rallies in Washington. On only one occasion did he condemn the wave of anti-abortion violence that began to mount during his administration, and then only at the end of an especially violent year, 1984, during which 29 abortion clinics or doctors offices were completely destroyed. The response of Reagan's Director of the FBI at the time, William F. Webster, was that the anti-abortion attacks were not terrorism because "we don't know who's doing it." Message to the anti-abortion vigilantes: Go for it. We won't do anything to stop you. Reagan pointedly declined or rejected requests to pardon anti-abortion bombers who were in jail in 1986 after he met in the White House with some of the most radical anti-abortion leaders.

At the 1986 annual meeting of the National Right To Life Committee, all four major candidates for the 1988 Republican Presidential nomination accepted invitations to speak at the anti-abortion convention. All came except George Bush, and all condemned abortion in the harshest possible terms.

In September 1988, during a presidential candidate debate with Michael Dukakis, in response to a question concerning abortion, George Bush stated clearly that somebody "should be punished" for having or performing an abortion, but that he, in 30 years of public life, hadn't "sorted it out" yet. The next day, at the urging of his managers, Bush issued a statement that women should not be punished, but doctors should be imprisoned for performing abortions. Bush received no substantial criticism from Democratic or Republican leaders, nor did he receive any serious published criticism from national pro-choice leaders. He won the election in a landslide. Bush continued the repressive Reagan policies concerning abortion including the filing of *amici* briefs opposing abortion in U.S. Supreme Court cases.

The policies and demagoguery of Reagan and Bush were accompanied, not coincidentally, by an unprecedented wave of anti-abortion violence across the United States.[16] While the violence began prior to 1981, the number and severity of incidents increased sharply after Ronald Reagan took office and were exacerbated with each Reagan anti-abortion pronouncement.

Through the end of 1992, hundreds of violent and aggressive anti-abortion incidents occurred, many of them unreported, many of the directed specifically at doctors. These took the form of gunshots fired and other unsuccessful assassination attempts, death threats, kidnapping, bombings, and arson. Dozens of clinics and doctors' offices were completely destroyed, some more than once. Several people, not physicians, have been critically injured and one remains a quadriplegic as the result of an anti-abortion attack.

Even in Boulder, Colorado, the most pro-choice community in the nation, we have not been immune from the organized national violence. The first attempt on my life was in 1978 in my own office parking lot; violent attacks, harassment, and death threats directed toward me, members of my staff, and my office increased dramatically in the mid-1980s; and five shots were fired through the front waiting room windows of my office in 1988, requiring the installation of bullet-proof windows.

Startlingly, the obvious and well-documented origin of this wave of political violence has been deliberately excluded from some of the most prominent reports presented by advocates of abortion services. One could read the 1991 report, "Who Will Provide Abortions?" and never know that abortion has been a major political controversy in the United States for 20 years and has been a principal organizing issue for gaining political power for the right wing, or that two Presidents of the United States over 12 years waged constant attacks on those who provide abortion services.

When asked about this glaring omission, officials reported that they deliberately excluded the political context and origins of anti-abortion violence because they did not want to "encourage" the violence by showing what catastrophic results it has had on the availability of physicians.

One must ask: could anything give anti-abortion fanatics more encouragement than they had from Ronald Reagan and George Bush on the Presidential campaign trail and in the White House? To ignore the massive effects of this powerful campaign of devaluation of physicians and those providing abortion services by the leader of the Free World for the previous ten years is simply whistling in the dark. It reduces the report to an exercise in hand-wringing and ineffective bleating.

The Grimes, et al, paper[17], while using epidemiologic methodology in an admirable and highly sophisticated way to document the pattern of violence, provides a reductionist conclusion that completely ignores the political context that is the obvious cause of the violence. In the paper, the authors identify "individuals" as responsible "multiple point source outbreaks" of the "epidemic." The fact that anti-abortion violence represents a wave of political terrorism and unofficial repression orchestrated by the highest political and governmental leaders in the country is completely ignored.

Taken together, the [previous] report, Grimes papers, and other reports, miss the "spear through the belly." The patient who is brought from the battlefield transfixed with a 6-foot spear and bleeding to death is examined carefully for nicks, cuts, and scratches with the conclusion that the cause of his enfeebled condition remains mysterious. The patient is advised to do sit-ups and run around the block to restore his health. The "hoofbeats in the night" are deemed to be zebras even though we are not in East Africa.

A response to the problem that seeks only to treat the symptoms, in some cases by accentuating the problems themselves, will not be sufficient to meet the need.

Without a diagnosis, we cannot recommend a treatment, and without a broad analysis, I cannot recommend a strategy.

Changes: good news and bad news

Fortunately, some of the political circumstances have changed as of January 21, 1993. We have a new President of the United States who supports reproductive freedom in general and abortion rights in particular. The Attorney General of the United States has pledged her support for the protection of abortion rights. We now have a new public health-oriented Surgeon General who strongly supports abortion rights. A major bill in Congress (S.B. 636) would protect those who seek access to abortion clinics either as patients or as staff members. Pro-choice organizations such as NARAL have begun recently to include physicians in their policy initiatives and to support pro-choice candidates with notable success in some areas, especially California and Colorado.

The bad news is that the anti-abortion movement has become even more violent. Dr. David Gunn was assassinated by his office in March, 1993, and an open attempt to assassinate Dr. George Tiller at his clinic occurred in August. These are only two of the most violent recent anti-abortion actions. The violent destruction of clinics continues across the country.

The American people, and the pro-choice movement in particular, must realize that we are dealing with a violent, terrorist political movement that is driven by a fascist ideology antithetical to everything this country stands for and which is a threat not only to women and doctors but to democratic institutions.

On August 12, 1993, my editorial entitled, "The Pope And My Right To Life" was published on the Op-Ed Page of the *New York Times*.[18] In the editorial, I denounced the fact that, because of the Pope's visit to Colorado in the company of hundreds of thousands of Christians, many of them anti-abortion fanatics, I now had to wear a bullet-proof vest to my medical office, Boulder Abortion Clinic. I also noted that Randall Terry, who came to Colorado the previous month to organize anti-abortion demonstrations, was last seen in Colorado a few years ago in front of my office as he prayed for my death with his followers. The afternoon the editorial was published, Randall Terry, in his national daily radio broadcast on the Christian Broadcasting Network (August 12, 1993) referring to me by name, called for either my "conversion" or "execution." Those who listened to the broadcast could draw no other conclusion but that Terry was inviting his followers to assassinate me. (Our clinic received numerous phone calls from listeners from all over the country.) The next day, a Catholic priest in Mobile, Alabama, attempted to publish a newspaper advertisement calling the assassination of doctors who perform abortions as "justifiable homicide." The following Thursday, August 19, a woman named Rachelle Shannon attempted to assassinate Dr. George Tiller by shooting him as he left his abortion clinic in Wichita, Kansas. Shannon, who had been arrested several times at anti-abortion demonstrations, had flown from Oregon to Oklahoma City where she rented a car to drive to Wichita; she edits an anti-abortion newsletter published by a man serving time in a federal penitentiary for felony arson of an abortion clinic.

The man who fatally shot Dr. Gunn on March 19, 1993, attended the church led by the Catholic priest in Mobile, Alabama who called such assassinations "justifiable homicide."

The authors of a new book, *Religious Violence and Abortion*, concluded after their study in Florida that violent anti-abortion acts are not the isolated acts of deranged loners but a national conspiracy of political violence.[19]

Conclusions

The first need is for the pro-choice community to recognize the serious political nature of the violent anti-abortion movement and the general long-term nature of its threat, and that it is part of a larger quest for power by the radical religious right .

The second need is to muster political leadership from the President of the United States on down, and to secure the public opposition of religious as well as other political leaders to the anti-abortion violence we are experiencing. This means the passage into law of serious protective legislation at the federal level, apprehension of the perpetrators of anti-abortion violence, and vigorous prosecution of the offenders.

The third need is to restore physicians who perform abortions to their historic role as respected members of society and as valued contributors to this activity. This means that their contributions must be actively and openly appreciated, and that their financial compensation for their services reflect the competence and sacrifices involved in providing them.

The [previous] report does contain some important and valuable recommendations concerning the strengthening of residency training programs with respect to abortion services in teaching hospitals and private outpatient abortion clinics. Unfortunately, realization of these goals depends on the political climate inside and outside the teaching programs. An anti-abortion chief of service can prevent all abortion training in a residency program that functions within a community climate that supports abortion rights. There are many instances, however, of Ob/Gyn faculties that wish to train resident physicians in abortion, but the public climate is unsupportive or apathetic. There are plenty of physicians who are expert in abortion service and want to teach but who currently have no or few opportunities to do so.

One of the ways these goals can be achieved is through training grants provided by private foundations interested in women's health care; these grant programs could be facilitated by pro-choice organizations could provide assistance both for trainees and for private physicians who can provide training. Another important potential source of support could be security grants provided to private practitioners for the purpose of protecting themselves against violent attacks. Private armed security guards, bullet-proof windows, electronic security, and bullet-proof vests are expensive and not usual costs of private medical practice.

Supporting the role of physicians also means that, while there are limited circumstances for the appropriate use of non-physicians to perform abortions, this avenue should not be offered as a panacea or substitute for the availability of physicians in performing abortions. My experience in performing thousands of abortions over a period of 20 years tells me that I often need every bit of medical education and experience I have to get a patient through a procedure safely. The problem is that the intraoperative problems sometimes are so dangerous that it is much better for the patient's safety that the person performing the abortion is the one with the skill and not the person simply "supervising". Even these physicians often pay exorbitant malpractice insurance premiums and have difficulty defending themselves in a malpractice action. The present malpractice legal climate does not lend encouragement to those who fantasize that lower-level practitioners can somehow solve the problem of the "lack" of abortion services while simultaneously lowering the already artificially low fees for services.

We used to have plenty of free abortion services by non-physician providers, of course. And many women died. We are reforming ourselves back to the nineteenth century.

I personally think that anyone who wants to perform abortions should be permitted to do so; but that person should first obtain a medical education and a medical license.[20]

We have worked for a century to bring abortion into the mainstream of medical care and to establish abortion as an operation that physicians should perform. We have worked to gain professional respectability among our colleagues. Now we are being told that we aren't needed. No. Wait. We are needed. To do what? To give "respectability", perhaps. Thanks. No thanks. No pain, no gain. No guts, no glory.

We might start by giving the physicians providing abortion services appreciation instead of the back of our hand. This means not merely an occasional ceremonial pat on the head but the minute-to-minute day-by-day week-by-week treatment with courtesy and respect. The contempt, indifference, and open hostility with which physicians performing abortions are often treated in the ordinary routine working situations and in public encounters says more than the grand public gesture about the true valuation given the physician. Sometimes the words of "support" lie, and it is a lie that cannot be concealed.

The pro-choice community has to decide how it really feels about physicians who perform abortions. I don't mean the physician who comes in from the regular practice or academic appointment for an occasional or even regular session at the local clinic or the physician who performs the odd abortion for a long-term patient or supplements the office income by adding a procedure session on Friday afternoon. These are all laudable and necessary activities and help many women. I am talking about the physician who puts it all on the line and says, "This is my specialty. This is what I do. This is who I am. This is what I live for. This is what my life means. I stand or fall on this." When we accord that physician the same value as the physician who is safely ensconced in the "respectable" orthodox Ob/Gyn or family practice or secure in the prestigious academic institution, we might get somewhere. And we might have more physicians willing to perform abortions and openly help women with this most difficult of life decisions.

If physicians are treated with respect and appreciation, and if they are adequately compensated for their work, they will provide abortions under circumstances that most people would consider to be barely tolerable. Physicians want to help. But they want to feel that they make a difference. If we want physicians to be involved in meaningful ways in the provision of abortion services, the message that they do make a difference and that we want them to make a difference must be conveyed by deeds more than words.

We start this job at the voting booth, not at the public relations expert's office.

Note: This paper was presented in 1993. Circumstances have changed in many ways: some things are better, and some are immeasurably worse. Some parts of this paper are redacted because it does not reflect these later improvements as this book is written in 2024. It is my snapshot of the contentious issues that we faced in 1993.

(Note: Although this paper was not published, my 1993 presentation of it and circulation of this draft did not improve my popularity in any the organizations mentioned.)

Notes

1 Kolata, G. Under pressures and stigma, more doctors shun abortion. *New York Times*, January 8, 1990.
2 Grimes, D.A., Forrest,J.D., Kirkman, A.L., and Radford, B. An epidemic of antiabortion violence in the United States. *American Journal of Obstetrics and Gynecology* 165:1263–68, 1991.
3 National Abortion Federation. Who Will Provide Abortions?: Ensuring the Availability of Qualified Practitioners. Recommendations from a National Symposium. Santa Barbara, California, October 25–26, 1990. Washington, DC: National Abortion Federation.

4 Rashbaum, W. Discussion remarks. In *Abortion in the Seventies*, W. Hern and B. Andrikopoulous (eds). New York: National Abortion Federation, 1977. p. 48.; Hern, W.M., and Andrikopoulous, B. (eds.). *Abortion in the Seventies*. New York: National Abortion Federation, 1977.

5 Grimes, D.A. Clinicians who provide abortions: The thinning ranks. Obstetrics and Gynecology 80:719–23, 1992.

6 Darney, P.D., Landy, U., MacPherson, S., and Sweet, R.L. Abortion training in U.S. obstetrics and gynecology residency programs. *Family Planning Perspectives* 19(4):158–62, 1987.; Westhoff, C., Mark, F., and Rosenfield, A. Residency training in contraception, sterilization, and abortion. *Obstetrics and Gynecology* 81:311–14, 1993.

7 Henshaw, S.K., and Van Vort, J. *Abortion Factbook*, 1992 Edition. New York: Alan Guttmacher Institute, 1992.

8 Potts, M., Diggory, P., and Peel, J. *Abortion*. Cambridge: University Press, 1977. Chapter 10, The American Revolution; Mohr, J.C. *Abortion in America*. New York: Oxford University Press, 1978.

9 Etzioni, A. *A Comparative Analysis of Complex Organizations*. New York: Free Press, 1961.; Hern, W.M., Gold, M., and Oakes, A. Administrative incongruence and authority conflict in four abortion clinics. *Human Organization* 35(4):376–83, 1977.

10 Hodgson, J.E., Smith, R., Milstein, D.: Menstrual extraction: Putting it and all its synonyms into proper perspective as pseudonyms. *JAMA* 228:849, 1974.

11 Bygdeman, M., VanLook, P.F.A. Anti-progesterones for the interruption of pregnancy. In: *Bailliere's Clinical Obstetrics and Gynaecology*, Vol. 2, pp. 617–29, 1988.

12 Darney, P.D., Landy, U., MacPherson, S., and Sweet, R.L. Abortion training in U.S. obstetrics and gynecology residency programs. *Family Planning Perspectives* 19(4):158–62, 1987.

13 Grimes, D.A. Clinicians who provide abortions: The thinning ranks. *Obstetrics and Gynecology* 80:719–23, 1992.

14 Baumol, W.J., and Blinder, A.S. *Economics: Principles and Policy*. New York: Harcourt Brace Jovanovitch, 1979. p. 608.

15 McKeegan, M. *Abortion Politics: Mutiny in the Ranks of the Right*. New York: The Free Press, 1992.

16 Blanchard, D.A., and Prewitt, T.J. *Religious Violence and Abortion: The Gideon Project*. Gainesville: University Press of Florida, 1993.

17 Grimes, D.A., Forrest, J.D., Kirkman, A.L., and Radford, B. An epidemic of antiabortion violence in the United States. *American Journal of Obstetrics and Gynecology* 165:1263–68, 1991.

18 Hern, W.M. The pope and my right to life. *New York Times*, op-ed page, August 12, 1993.

19 Blanchard, D.A., and Prewitt, T.J. *Religious Violence and Abortion: The Gideon Project*. Gainesville: University Press of Florida, 1993.

20 There are now instances (in 2024) in the United States where, to the benefit of many women, highly competent nurse-practitioners and physician assistants are performing safe surgical abortions.

18 The international role of abortion in women's health and population growth

In 1994, as Chair-Elect of the Population, Family Planning and Reproductive Health Section of the American Public Health Association, I was the American delegate from the APHA to the International Conference on Population and Development in Cairo. I presented the following paper to a packed audience of several hundred people at the beginning of the conference. As I finished my remarks, members of the Muslim Brotherhood, the people who assassinated Anwar Sadat, came to the microphone just in front of me and confronted me with their anger. They shook their fists at me and shouted "Are you ready to die?" It was terrifying. The police escorted me out of the back of the room. I was under armed guard for the rest of the conference.

Unfortunately, to my profound dismay, although I received an invitation from the editor to have this paper published in the *American Journal of Public Health*, I did not see the invitation until many years later. I was overwhelmed with other urgent matters in my medical practice when I returned home from the Cairo conference, such as taking care of patients. I was being stalked by an anti-abortion fanatic who was a marksman and survivalist. A national anti-abortion group had a press conference announcing their hit list of doctors to be assassinated, of which I was one. I did not get caught up with my mail (and still haven't). The original paper is published here for the first time.

Many of the facts presented in this paper are still true, but with the caveat that many of the worst numbers are worse. Women continue to die from unsafe abortion and unattended childbirth all over the world. Some countries, such as Mexico, have made abortion legal, whereas other countries, such as the United States, are increasingly making abortion illegal and as unsafe as it has been for thousands of years. Restrictions worldwide are generally the result of religious fanaticism (especially Christianity and Islam) and exploitation of abortion as a political issue to gain power, especially in the United States by the Republican Party.

The International Role of Abortion in Women's Health and Population Growth
Warren M. Hern, M.D., M.P.H., Ph.D.*
Chair-Elect
Population, Family Planning and Reproductive Health
Section, American Public Health Association**
Presented to the NGO FORUM 94
International Conference on Population and Development
United Nations
September 5–13, 1994 Cairo, Egypt

DOI: 10.4324/9781003514961-19

Abstract

Abortion, as well as other forms of fertility control, is an essential component of women's health care in the twentieth century. So when feminists argue that the health and educational needs of women must come first, they are right: no social goals are more important than liberating women from the tyranny of their own biology and giving them real control over their own lives and health. But there is another reason for doing what is right for women.

Every second, the human population grows by three persons, 180 per minute, 10,800 per hour, over a quarter of a million per day. For the past 10,000 years, the rate of increase has been increasing. Growth of the human population has averaged 1.9% per year for most of the past 45 years. Even if the rate has dropped to 1.7%, as some claim, it is the difference between going off a cliff at 45 miles per hour instead of 50 miles per hour. It would be better not to go off the cliff.

What does abortion have to do with this? Every year, about 55 million abortions are performed in the world. Unless those 55 million pregnancies are prevented by other means such as contraception, the world population would grow at up to 2.4% per year - much higher than it is, leading to a population of 10 billion by the year 2018. In order to stop population growth, safe abortion must be widely available to women. Better yet, all forms of contraception and sterilization must be available to all women and their partners. Doing the right thing for women is also the right thing for everyone else.

Introduction

Each year, at least 100,000 and as many as 250,000 women die needlessly from illegal or improperly performed abortions. The number may be as high as a half million. These deaths are unnecessary, preventable, and tragic for the women's families as well as for the women themselves. But they represent only a fraction of the 55 million women who obtain abortions each year, most under unsanitary and sordid circumstances that leave many hundreds of thousands of women with serious and permanent scars.

The most important reason to be concerned about these horrifying facts is because the health impact for women of illegal and unsafe abortion on their lives and the welfare of their families. But it is also necessary to examine the effects of the availability of abortion on the world population crisis.

Effects of abortion on women's health

Since earliest recorded history, and probably in prehistoric times, women have used abortion to control fertility.[1] Anthropologists have shown that women in nearly all tribal societies throughout the world use abortion as a means of preventing unplanned or unwanted births.[2]

In modern times, unsafe abortion has been repeatedly shown to be a leading cause of death for women in the child-bearing age range, principally where it is illegal.[3] Illegal abortion is everywhere associated with extremely high rates of morbidity for women seeking illegal abortion, high rates of hospitalization and blood transfusion resulting from the treatment of women for the complications of unsafe abortion, and incalculable suffering for the families of women who die from these preventable tragedies.

Legalization of abortion is associated with rapid drops in death rates among women having abortions and a decline in maternal mortality rates overall.[4] Women who are already at high risk for complications of pregnancy tend to seek abortions for their own reasons.[5] These include women who are very young, women who have recently experienced a term birth, women who have already experienced numerous term pregnancies, and women who are near the end of their reproductive careers. The women who at high risk for death and complications of pregnancy account for a large proportion of maternal mortality, and their access to safe abortion services results in a sharp decline in maternal mortality rates overall. These same women are at high risk, not only of having complicated pregnancies, but of delivering infants who are more likely to die or suffer permanent disability. Access to safe abortion thereby contributes to a similar reduction in infant and neonatal mortality rates. Children who are born as the result of desired pregnancies have a better chance of being born alive and healthy. Everybody benefits.

In the United States, prior to 1970, illegal abortion accounted for as much as half of all maternal mortality from 1920 to 1960.[6] These deaths were experienced more by members of minority groups than by others. For example, in 1965, black women were seven times as likely to die from unsafe abortion as white women.[7] In New York City, abortion accounted for 20% of the maternal mortality for white women, but it accounted for 55% of the maternal mortality for black women. Abortion accounted for 65% of the maternal mortality for Puerto Rican women living in New York City.[8] Access to safe abortion under the condition of illegality was more restricted for poor women and members of minority groups than for white women with money.

Following the legalization of abortion in the United States, both the maternal mortality rate and death rate due to illegal abortion declined sharply. In 1976, for the first time in the city's history, there were no deaths due to illegal abortion in New York City.[9] Since that time, the death rate due to abortion in the United States has dropped to about 3 per million procedures.[10] Death due to abortion has become an extremely small proportion of the overall maternal mortality rate in the United States because of access to safe abortion. A similar experience has been seen in other countries where abortion has become legal.

There are a number of reasons why death rates due to abortion drop when legal restrictions are removed. First, when abortion is legal, physicians can perform abortions in clean and medically safe facilities. Adequate preoperative evaluation and postoperative care can be provided. When minor complications occur, they can be treated promptly before they become major or fatal complications.[11] Physicians become experienced in performing abortions and can do so more safely. Women seek abortions early in pregnancy when it is safer to perform an abortion. Finally, there is no legal risk in making referrals for abortion or for the treatment of complications, and communications among professionals help women obtain proper services.

As the result of the widespread availability of safe abortion services in the United States, the death rate due to abortion is approximately 1/10th or less than the death rate due to term pregnancy under the best conditions. The U.S. maternal mortality rate is now in the range of 8 - 9 per 100,000 live births, although it is higher among the poor and some groups with limited access to good medical care, whereas the case fatality rate due to abortion is in the range of 1-3 per million procedures.[12] Under these conditions, there is no medical justification of any kind for restricting access to abortion services in any way. Efforts to impose restrictions flow from cultural, ideological, and political justifications and not from any basis in scientific fact.

The effects of abortion on population growth

In a study published in the National Academy of Science's 1971 report, *Rapid Population Growth*, Omran showed that developing countries cannot easily achieve a demographic transition to lower fertility without the widespread availability of abortion, legal or illegal.[13] Since a large proportion of population growth projected for the next century will occur in what are now developing countries, Omran's conclusions have special pertinence for policies affecting abortion in those countries.

At the present time, official projections state that the world population is growing at the rate of about 1.7% per year and that fertility rates are falling.[14] However, population growth rates have averaged 1.9% for several time spans beginning in 1950 and ending in 1990[15]. The 1993 population of 5.6 billion was half that size in 1956, giving a doubling time of 37 years and an average growth rate of 1.9% per year. An average of 100 million persons were added each year to the human population from 1987 to 1993 (5.0 to 5.6 billion), giving an average population growth rate of 1.8% per year, even though the official estimates are 94 million per year based on estimates of 144 million births minus an estimate of 50 million deaths. This yields an annual growth rate of 1.7%, providing a basis for optimistic reports that the growth rate is falling; but large numbers of marginal people in areas being colonized by young families with high fertility and a large excess of births over deaths are not included in official census reports. In some areas, census estimates may be low by 25% and growth rates low by 10%.

If the actually observed 1.8% growth rate is assumed for the next quarter century, and there is no strong evidence that this rate will decline, world population would reach 9.6 billion in 2025 and 10 billion in about 2027. Continuous growth at this rate, with a doubling time of 38.5 years, would mean a world population of about 15 billion in 2050 and 37 billion in the year 2100. We must ask: what would be the effect on these growth rates if 55 million women did not obtain abortions each year? Of the 55 million, we may assume that 20% (11 million) of the pregnancies would result in spontaneous abortion, or miscarriage, leaving a net number of additional births at 44 million. Further, we may assume a high infant mortality rate of 10%, or 4.4 million, which is higher than that experienced by most developing countries. We may not assume that each abortion averts one birth; the number is closer to .8 births averted per abortion[16], a factor which is accounted for by the estimated proportion (20%) of anticipated spontaneous abortions (miscarriages). Rounding off to a current average increase of 134 million per year on a base of the 1993 estimated population of 5.6 billion, we would experience a population growth rate of 2.4% per year with a population doubling time of 29 years. At this rate, we would reach a population of 10 billion by 2018, and the 1993 population of 5.6 billion would more than double to 11.25 billion by 2023. World population would reach 21.5 billion by 2050 and about 71 billion by the year 2100.

In its population estimates for the years up to 2150, the United Nations Department of International Economic and Social Affairs (1992) has projected that long-range projections may be as high as 19.2 billion for the year 2100, but this assumes a decline in total fertility rates from the current 2.5 overall to 2.17. There is only a 10 percent difference between the high estimate leading to a population of 19.2 billion in 2100 and a low estimate of 6 billion. UN forecasters state that the entire range of estimates is reasonable, and that there is great uncertainty in the population forecasts. The UN authors state, however, that a population of 28 billion in 2150 is likely to be beyond the carrying capacity of the planet.

If, however, a higher proportion of pregnancies could be prevented among those who wish to do so, and if a higher proportion of women seeking abortion for unwanted pregnancy were able to do so safely, the growth rates could be more easily brought to lower levels than are being observed at the present. Applying the US abortion ratio of 401 abortions per 1000 live births yields a total of 57 million, or an increase of 2 million abortions per year, which would, in itself, lower the overall population growth rate to a little over 1.6% per year. The objective, however, is not to increase the number of abortions performed but to decrease the need for them through sex education and contraception. By all accounts, the most powerful contraception, aside from actual fertility control methods, is education for women, which benefits women in many other ways. Education for women benefits society in innumerable ways. It is another happy case that doing the right thing for women also happens to be the right thing for everyone else.

Just the same, it is apparent that reaching the objective of lower population growth rates can only be achieved through the availability of all methods of fertility control, including abortion. No one method of fertility control will have sufficient impact to affect growth rates that are clearly out of control at the present time. It is also clear that, unless population growth rates are voluntarily brought lower, and eventually to zero, there is no hope of meeting the challenges of economic growth and reversing the otherwise fatal trend of irreversible destruction of the ecosphere in which we live. The time to focus on this fundamental challenge to survival of the human species is now, not when our fate is clearly sealed.

These observations also mean that some cherished cultural values concerning the inferior status of women and the desirability of large families must be abandoned for the sake of human survival.

Effects of restricting access to abortion services

In modern times, various governments have attempted to restrict women's access to abortion services. Reports of the effects of restrictive policies in Chile by Armijo and Monreal and by Requena were among the first in the world.[17] These and various other reports from Latin America have consistently indicated that complications from illegally induced abortion accounted for from 50 to 80% of blood transfusions in metropolitan hospitals in that region, a large proportion of hospital bed-days, and provide the leading cause of death for women in the child-bearing age range.[18]

The effects of Ceauşescu's notorious restrictive abortion policy in Romania are well known. When the Romanian government outlawed abortion in 1966 in order to increase the supply of able-bodied workers for Romanian factories, requiring women to have 5 children, the legal abortion rate went down and the birth rate went up briefly, but the maternal mortality rate went up dramatically. Most of the deaths were due to illegal abortion. By 1989, when Ceauşescu was deposed and the abortion law reversed, Romania had the highest maternal mortality rate in Europe (150 maternal deaths per 100,000 live births), and its abortion-related maternal mortality was ten times higher than its neighbors.[19] These hideous health consequences were accompanied by the activities of the "pregnancy police" of the Ceauşescu regime, who conducted a wide variety of police-state surveillances of women to detect pregnancy and abortion. The aim of controlling women's reproductive lives was revealed baldly for what it was - the use of women as reproductive machines to serve the state interests in economic production.

The effects of restrictive laws in the United States were not so dramatic because they were not, for the most part, accompanied by police-state tactics. On the contrary, few women were prosecuted for having abortions, but the effect of persecuting those who performed illegal abortions was to force women into "back-alley" procedures that often resulted in death or serious disability.[20] As noted previously, it has been estimated that, from 1920 through 1960, half of all U.S. maternal mortality was due to abortion.

Influences of abortion politics on United States government

Throughout the 20th century, social reformers such as Margaret Sanger fought to improve access to fertility control. But these efforts intensified during the 1960s and were directed toward easing restrictions on abortion.[21] In 1970, following recommendations by the Rockefeller Commission and Congressional hearings, Congress passed the Title X legislation providing significant support for domestic family planning programs. This was accompanied by the development of family planning programs, including voluntary sterilization services, in several US government programs such as the Office of Economic Opportunity.[22] Support for fertility control programs abroad was administered through the Agency for International Development. Abortion public health statistics and reproductive health program research in general flourished at the Centers for Disease Control in Atlanta, which made abortion services in the US the most highly monitored surgical activity in the world, and this aggressive evaluation helped make them among the safest. US support compared to total need for domestic and foreign fertility control programs was modest, but it was approached as a positive good and placed appropriately in a context of women's health care.

In 1976, however, the right wing of the Republican party and the religious right began strongly influencing the platform statements and nominating choices of the Republican party. By 1980, with the nomination of Ronald Reagan, moderates who supported reproductive choice were driven from influence. Reagan actively courted and benefitted politically from close association with the religious right and the anti-abortion movement in particular.[23] At his first press conference on the day after he was elected in 1980, the first thing Reagan said was, "I am going to make abortion illegal." He did not, but he and George Bush brought powerful forces to bear on the issue and imposed important restrictions on reproductive choice. Reagan and the Republican Party used the abortion issue with great effect in subsequent elections, and, combined with powerful conservative allies in Congress such as Henry Hyde and Jesse Helms, sought increasingly severe restrictions on both domestic and foreign fertility control programs. US assistance to programs such as the UNFPA were terminated on grounds that some money might be used by some programs for abortion or even abortion counseling.

In 1984, UN Ambassador James Buckley carried the Reagan administration's policy to the Mexico City Population Conference, saying, in effect: "Don't worry about population: At worst it's neutral. The way to solve the population growth problem is to give money to the capitalists."[24] By 1984, however, many representatives of developing countries realized that uncontrolled population growth was overwhelming all efforts at meaningful economic development, and they wanted help in the way of fertility control programs. In some Third-World countries, there was despair at US policy.

In 1988, when he was running for President, George Bush followed Reagan's lead in courting the radical right and anti-abortion movement. During the presidential debate of September, 1988, Bush said that he was inclined to punish women who had abortions, although (after 30 years in public life), he hadn't "sorted it all out yet." The next morning, after calculating the potential electoral damage, Bush's political handlers issued a statement in which he advocated the imprisonment of doctors who do abortions, but the women had suffered enough by having had them.[25] Bush was elected by a landslide. The next year, after Bush had vetoed Congressional legislation permitting Washington, D.C. to use its own funds to provide abortions for poor women who had been raped, US voters who claimed to support reproductive freedom were also found in a poll to support George Bush by a margin of 3 to 2. US government support for both domestic and foreign fertility-control assistance programs remained at levels lower than they were in the early 1970s in terms of real dollars.

The Bush administration remained opposed to support for UNFPA because of the controversy concerning China's abortion policies, and the House of Representatives repeatedly refused to appropriate $15 million for that program. During the election campaign of 1992, Bill Clinton actively sought the support of pro-choice groups and strongly supported reproductive freedom. Hillary Rodham Clinton was highly visible in these efforts. By January 24, 1993, Clinton had reversed a wide variety of Reagan-Bush administration domestic policies that had been aimed at restricting reproductive choice, and he nullified the Mexico City policy. He appointed former US Senator Tim Wirth as Counselor in the Department of State with a portfolio to include population policy. Wirth had a strong record of outspoken support of reproductive freedom as a member of the House of Representatives and as a Senator. Subsequent policy statements by Wirth and Clinton have consistently expanded this support, including a recent statement by Wirth that the goal should be the availability of fertility control methods to every couple on the planet who wants them. Abortion, however, is not included in this definition. There would be little Congressional support for such inclusion.

Policy considerations for the United States and for the International Conference on Population and Development

While the US policy position in 1994 concerning population and development as stated by Undersecretary for Global Affairs Tim Wirth is 180 degrees opposite of the 1984 US policy at Mexico City[26], it necessarily contains a conservative element due to conflicting political forces within the US Congress and electorate. The Clinton administration's view of abortion, for example, is that abortion should be "safe, legal, and rare." Even if it were inclined to do so - and it is not - this administration is not likely to advocate the removal of restrictions on abortion in other countries. The political backlash in the US would be serious, and the backlash from otherwise friendly countries would be serious. Additionally, legal abortion is under vigorous attack in the United States, and there is little support for public funding of abortion services in the US government, including the Clinton administration.

In public statements, Undersecretary Wirth has announced a goal of increasing US funding for foreign-assistance fertility control programs from a little over $500 million to $1.2 billion annually by the end of the century. These statements alone represent a dramatic departure from previous US policy. Wirth has also stated that a global budget of approximately $7 billion annually needs to be spent to meet the needs of some 300-400 million couples who need fertility control assistance at some level, with the US picking up a large share. It is difficult to imagine Congressional support for larger commitments than those stated by Undersecretary Wirth.

From the point of view of those who support reproductive freedom and who are also deeply concerned about the crushing effects of global population growth, however, the question must be asked: is it enough?

The policy debate – A chimera, a snare, and a delusion

A recent issue of The New York Times Magazine featured contrasting statements concerning population by a prominent demographer and feminist representative of the International Women's Health Coalition. The essence of the mini-debate was that a) controlling population growth has to be a major priority for everyone, and that b) no, women's rights and health issues must be first. A more troubling version of this "debate" was offered by Frances Kissling, head of Catholics For A Free Choice, at an April 6 press conference at PrepCom responding to a Vatican pronouncement in which she said, "As an American, I say no to population control. I say no to papal control."

At least three perspectives (or caricatures of perspectives) can be identified from this confusing array of positions: a) Control of population growth must be applied at all costs, including the sacrifice of individual rights, the least important of which are those of women; b) Population control is irrelevant and offensive; health care and justice for women is more important than any such misguided plan as population control, which is just another way to use women as the means of obtaining government objectives; population control is a Yankee imperialist plot to oppress women; c) (ostensibly by the Pope and the Vatican) The purpose of women is for childbearing, and they should have as many babies as possible, or at least as many as we can baptize, and they should stick to that noble activity instead of trying to run the world; and population growth is wonderful, we should have more of it.

The last of these positions, which is represented here perhaps more fairly than the others, has something to offend all adherents to the first two, and is really the only authentic contender in three-way contest. The Vatican really does believe that more is better and that women's reproductive rights are of no consequence.

As between the first two, stated fairly or not, there is no serious debate, or at least, there should be none. The feminists are absolutely correct to say that women's rights must be respected and advanced at every opportunity, that the health of women comes first, and that this includes all methods of fertility control as well as the context of better health care for women, more education and economic equity for women, and more opportunities for women to participate meaningfully in all societies. But I don't know any respectable demographers who disagree with this position.

It is, however, extremely myopic for anyone, including feminists, to deny that the juggernaut of population growth must be confronted. In order for us to survive as a species, we must stop population growth - not merely slow it down - as quickly as possible. This is a matter of utmost urgency, and it has been made more urgent by the regressive policies of the previous US administrations. If we do not stop population growth by exercising serious voluntary controls on fertility, it will stop because of rising death rates and fertility that is declining because of environmental pollution, starvation, and the metabolic effects of crowding. This is not merely a fantasy for the future; it is a reality with which many people now live.

Recommendations for U.S. Policy and for the ICPD statement

A U.S. policy that reflects the daily reality of people's lives and medical facts confronted by women and doctors around the world would look like this:

* Abortion is an essential component of women's health care in the twentieth century and should be widely available for all women without restrictions of any kind.
* Abortion gives women control over their own lives and reproductive decisions, and they are better prepared than any government to make decisions about whether or not to continue any particular pregnancy.
* Abortion is not rare now, it never has been, and it never will be. While abortion is not is safe and legal everywhere, and it should be. And for population growth to stop, abortion must be widely available on request everywhere.
* Where adequate and safe abortion services are not available, the US should vigorously support efforts to make them available.
* Abortion should be offered in the context of humane, dignified, and competent fertility control services and related health services that are geared to women's needs and coupled with strong education programs, especially for young girls and adolescents. Educational and economic opportunities and worthy life objectives other than reproduction are powerful contraceptives. Postponing the first pregnancy and delivery should be an especially important objective, mainly for medical reasons, but also because this has an exceptionally powerful effect on community fertility rates.
* US policies with respect to abortion should eliminate all barriers, including poverty, that limit access to abortion and other means of fertility control. Without this step, the US has no moral credibility in helping other nations with fertility reduction programs.
* The aim of all reproductive health programs should be to provide safe and effective fertility control and to reduce the number of both unplanned pregnancies and abortions to zero. These programs should occur in the context of broad maternal and child-health programs that reduce both maternal and infant mortality. To accomplish this end, it may be necessary to have a global expenditure by all governments of $150 billion annually; this amount is approximately half the US defense budget. Of this, $30 billion should be dedicated to all forms of fertility control, including safe abortion.

Concerning the ICPD Programme of Action, the following changes should be made in Chapter VIII (Health and Mortality) at [8.21]:

* Women should have unlimited access to safe abortion services...(DELETE "..in case of rape and incest." [8.21]
* Women who wish to terminate their pregnancies...humane treatment of complications of unsafe abortions. Abortion services should be safe and accessible. [8.21]

Action recommendation

The following changes should be made in Chapter VIII (Health and Mortality) at [8.21]:

* Women should have unlimited access to safe abortion services...(DELETE "..in case of rape and incest." [8.21]
* Women who wish to terminate their pregnancies...humane treatment of complications of unsafe abortions. Abortion services should be safe and accessible. [8.21]

Addendum (2024)

The maternal mortality ratio in the United States has risen from 8 per 100,000 live births in 1995 to 20.1 per 100,000 live births in 2019.[27] It is now about 33 per 100,000 live births. It is the worst of all industrialized countries. This has occurred while right-wing political repression of women and the criminalization of abortion has progressed under Republican political control. Worldwide, unsafe abortion is still the leading cause of maternal death and morbidity.

The world population has increased from 3.77 billion in 1971 to 5.6 billion in 1994 (the year of this conference) to over 8 billion at the beginning of 2024. We have reached completely unsustainable continued destruction of the global ecosystem, which cannot be halted or reversed as long as the human population is growing. All population and public health scientists agree that uncontrolled population growth cannot be stopped unless as many women and their families as possible have complete access to all forms of fertility control, including safe and effective contraception, safe abortion, voluntary sterilization, and integrated family planning services.[28]

Notes

1 Himes, NE. *A Medical History of Contraception*. New York: Schocken, 1970.
2 Devereux, G. *A Study of Abortion in Primitive Society*. New York: Julian Press, 1955; Early, J.D., and Peters, J.F. *The Population Dynamics of the Mucajai Yanomama*. San Diego: Academic Press, 1990; Weisbard, S.R. Indios Shamas de Peru. *Ethnographie* 53:19–74, 1957.
3 Armijo, R. and T. Monreal. The problem of induced abortion in Chile. *Milbank Memorial Fund Quarterly* 43(4): 263, 1965. Part 2; Requena, M. The problem of induced abortion in Latin America. *Demography* 5(2):785, 1968; Tietze, C. *Induced Abortion: A World Review, 1983*. 5th ed., p. 33. New York: The Population Council, 1983.; Hord, C, H.P. David, F. Donnay, and Wolf M. Reproductive health in Romania: Reversing the Ceaucescu legacy. *Studies in Family Planning* 22(4):231, 1991; Cates W., Jr. Legal abortion: The public health record. *Science* 215:1586, 1982; Pakter, J. The effects of liberalized abortion laws on abortion mortality and morbidity in New York City. In Hern W.M., and Andrikopolous, B. (eds), *Abortion in the Seventies. Proceedings of the Western Regional Conference on Abortion, Denver, February, 1976*. New York: National Abortion Federation, 1977.
4 Pakter, J. The effects of liberalized abortion laws on abortion mortality and morbidity in New York City. In Hern W.M., and Andrikopolous, B. (eds). *Abortion in the Seventies. Proceedings of the Western Regional Conference on Abortion, Denver, February, 1976*. New York: National Abortion Federation, 1977; Cates W., Jr. Legal abortion: The public health record. *Science* 215:1586, 1982.
5 Tietze, C. *Induced Abortion: A World Review, 1983*. 5th ed., p. 33. New York: The Population Council, 1983; Henshaw, S.K., and J. Van Vort. *Abortion Factbook, 1992 Edition*. New York: Alan Guttmacher Institute, 1992.
6 Lerner, M., and O.W. Anderson. *Health Progress in the United States:1900–1960*, chap 4, p. 34. Chicago: University of Chicago Press, 1963.
7 National Center for Health Statistics. *Vital Statistics of the United States, 1967*. Vol. 2 - Mortality, Part A, pp. 1–40, Table 1–15. 1967 mortality rates (per 100,000 live births) due to septic abortion: whites, 1.5; nonwhites, 10.2; overall, 3.

8 Gold, M., Erdhardt, C.L., Jacobziner, H., and Nelson, F.G. Therapeutic abortions in New York City: A 20-year review. *American Journal of Public Health and the Nation's Health* 55(7): 964–972, 1965.

9 Pakter, J. The effects of liberalized abortion laws on abortion mortality and morbidity in New York City. In Hern, W.M., and Andrikopolous, B. (eds). *Abortion in the Seventies. Proceedings of the Western Regional Conference on Abortion, Denver, February, 1976.* New York: National Abortion Federation, 1977.

10 Koonin, L.M., Smith, J.C., Ramick, M., et al.: Abortion Surveillance - United States, 1989. In: *CDC Surveillance Summaries*, September 4, 1992. *MMWR* 1992; 441 (No. SS-5).

11 Hern, W.M. The epidemiologic foundations of abortion practice. In *Abortion Practice.* Boulder, CO: Alpenglo Graphics, 1990.

12 Koonin, L.M., Atrash, H.K., Lawson, H.W., et al. Maternal mortality surveillance, United States, 1979–1986 (1991a). *CDC Surveillance Summaries, July, 1991. MMWR* 1991; 40 (No. SS-2):1–13.; Koonin, L.M., Kochanek, K.D., Smith, J.C., et al.: Abortion surveillance, United States, 1988 (1991b). *CDC Surveillance Summaries, July 1991, MMWR* 1991;40 (No. SS-2):15–42.

13 Omran, A.R. Abortion in the demographic transition. In *Rapid Population Growth: Consequences and Policy Implications.* Vol. 2. Baltimore: National Academy of Sciences and Johns Hopkins University Press, 1971.

14 Robey, B., Rutstein, S.O., and Morris, L. The fertility decline in developing countries. *Scientific American*, December, 1993; Bongaarts, J. Population policy options in the developing world. *Science* 263(5148):771–76, 1994.

15 United Nations, Department of International Economic and Social Affairs. *Long-Range World Population Projections.* New York: United Nations, 1992.

16 Keyfitz, N. *Applied Mathematical Demography.* 2nd ed. New York: Springer-Verlag, 1985.

17 Armijo, R., and Monreal, T. The problem of induced abortion in Chile. *Milbank Memorial Fund Quarterly* 43(4): 263, 1965. Part 2; Requena, M. Social and economic correlates of induced abortion in Santiago, Chile. *Demography*, 1965.

18 Casterline, J. Collecting data on abortion using national national surveys. In *Methodological Issues in Abortion Research.* New York: The Population Council, 1990.

19 Stephenson P., Wagner, M., Badea M., and Sebanescu F. (1992): Commentary: The public health consequences of restricted induced abortion - Lessons from Romania. *American Journal of Public Health* 82(10):1328.

20 Solinger, R. *The Abortionist: A Woman against The Law.* New York: The Free Press, 1994.

21 Garrow, D.J. *Liberty and Sexuality: The Right to Privacy and the Making of Roe vs. Wade.* New York: Macmillan, 1994.

22 Hern, W.M. Family planning and the poor. *The New Republic*, November 14, 1970; Hern, W.M. Biological tyranny. *The New Republic*, February 27, 1971.

23 Michelle McKeegan., *Fetal Politics: Abortion and the Making and Unmaking of a Conservative Majority.* New York: The Free Press, 1992.

24 *New York Times*, August 9, 1984. https://www.nytimes.com/1984/08/09/world/statement-by -us-delegate-to-the-conference-on-population-in-mexico-city.html Statement by U.S. Delegate to the Conference on Population in Mexico City.

25 *New York Times*, September 27. 1988 https://www.nytimes.com/1988/09/27/us/after-the -debate-bush-camp-offers-a-clarified-stand-about-abortions.html *NY Times* after the Debate; Bush Camp Offers a Clarified Stand about Abortions. By Gerald M. Boyd, Special to the *New York Times*.

26 Menken, J. (ed). *World Population and US Policy: The Choices Ahead.* New York: W.W. Norton, 1985.

27 Hoyert, D. Maternal mortality rates in the United States, 2021. *NCHS Report.* CDC. 2021.

28 Hern, W.M. *Homo Ecophagus: A Deep Diagnosis to Save the Earth.* London: Routledge Press, 2022; Speidel, J.J., and O'Sullivan, J.N. Advancing the welfare of people and the planet with a common agenda for reproductive justice, population, and the environment. *World*, 4:259–87, 2023. https://doi.org/10.3390/world4020018

19 Choice comments

To give the reader a sense of the tumultuous series of events and my responses to them in the public arena, I am including here the full texts of a few of the original publications of mine written for the general public that appeared in American newspapers and magazines during the past 50 years and an article by Bob Herbert in the *New York Times* about the hazards of my work brought by anti-abortion political terrorists.

Anti-abortion cemetery games

In January 2005, I received a call from a reporter for the *Denver Post* informing me that a local Catholic church had obtained the cremated remains of fetal tissue from my patients without my knowledge and planned to bury them in a ceremony at a Catholic cemetery on January 23, 2005, the day after the 32nd anniversary of the *Roe v. Wade* decision legalizing abortion in the United States. The incident became a national news story, and I began getting calls from women who were former patients of mine from all over the country and women coming to my office to express their concern and anguish over the invasion of their privacy and exploitation of their private grief for political purposes.

Each woman who has an abortion has different concerns and attitudes toward the tissue – and sometimes, fetus – that is removed from her at her request. For some who are terminating a desired pregnancy, a private burial or cremation service is needed. For others, for whom the pregnancy is the result of a sexual assault, no such service is wanted. On the contrary, the abortion may be a symbolic ending of a hideous personal experience and a relief from personal hell. The fact that others may want to exploit such a woman's grief and pain for political purposes only adds to the emotional trauma instead of allowing it to end and recede into the past.

Here is my article published in the *Daily Camera* following this incident:

Burial of ashes is an unethical spectacle[1]

Mortuary action was grievous and symbolic

Daily Camera *March 6, 2005 Guest Opinion*

It has been over a month since a reporter informed me that a local Catholic church had obtained the cremated remains of fetal tissue from my patients without my knowledge and planned to bury them in a ceremony at a Catholic cemetery on January 23, 2005. But I am still getting calls and questions about this

DOI: 10.4324/9781003514961-20

from former patients and women who come to me now seeking medical services, and the story is still getting national media attention.

Each woman who has an abortion has different concerns and attitudes toward the tissue – and sometimes, fetus – that is removed from her at her request. For some who are terminating a desired pregnancy, a private burial or cremation service is needed. For others, for whom the pregnancy is the result of a sexual assault, no such service is wanted. On the contrary, the abortion may be a symbolic ending of a hideous personal experience and a relief from personal hell. The fact that others may want to exploit such a woman's grief and pain for political purposes only adds to the emotional trauma instead of allowing it to end and recede into the past.

In the incident involving my office, Crist Mortuary, and the Sacred Heart of Mary Catholic Church, the basic facts are simple. In July, 2001, my representatives made a written and verbal agreement with officials of Crist Mortuary, using a contract provided by Crist, for the cremation of embryonic and fetal remains and burial of the ashes in Crist's non-sectarian Mountain View Cemetery. I paid Crist Mortuary $225 from September, 2001 through November, 2004 for this service on each of seven different occasions for a total of $1575. I had no reason to suspect that any other use would be made of these ashes. I was astounded and outraged to learn from the reporter and from news reports, including those in the Daily Camera, that all these ashes had been taken from the mortuary to the Catholic Church for burial. I was even more outraged to learn of the public spectacle that would occur at the church cemetery on January 23 in conjunction with the 32nd anniversary of the *Roe vs. Wade* decision of the Supreme Court.

In the days that followed the announcement of this event and the church's unauthorized use of these ashes, I received numerous telephone calls from former patients expressing distress at what was happening. Reactions ranged from re-awakened grief to towering anger. Every single patient who called felt that Crist Mortuary's violation of our agreement was unethical and that the actions of the church officials were inappropriate if not arrogant and hurtful.

Although I do not ask my patients to tell me their religion, many do tell me. Some request religious or traditional bereavement rituals according to their personal beliefs. More than 25 years ago, a Native American woman conducted her tribal bereavement ceremony in my office. The ceremony was extremely moving, and my entire staff was in tears by the time it was finished.

Some of our patients are members of the Orthodox and Conservative Jewish faiths and require specific burial rituals conducted by a rabbi. We have helped our Jewish patients have these ceremonies. We have had many patients who are Reform Jews, secular Jews, Protestant, Catholic, Mormon, Muslim, Hindu, Sikh, Buddhist, and Taoist; we have had some who were Coptic or Zoroastrian; and some of our patients are atheists who want no religious ritual of any kind. Most patients want no special arrangements. They choose not to be reminded of the pain they experienced with the loss of this pregnancy.

Other patients send us letters and joyful announcements for years showing us pictures of their living children and new babies. These patients and their families are grateful for the choice that we helped them make by being able to terminate a hopeless or dangerous pregnancy in a safe and dignified manner.

Abortion is almost certainly one of the most difficult, painful, and controversial issues in American society. The issue has been exploited by the Republican Party and by certain religious leaders for 30 years. Any public action taken with regard to this issue is a political statement. It cannot be interpreted otherwise. Any such action affects public opinion, public policy, and power arrangements. To deny this is preposterous.

In this particular instance, one side of the equation includes individuals and families that are attempting to resolve a life crisis involving a decision to reproduce, to form a family, and to make a lifetime commitment for which they may feel unprepared. This decision may be overlaid by tragic circumstances of catastrophic fetal disorder that seriously affect the quality of life not to mention financial burdens of the families involved, and it may affect the survival of the pregnant woman herself.

On the other side are religious fanatics and political zealots who are determined to prevent, at any cost, the others from exercising their own freedom and responsibility for their own lives. They know exactly how God thinks people should live, and they are willing to use the coercive power of the state to impose these rules.

They respect no boundaries, privacy, or rights of others.

When they cannot actively interfere with the free behavior of the others, this group engages in symbolic activity designed to inflict guilt, pain, shame, loss, and grief on those who do not submit to their imposed behavior.

It is a classic conflict between individual freedom and totalitarian rule. It is the difference between the Enlightenment and the Inquisition. It is the difference between a secular state that values individual expression and a theocracy that burns heretics at the stake. It is the kind of conflict that is at the origin of some recent wars. It is not an exaggeration to say that this is a struggle for the heart and soul of America.

Warren M. Hern, M.D., is director of the Boulder Abortion Clinic

---

Madness in the pursuit of fanaticism

The Human Life Statute: Will It Protect Life or Power?[2]

By Dr. Warren M. Hern

The *Denver Post,* Sunday, June 21, 1981

The Colorado legislature recently rejected two bills which would have made the human embryo a person from the moment of conception. If the bills had passed, any Colorado woman who had an abortion or miscarriage would be subject to prosecution for homicide. The "Human Life Statute" now before the U.S. Congress would have the same effect. It requires only a majority in both houses, plus the president's signature, to become law. Senate Bill 158 (HR 900 in the House), which is in the Senate subcommittee on separation of powers and is expected to pass the full Senate and be signed into law by President Reagan, seeks to impose a view of human existence on our society which is appealing in its apparent simplicity: Human life begins at conception.

On examination, however, this question proves to be more complex. Does conception mean "fertilization" or "implantation?" Which conception? Could it have been the one (which one?) that occurred three million years ago near Olduvai Gorge in Africa?

The view of a theoretical instant in which each individual comes into being is in conflict with the view of life as a continuous stream reaching back into the origins of life itself hundreds of millions of years ago. It is in conflict with the fact that each sperm and ovum is a human cell, that each diploid cell in the rest of the body has 46 chromosomes, and that, while the cells in each of our bodies are constantly dying and being replaced, our structures remain.

The idea that each fertilized ovum is a person is about the same thing as saying that each set of house plans is a house. Calling an ovum a person does not make it so. Calling a fetus an unborn person (and perhaps baptizing it) is as illogical as burying an undead body. This ruse perpetuates an illusion that is useful to some, but in the case of SB 158, the consequences to others may be catastrophic. Since the bill in question is aimed at making abortion illegal, it is worthwhile to examine some of the health and social consequences that such an action would have.

In 1920, the maternal mortality rate in the United States was 680 per 100,000 live births. By 1960, maternal mortality had fallen to around 38 per 100,000 live births. This reduction was brought about by a number of things: better prenatal care, better obstetrical care, the introduction of blood transfusion, antibiotics and other drugs; longer birth intervals, postponed first births, fewer total pregnancies per woman and better nutrition. Nearly half of all maternal deaths in both 1920 and 1960, however, were due to induced abortion in some areas of the country. In New York City, as late as 1965, 55 percent and 65 percent of maternal mortality among black and Puerto Rican women, respectively, was because of septic abortion.

Since 1970, however, abortion has become the safest surgical procedure – and the most heavily monitored – in the United States. The number of abortion deaths dropped from an average of 250 in the mid-1960s to less than 100 per year currently, while more than twice as many abortions are now being performed. A barrier contraceptive method backed up by early abortion is now the safest fertility control method available to women, and early abortion is now the safest of all possible outcomes for pregnant teenagers. This improved safety is almost entirely because of the legalization of abortion, first in Colorado and in other states, then nationally, which permitted the introduction of improved techniques and the accumulation of skills and experience by physicians performing abortions. The risk of death from early abortion is now less than one per million procedures.

Overall, the risk of death due to abortion is currently less than two per 100,000 procedures, whereas the risk of death due to term birth is approximately 14 per 100,000 live births under the best circumstances. The risk of major complications in abortion is 1/200th the risk a woman experiences in term birth. Caesarean section is one major complication, and if this is necessary, her risks are magnified many times. It is important to understand that these risks are experienced by women who are pregnant whether they wish to be pregnant or not, and whether they are rich or poor.

From a medical point of view, abortion should be the indicated treatment of pregnancy unless a woman has a desire to carry the pregnancy to term and reproduce. The effort to criminalize abortion through the mechanism of according the fetus the status of personhood, however, would have serious public health consequences not envisioned by its proponents. If interpreted literally by a zealous prosecutor, SB 158 would have the following consequences:

- It would proscribe all abortions, even if the woman's life is in immediate danger.
- It would criminalize the use of intrauterine devices.
- It would prevent the use of certain oral contraceptives and drugs such as diethylstilbesterol used in preventing pregnancy following unprotected intercourse, as in rape.
- It would prevent treatment, emergency or otherwise, of hydatidiform mole, chroioadenoma destruens, choriocarcinoma and unruptured ectopic pregnancy. The first three, including the third, which is a cancer, arise from conception to become an undifferentiated mass of cells or water sacs. These products of conception would be classified as "persons" under the law.
- It would prevent the treatment of women for conditions unrelated to pregnancy without absolute proof of non-pregnancy, which is impossible under most circumstances.
- It would result in the prosecution of women experiencing spontaneous abortion (miscarriage) for negligent homicide if evidence could be found that the woman engaged in any physical activity or substance use that might lead to spontaneous abortion.
- It would prohibit the use of amniocentesis for the diagnosis of genetic defects.
- It would probably interrupt current research on in-vitro fertilization (test-tube babies) for the benefit of infertile couples.
- It would prohibit evaluation of infertility in women since non-pregnancy would have to be proved before tests could be performed.
- It would prevent the use of x-rays on women who had suffered trauma and who were currently pregnant or might be.
- It would disrupt a confidential doctor-patient relationship in all cases of women in the reproductive age range.
- It would increase the number of unplanned pregnancies due to the criminalization of effective contraceptives.
- It would result in a catastrophic increase in the number of deaths and life-threatening complications due to improperly performed abortions.

As the result of criminalization, the number of abortions performed would probably drop to no less than half of the 1.5 million currently being performed nationally. An unknown number would be added to this fraction as the result of an increase in the number of unplanned pregnancies because of the criminalization of contraceptive methods. Women who experience "high risk" pregnancies – teenagers, older women, women who have recently delivered or who have had many pregnancies – would be forced to carry pregnancies to term whereas they are likely to choose abortion under the current circumstances for their own reasons. The result will be an increase in maternal mortality and complications due to pregnancy, increases in infant mortality, percentage of low birth weight infants, percentage of premature births, an increase in the proportion of developmental and functional abnormalities, an increase in the number of birth defects, and a higher neonatal mortality rate. The financial costs of these consequences will be met, in many cases, by the taxpayers.

One-third of all abortions currently are performed on teenagers. Most of these young women are unprepared for the emotional, intellectual, social and economic responsibilities of parenthood in a complex society and are unprepared to form stable families with their partners. The argument that they should be forced to continue unplanned pregnancies in order to increase the supply of adoptable babies is both cruel and delusional.

More than 90 percent of teenagers who continue unplanned pregnancies to term do not give up their babies for adoption. The technology of abortion is so widely available among physicians and non-physicians alike that enforcement would be hopeless, so what is the point of this exercise? Are we willing to have a police state and keep all women under constant surveillance to ensure the law is observed? Or will we simply put doctors in jail for performing abortions, leaving transgressions to the untutored?

In most societies throughout human existence, various fertility control measures have been used, including abortion. Laws have never prevented abortion, and they never will. SB 158 appears to be a response of a conservative minority to the relentless social change of the last 20 years. This social change has been fueled to a considerable degree by the introduction of highly effective, safe fertility control measures which are available on a wide scale for the first time in human history. From the point of view of cultural change, it is probably the equivalent in importance to the domestication of fire at the human hearth. An important consequence of this new availability of fertility control is the enhancement of the status and independence of women, which has been increasing over the past 50 years.

The new role of women, however, collides head on with the view that the principal function of women is to bear children. This view is no longer shared by a great many people. The view that women should confine their activities to reproduction, however, is held by a majority of the Congress, most of whom are men. Their logic, as expressed in SB 158, is that society must be protected against individuals (doctors who perform abortions; women who want them) to protect the embryos.

Could it be that there is a scarce supply of human embryos?: Could it be that we need a pronatalist public policy because of the shortage of people? Hardly. One important problem is that women are uppity: They vote, and they are now competing with men for jobs and power.

Fetuses, on the other hand, are apolitical, don't argue, present no economic threat, and may be defended along with the flag and motherhood before the voters at election time. They can be defended against sin and immorality, thereby throwing political opponents into disarray.

This conflict brings us clearly to an understanding of the struggle before us. The issue is not the protection of human life. We are already doing that by providing safe abortions for women. The real issue posed by SB 158 is the definition of power: who has it and who doesn't.

The issue is whether power in America will be wielded absolutely by those who cannot get pregnant or whether it will be shared by those who can.

A more basic question before our society is not when life begins, but who is best prepared to decide when to transmit life to a new generation – the individual or the state? The right of the individual woman to make this choice should be supported. In this matter, she is more competent than any government.

Warren M. Hern, M.D., M.P.H., is director of the Boulder Abortion Clinic

---

Killing for life

"Killing for life" is senseless[3]

By Warren Hern

Denver Post *Guest Opinion, Saturday, April 8, 1995*

What kind of person is driven to kill another human being in the name of "life?" That doesn't make sense.

What makes some people in our society absolutely determined to control the most personal, intimate and private aspects of the lives and bodies of fellow citizens whom they do not even know? That doesn't make sense, either.

What brings members of the anti-abortion movement to the belief that they have the right to use the coercive power of the state to force others to behave according to their peculiar moral principles: which supposedly include Christian love and forgiveness? Why does the religion with a message of peace provoke violent attacks on the property and lives of those who disagree?

How can anti-abortion fanatics justify using freedom of speech and religious expression to urge the murder of others?

There is an answer to these questions, but the first step in finding it is to recognize that the agonizingly painful conflict about abortion is not about facts, reason or persuasion: it is about power.

People who think that the abortion controversy doesn't affect them should look again. It affects election results, Supreme Court and surgeon general nominations, control of Congress, foreign policy, the national budget, and the ability of Congress to conduct the nation's business. Anti-abortion terrorism is diminishing the availability of an essential component of health care used by millions of women. The most insidious thing about the anti-abortion movement, however, is its militant attack on things that Americans cherish most – privacy and free speech.

A woman approaching a doctor's office or abortion clinic, whether she is alone or accompanied by her partner or family member, is there to seek a private medical service that has been stigmatized for centuries.

Her condition is the result of her most private, intimate needs and actions and her most important private relationship. It is not only inappropriate, it is insane behavior for anti-abortion fanatics to attempt to give her unwelcome moral messages at that point. It is, in fact, a form of psychological rape. It is an assault. The purpose of anti-abortion demonstrations is not to express an opinion or to convince but to inflict pain, guilt, shame, terror – and now, death. It is intolerable behavior, not free speech.

The assault on free speech by the anti-abortion fanatics produces an even graver danger, which is that their activities will, if unchecked, lead inevitably to a loss of freedom for all of us.

Partly because of the Jan. 22 announcement of the American Coalition of Life Activists of a hit list of doctors it wants eliminated (including me), I am now under the 24-hour protection of armed federal marshals for the third time in two months. That announcement has seriously diminished my freedom. On several occasions, Denver-based anti-abortion TV talk show host Bob Enyart has viciously attacked me over 750 cable channels. Viewers report their concern that he is inciting someone – anyone – to kill me. He even did this on Dec. 30, the evening of the Brookline abortion clinic killings.

Randall Terry, the Christian minister who leads Operation Rescue, has publicly prayed for my death (Oct 7, 1990). During his Aug. 13, 1993, live program on the Christian Broadcasting network, quoting the Bible, he invited his radio listeners to assassinate me.

What is more at stake than the lives of a few doctors is the issue of whether Americans now accept the level of violence and terrorism embraced by the anti-abortion movement as a means of political expression. When the anti-abortion movement gets through with us, who's next? Supreme Court Justices? Yes, says Roy McMillan.

Neither the anti-abortion demagogues nor those they hope to inspire care about me as a person or about the women whose lives I save as a physician. What they care about is power. So does the Republican Party, which has been the chief beneficiary of the 20 years of anti-abortion rhetoric that has led to this terrorism.

Republican leaders have encouraged and used anti-abortion activists to win many important elections since 1980. Bob Dole and three other Republican presidential candidates (including George Bush) accepted invitations to the 1986

National Right to Life Committee annual meeting in Denver. Phil Gramm gave $175,000 of Republican Senate Campaign funds to the NRLC to make last-minute anti-abortion ads against Democratic opponents in 1994.

Now, the Republicans are impaled on this ideology, and the rest of us are impaled on anti-abortion violence.

Warren M. Hern, a physician, is director of the Boulder Abortion Clinic

---

The first assassination

Anti-abortion movement put weapon in slayer's hand[4]

By Warren M. Hern

Daily Camera *Guest Opinion, Sunday, March 20, 1994*

The news that Dr. David Gunn's assassin is going to jail for a long time is welcome. But we who provide abortion services would rather have Dr. Gunn back than see Michael Griffin go to jail.

And we are not comforted. We know that many people in the anti-abortion movement see Griffin as a political hero, and that his act inspires others, as it did the woman who shot Dr. George Tiller last August. No sooner had Griffin's verdict been announced than the fanatics who support him declared that he did the right thing. To them, killing a doctor who does abortions is "justifiable homicide." It isn't. Why is it necessary to say that?

We are beginning to emerge from the long night of terror under the Reagan and Bush administrations, when we knew we had no tribunal at the highest levels of government. We now have a president and administration that supports the right to choose and that upholds the Constitution in these matters, we have legislation passed by both houses of Congress that will help protect us, and even the Supreme Court has ruled that we may seek redress against those who would use force to close and obstruct abortion clinics.

But we ask: How many more Michael Griffins are out there who believe they have such a monopoly on the truth that they may use deadly force to kill those who disagree? A lot, we think.

While I am encouraged by the jury's verdict and grateful that justice has been done, and while I am confident that the vast majority of Americans reject the ruthless violence of the anti-abortion movement, I have just finished installing a high fence with electric controls around my office to protect us from people like Griffin. It cost nearly $20,000. That is not a normal cost of medical practice, but it is a normal cost of providing abortion services. And that doesn't include all the other tens of thousands of dollars we are forced to spend to protect ourselves and our patients from a political terrorist movement.

One federal judge stated to me recently that the problem is now solved with the passage of federal legislation and court rulings that are beginning to open the way for legal attacks on the anti-abortion movement.

Some people may think the problem is solved. We do not, and we may not dare assume that in our daily lives. We watch, we take precautions, and we live our lives more carefully, because now everyone knows what we have known for years: The anti-abortion movement will stop at nothing to achieve its ends and to gain power. Part of the reason is that it is linked to other forces of extremism and reaction in this country that threaten democratic society.

Why must we work behind bullet-proof windows, high steel fences, and wear bullet-proof vests? Because what we do gives freedom to women, and that helps secure freedom for all of us. The anti-abortion movement hates freedom in any form.

That's why it is so dangerous.

How ironic it was that Griffin's defense team tried to get him off by claiming that his mind had been warped by anti-abortion propaganda films. It had been, of course. And they claimed that he should not be held responsible for the results of letting his mind be warped. He should be, of course. But it illustrates that the consequence of their propaganda and hate literature had exactly the effect intended. Their delusion was fulfilled.

It is a dangerous delusion, America, and you had better listen and understand that it hates all you stand for: individual freedom as distinguished from state control of human lives; free thought instead of ignorance; and personal responsibility for one's own actions instead of mindless totalitarianism.

Michael Griffin tried to kill a thought – freedom. He did not succeed.

Dr. Warren Hern is director of the Boulder Abortion Clinic

The Politics of Abortion[5]

Warren M. Hern, M.D.

The Progressive, *November 1972*

Volume 36, Number 11 Copyright © 1972

A year ago, New York City Councilwoman Carol Greitzer told the annual meeting of the National Association for Repeal of Abortion Laws (NARAL), of which she is president, that American women were determined to make abortion an issue in the 1972 elections. No politician who opposed the availability of safe abortions for all women would have women's support in 1972, she warned candidates in emphasizing the political arithmetic that women are a majority of the electorate.

If there was any doubt then that abortion would be an issue in 1972, President Nixon's unprecedented letter last May to Terence Cardinal Cooke, supporting the Catholic hierarchy's effort to repeal the liberal New York abortion law, tossed the issue into the political arena. George McGovern, who was assailed in some of the primaries, particularly in Nebraska and New York, as a supporter of abortion, maintains the issue is a matter for state - not Federal - laws.

Legislatures are in a ferment over abortion legislation, and. court dockets are crowded with challenges to old abortion statutes and to new ones devised to replace those declared unconstitutional, such as Connecticut's new and restrictive law which in turn has been upset by a Federal district court. The New York legislature, spurred on by Cardinal Cooke's forces and President Nixon's encouraging letter, repealed its own landmark 1970 statute only to have the repeal bill vetoed by Governor Nelson Rockefeller.

Because most legislators and candidates are men, usually of comfortable means, many of them refuse to face up to the grim fact that those who pay the heaviest price with their health and very lives for the failure to liberalize or repeal state abortion laws are women too poor to afford the safe abortions available to women in better financial circumstances.

It has been estimated that between one million and a million and a half abortions occur annually in the United States. This means that about one-fourth of all pregnancies end in abortion.

In the March, 1971, issue of the *American Journal of Public Health,* Drs. Ian Schneider and Carl Tyler, both obstetricians, predicted that one out of every three U.S. pregnancies will end in abortion if all laws restricting abortion are removed.

Abortion is the only area of medical practice hampered by criminal penalties. This restriction interferes with the patient-physician relationship in a fundamental way. The point was explored in the *Belous* case in California in 1969 in which 80 leading obstetricians from medical schools across the country, in defending Dr. Leon Belous' right to perform an abortion, joined in an eloquent *amici curiae* brief. The brief contended that the criminal penalties attached to abortion force the patient to plead her case and become an adversary of her doctor. By asking him to exercise his professional judgment, she endangers his right to practice medicine and perhaps his very freedom. If he performs the abortion, he is subject to prosecution and must justify his action by testifying in his own behalf. If he refuses to perform the abortion, he is not subject to prosecution and does not have to justify his decision.

Even if the doctor's medical judgment tells him that the best treatment for a particular patient's pregnancy is an abortion as she has requested, proceeding to that treatment may cause him to lose his license to practice medicine and may *even* send him to jail. The physician therefore has a personal stake in the outcome and cannot render a truly objective medical opinion about the proper treatment of his patient. Her rights are thereby also jeopardized, especially if she does not have the money to pay the added costs of extralegal stratagems such as "psychiatric consultation" which might provide "mental health" grounds for a legal abortion.

The inevitable result of all this is that few doctors are willing to perform abortions, and a simple operation is made both expensive and hard to get. Desperate women are driven to clandestine abortions, many of them done under unsafe and unhygienic conditions.

Of approximately one million abortions performed in 1967, fewer than 10,000 were reported in the Federal Government's *Vital Statistics* as done legally in hospitals as "therapeutic abortions"- that is, done to preserve the life, or health, of the mother. The other 990,000 abortions were done illegally by persons ranging in competence from skilled physicians to unskilled and unscrupulous quacks. Some of the women attempted to perform abortion on themselves, using such instruments as coat hangers and knitting needles, often with fatal results. Women who have experienced unsafe abortion attempts frequently develop massive infection, or "sepsis," and arrive at the emergency room in critical condition with fever, hemorrhage, and mul tiple complications. The hospital stays of those who survive are long, expensive, and disruptive of their family lives.

Septic abortion has been one of the leading causes of death among child-bearing women for many years, with a disproportionate share of the deaths falling among the poor and minority groups who cannot afford safe abortions. In 1967, for example, the death rate attributed to septic abortion, as reported in the Government's *Vital Statistics,* was nearly seven times as high among non-whites as among whites. For a five year period from 1957 to 1962, Drs. Edwin Gold and Carl Erhardt found that more than half of all maternal deaths (deaths related to pregnancy and childbirth) among Puerto Ricans and blacks living in New York City were caused by septic abortion.

Recent changes in the laws of a few states have resulted in an increase in the number of reported legal abortions. The Department of Health, Education and Welfare Center for Disease Control has stated that more than 180,000 such abortions were reported in 1970. According to Dr. Christopher Tietze of the Population Council, as many as 500,000 legal abortions may have been performed in 1971. The increase in the legal availability of safe, competently performed abortions has been directly associated with a decline in deaths from clandestine abortion in many of these states, especially New York and California. For example, Dr. Jean Pakter of the New York City Health Department reported that the rate of abortion-related deaths in New York City during the first four months of 1971 was less than one-fourth of what it was in the 1960-1962 period. Meanwhile, the ratio of legal abortions to live births has risen from 1.8 per 1,000 to 447.7 since 1967.

Following the implementation in 1968 of a liberalized abortion law in California, the rate of maternal deaths stemming from abortion decreased nearly 63 per cent by the end of 1969. In a report published in an April, 1971, issue of *Obstetrics and Gynecology,* Drs. Gary Stewart and Philip Goldstein stated that abortion-related deaths decreased dramatically in the San Francisco Bay Area while the therapeutic (legal) abortion rate rose. In 1969, there were no abortionrelated deaths in the Bay Area.

The severely restrictive laws of most states have been the greatest obstacle to safe abortion services. Professor Cyril Means of New York Law School has pointed out that these Nineteenth Century laws were primarily intended to protect women from an operation which was far more dangerous at that time than full-term pregnancy. Subsequent advances in medical technology have made an abortion performed during the first two months following conception six to ten times safer than a full-term uncomplicated pregnancy, according to statistics published by Dr. Tietze of the Population Council. Means cited a common-law principle in arguing against the previous restrictive New York abortion law: *"Cessante ratione legis cessat et ipsa lex"* (Once the reason for a law has ceased to exist, the law itself ceases to exist).

Means regards the discriminatory effect of state abortion laws in favor of the rich, and against the poor, as one of their worst aspects. He points out that, as administered, restrictive abortion laws exempt the rich and penalize the poor more than perhaps any other type of legislation.

Since 1967, 17 states Arkansas, California, Colorado, Delaware, Georgia, Kansas, Maryland, Mis sissippi, New Mexico, North Carolina, South Carolina, Virginia, Oregon, Alaska, Hawaii, New York, and Washington have revised or repealed their abortion laws, and four of these-Alaska, Hawaii, New York, and Washington-have done away with all but a few restrictions such as the patient's residency, duration of pregnancy, and performance by a physician.

These liberalizations have been effected against a background of rising public acceptance of abortion. A recent Harris poll disclosed that 48 per cent of those likely to vote this November favor a Federal law legalizing abortions up to four months of pregnancy, and 43 per cent oppose it. A Gallup poll following the Harris findings disclosed the rapid rise in support for liberalizing abortion laws. Gallup found 64 per cent of the public, including 56 per cent of Roman Catholics, now believe the decision to have an abortion should be left solely to the woman and her doctor. This two out of three ratio of public approval compares to 40 per cent approval reported by Gallup in a November, 1969, poll.

Where state restrictions have merely been modified, access to abortion has been made easier for the wealthy but not for the poor. Along with economic discrimination, pregnant women who are poor and seeking an abortion face bureaucratic delays, unnecessary anguish, and serious medical complications. These delays often result in the abortion being performed during the second "trimester" of pregnancy (months four-six), requiring hospitalization and higher costs. The Joint Program for the Study of Abortion (JPSA), conducted by Dr. Tietze for the Population Council, shows much higher risks for women having second trimester abortions.

This discrimination was recognized by U.S. District Court Judge Gerhard A. Gesell in 1969 when he declared the District of Columbia's abortion statute to be unconstitutional. Citing the equal protection clause of the Fourteenth Amendment, Judge Gesell ruled that it was necessary for the community to make abortions available to the poor as well as the rich. The Supreme Court later reversed Judge Gesell in handing down its first decision on the subject of abortion, declaring in *Vuitch* that the D.C. statute was constitutional.

In another decision now under appeal to the Supreme Court, a U.S. District Court in Georgia clearly recognized the fact that "...physicians and psychiatrists are more accessible to rich people than to poor people, making abortions more available to the wealthy than to the indigent ..." but declared this not to be a violation of the equal protection clause.

As alluded to in the Georgia decision, a significant part of the discrimination experienced by the poor under restrictive abortion laws is the requirement, in most states, of obtaining declarations from one or two psychiatrists that an abortion is necessary to preserve or restore the mental health of the woman seeking an abortion.

This peculiar situation is the direct result of the traditional medical view that pregnancy is "normal." The profession clings to this view in spite of the fact that pregnant women experience a variety of recognized signs and symptoms, undergo important physiological changes, are exposed to a significantly increased risk of death as the direct consequence of being pregnant, and seek medical attention whether the pregnancy is desired or not.

However, the view that pregnancy is "normal" means that there must be some justification for interrupting the pregnancy with a "therapeutic" abortion. Since modem medical technology has made it possible, in most cases, to get a woman with even severe heart or kidney disease through the stresses of pregnancy, the burden of "justification" has fallen on the chimera of "mental illness." This is consistent with the traditional medical attitude that, in the words of psychoanalyst May Romm, intense conflict about a pregnancy or about giving birth to a child is "psychopathological."

Under the ground rules of this situation, the woman must feign mental illness, threaten suicide or other catastrophe, and the psychiatrist must ascertain that the woman will be in danger to herself and/or others if she does not obtain the abortion. Such a prediction is impossible to make, and as much has been admitted by prominent psychiatrists on both sides of the question. In addition to being a demoralizing and degrading experience for the woman, mandatory psychiatric justification for abortion is a waste of the psychiatrist's time and a prostitution of psychiatry. The additional costs it imposes on the performance of a 15 minute operation add another burden to the economic discrimination experienced by the poor, to say nothing of the barrier of sophistication required in acting through a psychiatric encounter. The charade of routine psychiatric consultation, however, is only one of the obstacles to safe abortion for the poor.

The cost of a safe but illegal abortion in most places is in the range of $600-$1,000, and even this much does not always guarantee a safe abortion. But in New York and Washington, D.C., the price of a safe, legal abortion during the first trimester (three months) of pregnancy has fallen to around $150-$200. This decreased price level was predicted last year by Dr. Louis Hellman, HEW Deputy Assistant Secretary for Population Affairs, at a national conference on abortion held in New York City: "We are in the marketplace, and the thing that will bring the rates down quicker than anything I know of is for states other than New York to have liberal abortion laws."

The lowered prices, however, are still beyond the reach of many women who desire abortions. Dr. Jean Pakter of the New York City Health Department reported that during the last six months of 1970, nearly half the abortions performed in New York municipal hospitals and in the service wards of voluntary hospitals were paid for with Medicaid funds. Most of the rest were paid through private insurance plans such as Blue Cross. Abortions are being paid for with **HEW** funds under sections of the Social Security legislation in those states where abortions are not restricted by law. Even in New York, however, where this payment practice has been well established and is continuing, a see-saw court battle has developed over the use of Medicaid funds for abortion. Those favoring such use won a major round recently when a panel of three Federal judges upheld Medicaid payments for abortions, saying that to refuse aid "would deny indigent women the equal protection of the laws to which they are constitutionally entitled."

The Office of Economic Opportunity, which is providing Federally subsidized family planning services for approximately 500,000 low-income women across the nation, has an internal policy prohibiting the use of OEO funds for abortions. Even if this restriction were removed, most state laws would prevent the use of this money for abortion services. Nonetheless, a management survey of OEO family planning programs completed in early 1971 revealed that 60 per cent of the project directors wanted this restriction removed to be able to provide abortions for women requesting them.

There seems to be little doubt that the poor and disadvantaged minority groups are taking advantage of the greater availability of abortions where legal restrictions have been removed. The ratio of abortions to live births was higher among New York City nonwhite women between July, 1970, and March, 1971, for example, than it was for whites. More than half of all abortions among New York City residents during the same period were experienced by nonwhites and Puerto Ricans. During the second year of the operation of Colorado's new liberalized abortion law, more than half the patients had yearly family incomes of less than $6,000.

Nationwide, about two-thirds of the abortions reported to the Population Council's Joint Program for the Study of Abortion (JPSA) from July 1, 1970, to June 30, 1971, were performed on white women. Twenty-six per cent of the abortions were performed on black women. Nearly 60 per cent of the abortions were performed on private patients, but only 13 per cent of the private patients were black. While more detailed analysis is not yet available, the significance of these data can be inferred tentatively from the fact that the complication rate for nonprivate patients was approximately twice as high as that experienced by private patients. This phenomenon is probably explained by the clinical impression that private patients tend to appear earlier for abortion, when it is safer, are in better health to begin with, and are more likely to have a private physician to return to for assistance should any complications develop.

In a recent issue of the *American Journal of Obstetrics and Gynecology*, 100 professors of obstetrics joined in making an unprecedented "statement on abortion." The professors, many of them chairmen of obstetrics departments at leading U.S. medical schools, strongly recommended that most abortions be performed during the first three months of pregnancy on an outpatient basis. In clear recognition of the issue of economic discrimination, they stated, "Abortion should be made equally available to the rich and the poor."

The report of the President's Commission on Population Growth and the American Future emphasized the discriminatory effect of abortion laws and their effect on the health of the poor. The Commission recommended that state laws be liberalized to conform with the New York State statute, allowing abortions to be performed by licensed physicians on request. The Commission also recommended greater public and private financial support of abortion services.

The Population Commission recommendations are consistent with an earlier statement by the American Public Health Association. APHA's "Recommended Standards for Abortion Services," adopted in November, 1970, state: "Abortion services are an integral part of comprehensive family planning and maternal and child care. . . . The public interest requires that health agencies . . . make every effort to provide safe, accessible abortion services at reasonable fees for all who are in need of such services."

In his rejection of the conclusions of the Population Commission report, President Nixon made it clear that he does not think that abortion should be available to either the poor or rich, even though it is available to both-with different risks and costs. It is not clear to what extent Mr. Nixon's opposition to abortion is personal, or the result of his assessment of the political effect of his opposition on Catholic voters.

Those who grasp the abortion issue with an eye toward winning the Catholic vote, however, may find it a two-edged sword. The Women's National Abortion Action Coalition (WONAAC), a militant young organization dedicated to political action to end barriers to safe abortion, has gathered strength and momentum steadily in recent months. It must be remembered that most of the 500,000 reported legal abortions performed in 1971 were experienced by young single women, some of them Catholic, many of them well-educated or in college, politically active or able to vote, and acutely conscious of the difficulties encountered in obtaining a safe abortion.

In July, 1972, WONAAC sponsored the third Women's National Abortion Action Conference at Hunter College in New York City, which drew more than 800 local representatives from all over the country. WONAAC's goals include the repeal of all abortion laws and restrictive contraceptive laws. WONAAC is also supporting Congresswoman Bella Abzug's proposed Federal Abortion Rights Bill. Its leaders have organized their activities with a view to fall elections. While WONAAC does not support or oppose individual candidates, its members are pressing candidates at all levels for commitments to repeal outdated and inequitable abortion laws.

As Carol Greitzer said, somebody had better start counting the women.

Warren M. Hern is a physician and epidemiologist who recently resigned from the national headquarters staff of the Office of Economic Opportunity's family planning program. He now teaches public health and does private consulting work.

Reprinted by permission of *The Progressive*

Anti-abortion atrocity in Alabama

Pregnancy Kills. Abortion Saves Lives.[6]

> Every pregnancy poses a "serious health risk" to the mother.

By Warren M. Hern

New York Times *May 21, 2019 Opinion Op-Ed Page*

Dr. Hern is a physician and epidemiologist who specializes in late-abortion services.

Pregnancy is a life-threatening condition. Women die from being pregnant. We have known that for thousands of years.

They die from hemorrhage, infection, pre-eclampsia (which can lead to fatal seizures), obstructed labor, amniotic fluid embolism, thromboembolism, a ruptured uterus, retained placenta, hydatidiform mole, choriocarcinoma and many other causes that fill the obstetrics textbooks. Modern medicine can prevent and treat many, but not all, of these conditions. Some potentially fatal problems cannot be foreseen or prevented.

Pregnancy always comes with some irreducible risk of death.

There are factors that put some women at higher-than-average risk of death from pregnancy: age (to be an early adolescent is more dangerous), high blood pressure, many previous pregnancies, diabetes, obesity, a history of cesarean delivery, uterine abnormalities, a scarred cervix, a placenta previa (in which the placenta covers the cervix). A placenta previa can result in sudden, catastrophic hemorrhage that is fatal, and it can require a cesarean delivery — which carries its own risks — since a normal vaginal delivery is impossible.

The measure of risk to a woman's life from pregnancy itself is called the "maternal mortality ratio." That is the number of women who die of causes related to or aggravated by pregnancy per 100,000 live births.

In Alabama, the overall maternal mortality ratio in 2018 was 11.9 per 100,000. Among white women, the 2018 maternal mortality ratio was 5.6; among black women, it was 27.6, making black women in Alabama almost five times more likely to die as a result of pregnancy than white women. For the United States overall, the maternal mortality ratio was 20.7.

By comparison, a study in the journal Obstetrics & Gynecology on abortion mortality from 1998 to 2010 found that for the 16.1 million abortions performed during that time, the overall death rate was 0.7 per 100,000 procedures. The death rate for early-abortion procedures — those that took place within the first eight weeks of the pregnancy — was less: 0.3 per 100,000.

Pregnancy is dangerous; abortion can be lifesaving.

Alabama's new law claims that it does not prohibit abortion if there is a "reasonable medical judgment" that the pregnancy poses a "serious health risk" to the woman. An abortion may be performed if a "reasonable medical judgment" "necessitates" that a pregnancy be terminated to "avert her death or to avert serious risk of substantial physical impairment of a major bodily function."

The definition of a "major bodily function" is not given, nor is it distinguished from a minor bodily function.

But pregnancy itself poses a "serious health risk" — including the risk of dying and losing *all* bodily functions. A woman's life and health are at risk from the moment that a pregnancy exists in her body, whether she wants to be pregnant or not.

All of the above raises multiple important questions: Could a doctor who determines that a woman is pregnant also determine, as a consequence of that pregnancy, that a "serious health risk" exists? Could that doctor then end her pregnancy without fear of prosecution? Who decides what a "reasonable medical judgment" is or what a "major bodily function" is? What are the criteria for these judgments?

Does the Alabama legislature recognize that the effects of its new law, depending on how it is enforced, are unequal, since black women are more likely to die from pregnancy in Alabama than white women and so are more likely to benefit from the availability of safe abortion?

Surely the Alabama legislature has carefully considered all of the above in drafting this law, which affects more than 2.5 million women in that state, some of them more than others.

Or perhaps not. Maybe all of this is moot. Perhaps the goal of the Alabama law, in addition to triggering a legal challenge to Roe v. Wade, may be to discourage doctors from even practicing medicine in that state, lest they be accused of performing an illegal abortion and sentenced to prison for the rest of their lives. Perhaps the vagueness of the law and the confusion is the point. Vagueness and confusion are tools of tyranny.

The intent of the Alabama legislature and its new law is clearly to prohibit and prevent abortions from being performed. But does it?

Warren M. Hern, a physician and epidemiologist, is director of the Boulder Abortion Clinic in Boulder, Colo., where he specializes in late-abortion services. He is the author of the medical textbook "Abortion Practice," a comprehensive guide to performing safe abortions.

A philosophical reflection

Religion, Power and Reproductive Freedom

A checkered history of conflict[7]

Warren M. Hern, M.D., M.P.H., Ph.D.

Director, Boulder Abortion Clinic

Recipient, 2018 Faith and Freedom Award

Presented at the Faith and Freedom Awards Ceremony

Religious Coalition for Reproductive Rights.

Temple Emanuel, Denver, May 3, 2018

Thank you for inviting me to be here this evening and receive this award. It is a great honor, and it is a privilege to be here. It is also a privilege to do the work we do to help women and their families. It is my definition of practicing medicine.

It is ironic from my point of view that you are bestowing this honor on an apostate Methodist who gave up on Christianity nearly 60 years ago after reading Sir James Frazer's *The Golden Bough*, Bertrand Russell's *History of Western Philosophy*, *Why I Am Not A Christian*, and *Unpopular Essays*, Erich Fromm's *Escape From Freedom*, R.H. Tawney's *Religion and The Rise Of Capitalism*, Charles Guignebert's *Jesus* with Greek footnotes that I learned to read, *The Consolation of Philosophy* by Boethius, *A Guide for the Perplexed* by Maimonides, *In Praise of Folly* by Erasmus, the works of Baruch Spinoza, Plato's **Απολογία** concerning the persecution of Socrates, Aristophanes' satire of sophistry in *The Clouds*, Lessa and Vogt's *Reader in Comparative Religion*, *Man and His Gods* by Homer Smith, *The Imitation of Christ* by Thomas á Kempis, the works of Paul Tillich and Reinhold Niebuhr, and several times through The King James Version of *The Bible*.

I read some of these on my lunch time while sitting under my water truck on a construction job and while camped out in the mountains during another construction job. I had the heart of a believer and the mind of a skeptic. The skeptic won. I enjoyed the Unitarians at Dick Henry's church on 14th & Lafayette, and the ritual was comfortable, but I found it disconcerting to go from "Our Father, Who Art In Heaven" to "To Whom It May Concern." I had sung enthusiastically and joyfully in *The Messiah* every Christmas in excellent choirs from junior high through medical school, and I loved the music. I still do. But skiing and hiking in the mountains – my real cathedral – got to be more important than going to any church. I was baptized when I was very young, but it obviously didn't have much effect.

In my work as a physician helping women by performing abortions, I have been confronted with the conflict among religions about this issue and, further, the checkered history of religion in matters of truth and power.

While religious traditions may offer important insights into our relationship with the cosmos and our ethical relationships with fellow humans, I could not help noticing that religion has been sometimes on the side of truth and freedom, but at other times, it has been on the side of brutal power and repression.

Socrates was prosecuted for doubting the gods of theocratic Athens and thereby corrupting the youth. The message was: "Believe this or die." Two thousand years later, the medieval Catholic church carried out the Inquisition, whose victims included Galileo and Giordano Bruno, whose crimes were independent thought. Martin Luther, although cruelly anti-semitic, challenged the dogmatism and authoritarianism of the Catholic Church. Hitler described Christianity as the foundation of German values, which embraced anti-semitism for many, but not all, German Christians. Christianity was used to defend apartheid in

South Africa and slavery in the United States, torture in the Inquisition, and the slaughter of Native Americans by both the *Conquistadores* and our own fellow citizens.

Then we have the awakening of the Christian community in the struggle for civil rights in the 1960s in this country. The moral leadership of Dr. Martin Luther King and his associates is an historic beacon for all time.

In the 1960s, tens of thousands of women throughout the country were given critical help in finding safe abortions by the Clergy Counseling Service. Those religious leaders held that having an abortion was a moral choice, and they gave women the support they needed to effect that choice.

Now, we have the radical religious right in the United States, which has joined with the radical political right in its effort to fight and destroy the reproductive rights of women and to make women servants of the fascist state. In 1986, TV evangelist and Republican candidate for President, Pat Robertson, said in Denver during a National Right To Life meeting that we must oppose abortion so that "we will have enough soldiers to fight the wars and people to pay the taxes." Joseph Scheidler, a defrocked Catholic monk, went around the country urging violence against abortion clinics and doctors, and he came to my office several times in 1985 and 1986. One of his followers threw a stone through the front window of my office a few days after I had seen the flame scars on the Jewish Community Center and synagogue left from the 1938 *Kristallnacht* in East Berlin.

In March, 1988, five shots were fired through the front windows of my waiting room, narrowly missing a member of my staff. I had just walked through the room. It was one of several attempts on my life. Randall Terry, surrounded by his followers, stood in the street in front of my office in 1991 and prayed for my execution. In March, 1993, Dr. David Gunn was assassinated in Pensacola, Florida by Michael Griffin, who was defended by Joe Scarborough, for whom this was a springboard to political stardom in the Republican Party, a seat in Congress, and a lucrative morning TV show. Later in 1993, Rev. David Trosch, a Catholic priest in Alabama, declared that killing doctors who perform abortions is "justifiable homicide." A few days after his announcement, Randall Terry went on National Christian Radio Network, and, naming me and quoting scripture, invited his listers to assassinate me. The next day, Shelly Shannon tried to assassinate Dr. George Tiller in Wichita. Reverend Trosch formed the "American Coalition of Life [sic] Activists" and advocated the assassination of abortion doctors. Paul Hill, a member of the group, then assassinated Dr. John Britton along with Dr. Britton's bodyguard, also in Pensacola. The "American Coalition of Life Activists" had a national press conference on January 22, 1995 and announced the hit list of the first 13 abortion doctors they wanted eliminated. I was on the list, and so was Dr. Tiller. Dr. Barnett Slepian was assassinated in 1998, and Dr. George Tiller, a close friend of mine, was assassinated in his Lutheran Church in 2009.

The Mafia has the decency to keep its hit lists private.

The last time I was privileged to visit this temple was in June, 2009, a few days after Dr. Tiller's assassination, when I was invited by Rabbi Stephen Foster and Betty Serotta to speak here about my friend. During that month, an anti-abortion fanatic threatened the lives of my family. I received a letter from Shelly Shannon from her cell in Kansas state prison telling me that I'm next.

Quoting now from something about this subject that I wrote earlier:

"The murder of Dr. David Gunn [the first of the abortion doctors to be assassinated] was not the isolated act of a deranged loner. It was the inevitable consequence of 20 years of violent and inflammatory rhetoric from the radical Christian right that paints abortion as a "Holocaust" and doctors who perform abortions as "baby killers," "murderers," "Nazi doctors," and other hateful epithets.

Dr. Gunn's assassination culminated 20 years of violent terrorist acts that included stalking and harassment of patients and staff members and the bombing of clinics. The idea that a six-week embryo is equal to or more important than the life of a cantankerous adult doctor is no longer a sick private delusion. **It is a collective psychosis masquerading as religion that has become a political force threatening democratic society."**

I wrote those words in an editorial published in the *Denver Post* in 1993.

Guess who's running the country now?

It is difficult for me to be neutral and objective about Christianity's contribution to this frightening fanaticism. There is much more to this story.

As personified by Pat Robertson and others such as Jesse Helms and Jerry Falwell, the Republican Party has been taken over by Christian anti-abortion fanatics. The policy of the Republican Party is that women are for pleasure and having babies, and they should have as many as possible. The philosophy is clearly that individuals are here to serve the state and not the other way around. Individual freedom is subject to cancellation because it does not serve the needs of the state.

That is the current Republican philosophy, and it is a fascist philosophy. The underpinnings are both Protestant Evangelical and Catholic theology, and its advocates are in complete control of all three branches of the federal government of the United States at this time. Fanatic opposition to abortion has helped to elect Republicans across the country. It was critical to the success of Robert Dole, Ronald Reagan, George H.W. Bush, Newt Gingrich, George W. Bush, and Donald J. Trump, who had the overwhelming political support of Christian evangelicals. For 40 years, for the Republicans, abortion has been the hammer and tongs to power.

What is the response of religious leadership in this crisis of not only reproductive freedom but democracy itself? Where is the high ground of moral leadership for Christians who support the rights of women to be healthy and to be free from the tyranny of their own biology? The Jewish community has been outspoken in support of reproductive rights in harmony with rabbinic law, which values the life of the woman over the life or potential life of the fetus. Since I am an admirer of

Talmudic teachings but am not a Talmudic scholar, I refer you to Rabbi Foster and others who are experts on this. But I sympathize with pro-choice Christians whose faith is being given a bad name by the totalitarians who oppose us.

Whose morality? Whose "family values?" Whose virtues? It is not only a religious question. It is a matter of power. Who has the power to make the decision to transmit life to a new generation: the individual or the state? You and I know that no government has the capacity, nor should it have the right, to make that decision for any woman, and that any woman is more competent to make that decision than any government. You and I know that safe abortion is a fundamental component of health care for women in the twenty-first century, and that affirming that during the past 50 years has been one of the great public health successes of all time. But those who lust for power and who are willing to walk on the bodies of women to get it are determined to eliminate that great step forward for humanity.

This, then, at this moment, is completely about power: Who has it, and who doesn't? Which way are the guns pointed? That's a matter we decide at the polls in a democracy. But we are now faced with an ignorant, cruel, corrupt, autocratic, racist, misogynist, authoritarian criminal regime in Washington, D.C., that hates individual freedom, the rule of law, civil rights, voting rights, any part of the natural world not being exploited for profit, democracy, the free press, facts, and thought itself. We have an existential threat to democracy in America. Unless we secure it by our voices and votes, and with the help of this religious community, women will not have reproductive freedom, and if women are not free, none of us are free.

[*end of speech*]

***

'Abortionist' Carries A Charged Meaning[8]

Sept. 7, 1993 Letter to the Editor, *New York Times*

To the Editor:

The use of the word "abortionist" in the headline of your Aug. 21 report on the return to work of Dr. George Tiller, who was shot and wounded outside his clinic two days earlier, was highly offensive to many physicians such as myself who provide abortion services.

Aside from the fact that the word "abortionist" does not appear in the article, it is a highly charged word that is pejorative, derogatory and defamatory. It is most often used by antiabortion fanatics in close company with words like "murderer," "baby-killer" and other slanderous phrases to describe physicians who perform abortions.

There are some words that are so laden with historically stigmatized meanings that they cannot be separated from that context, no matter how hard people may try to bring them into accepted use. Examples are "final solution," "ethnic purity" or "racial purity" and other terms associated with political totalitarianism or group discrimination.

The term abortionist has been used most often to describe illegal actors in a sleazy world of avaricious, incompetent criminals exploiting immoral women in a sordid and hazardous procedure. The world has changed, and I would hope your usage reflected that.

For myself, I am proud to be a physician who specializes in providing safe abortion services for women who need them, and I will continue to do so.

WARREN M. HERN, M.D. Director, Boulder Abortion Clinic

Boulder, Colo., Aug. 25, 1993 https://www.nytimes.com/1993/09/07/opinion/l -abortionist-carries-a-charged-meaning-856193.html?searchResultPosition=6

Who Gets to Speak In Abortion Debate?[9]

Dec. 2, 2003 Letter to the Editor, *New York Times*

To the Editor:

Re "Frank Talk About Abortion" (editorial, Nov. 30):

As a physician providing abortion services, I am appalled by what our nation's leaders are doing about this extremely difficult and complicated matter. It does usually seem that the knowledge and opinions of the doctors and the patients are not significant determinants in the formulation of this public policy.

In my medical practice, which has increasingly specialized in helping women who have decided to terminate desired pregnancies complicated by catastrophic fetal disorders or other medical issues, both we and the patients are alarmed by the "partial birth" abortion ban recently passed by Congress and signed by President Bush. There is no solid evidence that the procedure as specified and described in the legislation is being performed by anyone or, if so, by whom, where or how often. But we ask: will we be prosecuted?

We fear President Bush and John Ashcroft.

WARREN M. HERN, M.D.

Boulder, Colo., Nov. 30, 2003

The writer is director of the Boulder Abortion Clinic.

https://www.nytimes.com/2003/12/02/opinion/l-who-gets-to-speak-in-abortion -debate-382086.html?searchResultPosition=8

A Doctor's Fear.[10] *New York Times*, Letters to the Editor,

Jan. 31, 2001

To the Editor:

As a doctor who has been on the assassination hit lists of anti-abortion fanatics for many years, I am alarmed at the prospect of having John Ashcroft as attorney general (news article, Jan. 30).

I cannot imagine an otherwise formally qualified person who would be a greater danger to me, to my freedom, to the welfare of my patients and to the freedom of women to make basic personal choices in their lives.

I do not believe Mr. Ashcroft's statements that he accepts Roe v. Wade as "settled law," or that he would respect this constitutional right. I do not believe that he will enforce the Freedom of Access to Clinic Entrances Act, nor do I believe that he will prosecute anti-abortion violence under any other law. His nomination is an affront to the public trust.

WARREN M. HERN, M.D.

Boulder, Colo., Jan. 30, 2001

The writer is director of the Boulder Abortion Clinic.

Opinion - Letters to the Editor, *The New York Times*

How It Feels to Be on Anti-Abortion Hit List[11]

Feb. 4, 1995

To the Editor:

While I feel ambivalent about your decision not to report the American Coalition of Life Activists' hit list of a dozen doctors it wants eliminated, I am grateful for "The Escalating War on Legal Abortion," your Jan. 28 editorial criticizing this announcement. Not a bullet has been fired at any of us since then, as far as I know. But speaking as one of those physicians, I can testify that such an announcement goes a long way toward destroying one's life. That, of course, is the intended effect.

I am grateful also for the protection of Federal marshals, who were assigned to me and my colleagues after this announcement. But why should it be necessary for doctors who help women to be protected by armed guards?

What is more at stake than the lives of a few doctors is the issue of whether Americans now accept the level of violence and terrorism embraced by the anti-abortion movement as a means of political expression. When the anti-abortion movement gets through with us, who's next? People who write books?

We must surely ask whether it is beyond the limits of free speech that a group operating under the laws of the United States can stand up at a press conference, identify targets among people who belong to a category already marked for assassination by ideological colleagues of the announcing group, and then sit back and wait for the inevitable results.

In a society awash in the glorification of violence, notorious for unlimited access to lethal military weapons and diffused with people suffering from untreated severe mental illness, the probabilities are excellent that one or more of us will be assassinated. It is a new form of electronic fascism.

Assassination has been a tool of tyrants for thousands of years. The technology and the degree of "plausible deniability" have improved over time.

Neither the American Coalition of Life Activists nor those it hopes to inspire care about me as a person, or about the women whose lives I save as a physician. What they care about is power. So does the Republican Party, which has been the chief beneficiary of 20 years of anti-abortion rhetoric leading to this terrorism.

How many more doctors, receptionists and other abortion clinic workers have to be killed before the American people and their Government step in and stop this insanity? When will Americans see that the anti-abortion ideology is a collective psychosis masquerading as religion, which has become a political force threatening democratic society?

WARREN M. HERN, M.D. Director Boulder Abortion Clinic Boulder, Colo., Jan. 29, 1995

https://www.nytimes.com/1995/02/04/opinion/l-how-it-feels-to-be-on-anti -abortion-hit-list-286895.html?searchResultPosition=10

Opinion Op-Ed page, *New York Times*

Hunted by the Right, Forgotten by the Left[12]

By Warren M. Hern

March 13, 1993

The right to a safe, legal abortion is meaningless if no one is able or willing to perform it. A woman's power to control her own body does not bring with it a capacity for self-abortion without assistance. Yet for much of the last two decades, the public and the women's movement seemed to forget that doctors are a necessary -- and vulnerable -- part of this equation. The anti-abortion movement -- in part a violent, national terrorist movement -- never forgot it. That's why a Florida doctor who performed abortions, David Gunn, was assassinated on Wednesday.

For three years, there have been numerous reports about the lack of doctors and facilities for abortions. These complaints have largely been true. But some of the reasons behind them are not well known.

In the 1960s, doctors were active in making abortion legal. Their help was critical in the years following legalization both in performing abortions and in mobilizing public support for them. Doctors have performed more than 30 million abortions in the U.S. since 1970. But many have stopped doing so and few are learning how to do them properly.

Increasingly, doctors have been made to feel irrelevant. Feminist abortion clinics treat doctors like technicians and are especially contemptuous of male physicians. Entrepreneurs who treat abortion strictly as a retail business also tend to treat doctors as technicians. Doctors who perform abortions have usually acquiesced in these roles, and their status has plummeted lower than that of physicians who do insurance company examinations.

Abortion doctors' only ally has been bullet-proof glass

I know of clinics that don't allow doctors to speak with patients, and of others where medical policy is set and changed by administrators without consulting physicians. Pro-choice organizations often ignore, patronize and disparage the contributions of physicians who specialize in abortions, in contrast with their support for well-known physicians in conventional specialties who perform some abortions.

Abortion has become a commodity, like soap, and its social value has dropped. Competition has become intense and fees have been cut, resulting in reduced income for doctors and others who provide the services as well as poorer treatment.

Insurance costs, particularly for coverage from property destruction by anti-abortion vigilantes, have gone up. There were more than 180 acts of violence against abortion providers last year, double the amount in 1991. Security expenses have gone through the roof: It costs a lot of money to surround one's office and home with armed security guards and to install bulletproof windows and electronic security systems. These are not normal costs of medical practice.

Does all this mean that there will be a shortage of people to do abortions? Not necessarily. But it may mean that women will suffer or die as skilled practitioners become scarce. The Wall Street Journal reported yesterday that only 7 percent of residency programs offer training in second-trimester abortions as against 23 percent in 1985.

The main reason doctors have become unwilling to perform abortions is of course political. When George Bush was elected in 1988 after advocating the imprisonment of doctors who performed abortions, it did not encourage many physicians to dedicate their careers to this specialty

Warren M. Hern, a physician, is Director of the Boulder Abortion Clinic

https://www.nytimes.com/1993/03/13/opinion/hunted-by-the-right-forgotten -by-the-left.html?searchResultPosition=11

https://timesmachine.nytimes.com/timesmachine/1993/03/13/issue.html

---

In America; In the War Zone[13]

By Bob Herbert The *New York Times Nov. 8, 1998*

There are times when Dr. Warren Hern feels more like a combat veteran than a physician. Here is what he says about a normal workday: "I walk out of my office and the first thing I do is look at the parking garage that the hospital built two doors away and see if there is a sniper on the roof. I basically expect to be shot any day."

Two of his close friends have been shot. "My dear friend, Garson Romalis in Vancouver -- he was the first of the Canadian doctors to be shot. They almost shot off his leg. He nearly died on his kitchen floor."

That was in the fall of 1994. Dr. George Tiller was another friend. He was shot in both arms in Wichita, Kan., in 1993.

Other doctors have fallen. Dr. David Gunn was shot to death in Pensacola, Fla., in 1993, and Dr. John Britton was shot to death, also in Pensacola, in 1994. Dr. Barnett Slepian was shot to death in the Buffalo suburb of Amherst a little over two weeks ago.

There are big headlines whenever a doctor who performs abortions is killed, but the relentless terror and gruesome violence that continue to plague abortion providers and the people who assist them take place below the level of consciousness of most Americans.

Few people know about Robert Sanderson, the Birmingham, Ala., police officer moonlighting as a security guard whose body literally was blown to pieces in the bombing of a clinic last January. Or about the widely circulated "Army of God" manual that gives detailed information on the construction and use of bombs and other murderous devices, and recommends that if you don't kill doctors who perform abortions you should at least render their hands useless.

"It's a war zone," said Dr. Hern, who runs the Boulder Abortion Clinic in Boulder, Colo. "It's very frightening and it ruins your life."

The terror frightens everyone. Dr. Hern said: "We had this absolutely fantastic candidate for a front-desk job in my office. She was ready to accept, but because of the assassination of Dr. Slepian she decided not to work here. She talked to her friends and family and decided she could not live with that kind of fear. I didn't blame her. That has happened on numerous occasions. We've had people leave here because of the violence."

What that means, said Dr. Hern, is that the violence and the terror are working.

"How do we provide these services to women," he asked, "if those who would help us are terrified?"

The anti-abortion terrorists get much aid and comfort -- sometimes openly, sometimes covertly -- from various right-wing political elements, including members of the Christian right, the militia movement and the white supremacy movement. The moral fervor of the right, so loudly proclaimed, is selective indeed. The feeling of many on the right is that if violence and terror result in the curtailment of abortion, so be it.

Dr. Hern is the author of *Abortion Practice*, the principal textbook on abortion for doctors in the U.S. and a number of other countries. He is also an associate clinical professor of obstetrics and gynecology at the University of Colorado.

He lost count of the death threats against him many years ago. They started as soon as he began doing abortions back in the early 1970's. "I slept with a rifle beside my bed," he said, "because I lived up in the mountains and was afraid I would be attacked."

He wears a bulletproof vest at some of his public appearances. In 1988 someone fired five shots into his office. "I had to install bulletproof windows," he said. He'd already hired private, armed security guards. The harassment, the demonstrations and the terror continued. The office at times was surrounded by 50 to 100 peace officers of one kind or another.

"It was," said Dr. Hern, "a nightmare."

Now the hard right has been dealt a setback. The extremists have faltered, at least momentarily. Newt Gingrich is packing his bags and the Republican Party is searching frantically for a friendlier demeanor. This can only help.

"It seems that the radical right lost a lot of ground in the election and that's very encouraging," said Dr. Hern. "There clearly are Republicans out there who don't agree with that agenda and they should be running the party. Then people can get a little balance back."

https://www.nytimes.com/1998/11/08/opinion/in-america-in-the-war-zone.html ?searchResultPosition=4

No Headline[14] **The** *New York Times* **March 12, 1993**

"I work in four layers of bullet-proof windows. Death threats are so common they are not remarkable. I went to a pro-choice meeting in Denver recently, and as I walked through the picket line, someone said, 'You should die."

–DR. WARREN HERN, – medical director of the Boulder Abortion Clinic.

Abortion Protesters Outnumbered in Denver

By <u>Dirk Johnson</u> **The** *New York Times* **Aug. 14, 1993[15]**

Hoisting placards that reviled a doctor who performs abortions here as a killer, about 40 members of Operation Rescue marched and kneeled in prayer on the sidewalks outside the Swedish Medical Center here today.

But they were outnumbered by more than 2 to 1 by others with signs that declared, "This clinic stays open."

The anti-abortion group had relished the visit by Pope John Paul II and 150,000 Roman Catholics as a rare chance to muster huge protests at clinics in the Denver area.

Instead, the rather lonely protest today amounted to the latest setback for Operation Rescue, whose demonstrations around the country this summer were also poorly attended.

Cold Shoulder From Catholics

Even the Roman Catholic organizers of World Youth Day turned a cold shoulder to the anti-abortion protesters. "There is no more eloquent speaker for pro-life than John Paul II," said Sister Mary Ann Walsh, a spokeswoman for the event. "And we would not want to see anyone distract from his message."

But the failure of Operation Rescue to recruit large numbers of Catholics to protest against abortion should probably come as no surprise.

Despite the Vatican's edict against abortion, followers of the church are hardly uniform in their views on the subject. And among those who do oppose abortion, many are uncomfortable with the zeal of Operation Rescue and its fundamentalist tenets, which are not part of the Catholic tradition.

The group has also suffered from the publicity surrounding the killing of a doctor outside a Pensacola, Fla., clinic where abortions are performed.

When he arrived in Denver on Thursday, the Pope referred to "the right to life," an unmistakable statement against abortion. But the Pontiff does not lace his speeches with threats of damnation in the manner of Operation Rescue.

Referring to the failure of Operation Rescue to attract large numbers of Catholics to join its protest, Philip Faustin, a spokesman for the group in Denver, said: "We'd love to have thousands, but this is who's here. That's the reality of the situation."

The leader of the anti-abortion group, Randall Terry, appeared on Christian radio stations this week to assail a Boulder doctor, Warren Hern, as a "baby killer" and issued what Dr. Hern considered a dangerous threat. Dr. Hern has criticized the tactics of the anti-abortionist protesters.

In his radio appearances, Mr. Terry said of Dr. Hern: "I hope someday he is tried for crimes against humanity, and I hope he is executed. I make no bones about it friends, it is a biblical part of Christianity that we pray for either the conversion or the judgment of the enemies of God."

Coming just five months after an anti-abortion protester shot and killed the doctor in Florida, Mr. Terry's words were construed by many abortion rights groups as a call to violence.

Dr. Hern said in an interview today that he was considering filing criminal charges. "He's clearly inciting someone, anyone, to kill me," Dr. Hern said.

Mr. Terry, who is traveling to promote a new book, could not be reached for comment. But Mr. Faustin said Mr. Terry did not mean that anyone should harm Dr. Hern.

"He meant only that God would deal with him," Mr. Faustin said.

Expose the Killer

About 150 anti-abortion protesters gathered Thursday night in a suburban Denver church, where leaflets were distributed under the title "Expose the Killer" along with a map showing the location of the Swedish Medical Center, where Dr. Hern works.

Abortion clinics here had expected much larger protests during the Pope's visit. Katherine Spillar, a coordinator for the Feminist Majority, an abortion rights group, said more than 2,000 Denver residents had been recruited to "protect the clinics."

Groups that support the right to choose abortions say the low turnout illustrates the shifting views of most Americans.

"The country is growing tired of their street theater," said Celeste Lacy Davis, a lawyer with the Planned Parenthood Federation in New York, referring to the anti-abortion groups. "But we are very concerned that they will turn to even more extremist acts."

Man Arrested in Threats to Colorado Abortion Clinic[16]

By Kirk Johnson, *New York Times* Aug. 27, 2009

DENVER Threats telephoned to an abortion clinic in Boulder, Colo., have led to the arrest of a man who, according to a federal indictment, gave chilling details about how two people would be dispatched to kill the family of the clinic's director.

The man, Donald Hertz, 70, of Spokane, Wash., was arrested Wednesday in Spokane. He was charged with transmitting a threat in interstate commerce and violating the Freedom of Access to Clinic Entrances Act.

Mr. Hertz's indictment was the first in an abortion case since the killing of Dr. George R. Tiller, an abortion provider from Wichita, Kan., who was shot to death in May while attending church, a Department of Justice spokesman said.

Mr. Hertz's lawyer, W. Russell Van Camp, said Mr. Hertz, a retired real-estate and insurance broker who was released without bail Wednesday after a court appearance, would plead not guilty.

"I've known him 30 years, and he's never been in any trouble whatsoever," Mr. Van Camp said in a telephone interview from Spokane. "He's very pro-life, I can tell you that, but he's not a member of any radical organizations and never been arrested for picketing or any pro-life activity."

Mr. Hertz faces a maximum prison sentence of up to six years and a fine of up to $350,000 if convicted.

The investigation was set off on June 23, after the Boulder Abortion Clinic, about 40 minutes from Denver, received a call from someone who threatened the family of Dr. Warren M. Hern, the clinic's director. The threat, according to the indictment, was specific: two men from Utah would carry out the killings.

Dr. Hern, who said he had been providing abortions in Colorado since 1973, said that he had received numerous death threats over the years, but that since the killing of Dr. Tiller, he took every threat more seriously. A Kansas man, Scott Roeder, has been charged with the killing of Dr. Tiller, who was described by Dr. Hern as "a good friend and a medical colleague."

The Freedom of Access to Clinic Entrances Act, passed by Congress in 1994, makes it a federal crime to injure, intimidate or interfere with, by force or threat of force, employees of a facility that provides reproductive health services.

Abortion Clinics Preparing for More Violence

By Felicity Barringer, *New York Times March 12, 1993*[17]

The low-rise suburban landscape that is the setting of most abortion clinics is an unlikely backdrop for martial metaphors and discussions of how to block bullets. But in one small city after another, abortion providers said today that they saw the fatal shooting of their colleague, Dr. David Gunn, on Wednesday as the inevitable result of a moral battle that long ago turned physical.

If abortion opponents see the shooting as an "isolated incident" and the work of a "nutcake," abortion rights advocates -- both feminists and the obstetricians who perform 1.6 million abortions each year in the United States -- see it as the culmination of a decade or more of blockades, fire bombings, chemical attacks and nighttime gunfire.

Given that history, the slaying of Dr. Gunn in Pensacola, Fla., has become a call to arms among abortion providers who say it is past time to defend themselves and each other.

In Boulder, Colo., it is bullet-proof windows. In Santa Rosa, Calif., abortion rights volunteers are organizing 24-hour watches at clinics. In Fort Wayne, Ind., and Wichita, Kan., abortion clinics employ security guards, as does the Planned Parenthood clinic in Des Moines. The clinic in Kansas City, Mo., hired armed guards today.

Dr. G. W. Orr, an obstetrician who performs abortions in Omaha is getting a bullet-proof vest. So is Dr. Buck Williams in Sioux Falls, S.D., and he is not stopping at that. "Overnight I changed handguns and went from a .38-caliber to a .45," he said. "That'll just make a bigger hole in somebody.

In Milwaukee, Dr. George Woodward went public at a news conference today about the threats he had received as an abortion provider, figuring that high visibility was safer than a low profile. In a later telephone interview he said: "I'm working hand in glove with Planned Parenthood and the Milwaukee and Brookfield, Wis., police departments, doing everything I can to take every precaution I can. I haven't become a Salman Rushdie yet, but I may."

On the other hand, some abortion providers said there was little more they could realistically hope to do to protect themselves.

In Colorado, Dr. Warren Hern, medical director of the Boulder Abortion Clinic, said: "I am sitting here behind my desk, looking out a bullet-proof window. I work in four layers of bullet-proof windows. Death threats are so common they are not remarkable. I went to a pro-choice meeting in Denver recently, and as I walked through the picket line, someone said, 'You should die.' "

The news of Dr. Gunn's shooting was a wrenching departure from the script of the nation's longest-running public morality play, one that forced the players to rethink their own rote approaches to their roles. While the focus of abortion rights activists was the need for protection and resistance, many abortion opponents, whose movement had been built on appeals to morality, showed palpable anguish over an act of violence in the name of their cause.

Abortion Foes React

Such anguish was not evident in the earliest reactions from groups like Operation Rescue, Rescue America and Missionaries to the Preborn, which mixed often-pallid condemnations of the murder with calls for support funds for the family of Michael F. Griffin, the man accused of killing Dr. Gunn.

In an interview with CBS News, Randall Terry, director of Operation Rescue, said of Dr. Gunn, "While we grieve for him and for his widow and for his children, we must also grieve for the thousands of children that he has murdered."

Debbie Dykes, a member of the American Family Association in Bradenton, said, "I think the man that was killed -- and it was unfortunate -- he should be glad he was not killed the same way that he has killed other people, which is limb by limb."

By contrast, the United States Catholic Conference and some other longtime abortion opponents reacted with rage tempered with sorrow at an act that some felt threatened the moral foundation of their cause.

"The violence of killing in the name of pro-life makes a mockery of the pro-life cause," the conference said in a statement. "As we abhor the violence of abortion, we abhor violence as a dangerous and deplorable means to stop abortion."

The statement added, "It is not enough to say, 'We sympathize with Mr. Griffin's motivations but disagree with his actions.' In the name and in the true spirit of pro-life, we call on all in the pro-life movement to condemn such violence in no uncertain terms."

A Shared Term: 'Terrorist'

Bill Price, president of Texans United for Life, sounded a similar theme. "I'm a little bit disturbed by comments and quotes from colleagues in the pro-life movement which appear to be rationalizing or justifying or minimizing this horrific act," he said.

"I think, frankly, there has been a philosophical or even moral groundwork laid for assassinating abortionists by certain people in the pro-life movement, and I think they bear some of the blame. If they don't stop it, there will be an increase in these kinds of acts. You don't win a moral war through force or coercion or intimidation. You win through reason.

"I think it is a defining point in the history of this struggle," he added. "Responsible leaders have to speak out against this. If they don't, we will just become a bunch of terrorists."

While Douglas Johnson, a spokesman for the National Right to Life Committee, dismissed Mr. Griffin as "a nutcake," abortion rights advocates used Mr. Price's word, "terrorists," in their calls for help from local and state officials and from President Clinton, Congress and the Federal Bureau of Investigation.

Clinton Condemns Shooting

In a statement today, President Clinton said: "I was saddened and angered by the fatal shooting in Pensacola yesterday of Dr. David Gunn. The violence against clinics must stop."

Abortion rights advocates argued that the shooting should give renewed impetus to efforts to pass legislation like the Freedom of Choice Act, which would codify into law the provisions of the Supreme Court's 1973 Roe v. Wade decision legalizing most abortions. They also pushed for passage of a bill now in the House that would make it a Federal crime to interfere with abortion clinics' services to their patients.

Several states are considering similar laws to protect access, and legislators in Tallahassee, Fla., said today that they would speed up consideration of a measure in that state.

Some abortion rights activists argue that the need for such laws increased recently when the Supreme Court ruled that abortion protesters could not be enjoined from blocking access to clinics under a 19th Century law known as the Ku Klux Klan Act, which prohibits conspiracies to deny citizens their constitutional rights. Injunctions under state laws, like those governing trespass, remain in force, though it is not known how many such laws there are.

'Huddling Together for Warmth'

Telephones at clinics rang constantly today, with calls from reporters, from groups like Planned Parenthood and the National Abortion Federation, and from other clinics expressing sympathy and support. "It's mostly huddling together for warmth," said Peg Johnston, an administrator at Southern Tier Women's Services near Binghamton, N.Y., the hometown of Mr. Terry.

Although her clinic has put up a perimeter fence to keep protesters off the property, she said: "I don't think there's any real way to protect yourself against this kind of terrorism. We've all been saying and worrying that the violence was going to escalate."

During a break in a hearing at State District Court in Dallas, where Roe v. Wade was first heard, Dr. Norman Tompkins said he is "very much" concerned about his safety and that of his family after the Florida killing. "It scares the living daylights out of me," he said.

Notes

1 Hern, W.M. Burial of ashes an unethical spectacle. *Daily Camera*, March 6, 2005. https://www.academia.edu/45269675/BURIAL_OF_ASHES_AN_UNETHICAL_SPECTACLE_Mortuary_action_was_grievous_and_symbolic

2 Hern, W.M. The human life statute: Will it protect life or power? *Denver Post*, Sunday, June 21, 1981. https://www.drhern.com/wp-content/uploads/2018/05/human-life-statute.pdf

3 Hern, W.M. "Killing for life" is senseless. *Denver Post*, Saturday, April 8, 1995. https://www.academia.edu/45269705/Killing_for_life_is_senseless

4 Hern, W.M. Anti-abortion movement put weapon in slayer's hand. *Daily Camera* Guest Opinion Sunday, March 20, 1994. https://www.drhern.com/wp-content/uploads/2018/05/anti-abortion-movement.pdf

5 Hern, W.M. The politics of abortion. *The Progressive* 36(11), November 1972. https://www.drhern.com/wp-content/uploads/2018/06/Politicsab72.pdf

6 Hern, W.M. Pregnancy kills. Abortions save lives. Every pregnancy poses a "serious health risk" to the mother. *New York Times,* May 21, 2019, opinion op-ed page. https://www.nytimes.com/2019/05/21/opinion/alabama-law-abortion.html

7 Hern, W.M. *Religion, Power and Reproductive Freedom: A Checkered History of Conflict.* Presented at the Faith and Freedom Awards Ceremony Religious Coalition for Reproductive Rights. Temple Emanuel, Denver, May 3, 2018. https://www.drhern.com/wp-content/uploads/2023/06/religion-power-and-reproductive-freedom-warren-hern-md.pdf

8 Hern, W.M. "Abortionist" Carries a Charged Meaning. Letter to the Editor, *New York Times.* September 7, 1993. https://www.nytimes.com/1993/09/07/opinion/l-abortionist-carries-a-charged-meaning-856193.html?searchResultPosition=6

9 Hern, W.M. Who gets to speak in the abortion debate? *New York Times.* Letter to the Editor, December 2, 2003. https://www.nytimes.com/2003/12/02/opinion/l-who-gets-to-speak-in-abortion-debate-382086.html?searchResultPosition=8

10 Hern, W.M. A doctor's fear. *New York Times*, Letter to the Editor, January 31, 2001. https://www.nytimes.com/2001/01/31/opinion/l-a-doctor-s-fear-687693.html?searchResultPosition=9

11 Hern, W.M. How it feels to be on anti-abortion hit list, Opinion – Letters to the Editor, *New York Times*, February 4, 1995. https://www.nytimes.com/1995/02/04/opinion/l-how-it-feels-to -be-on-anti-abortion-hit-list-286895.html?searchResultPosition=10

12 Hern, W.M. Hunted by the right, forgotten by the left. *New York Times*, op-ed page, February 13, 1993. https://www.nytimes.com/1993/03/13/opinion/hunted-by-the-right-forgotten-by-the -left.html?searchResultPosition=11   https://timesmachine.nytimes.com/timesmachine/1993/03 /13/issue.html

13 Herbert, B. In America, in the war zone. By Bob Herbert *New York Times*, November 8, 1998. https://www.nytimes.com/1998/11/08/opinion/in-america-in-the-war-zone.html

14 Barringer. F. Abortion Clinics Expect Violence, *New York Times*, March 12, 1993. https://times-machine.nytimes.com/timesmachine/1993/03/12/issue.html

15 Johnson, K. Abortion protesters outnumbered in Denver, *New York Times*, August 14, 1993 https://www.nytimes.com/1993/08/14/us/abortion-protesters-outnumbered-in-denver.html?sea rchResultPosition=13

16 Johnson, K. Man arrested in threats to Colorado abortion clinic, *New York Times*, August 27, 2009, https://www.nytimes.com/2009/08/28/us/28abort.html?searchResultPosition=24

17 Barringer, F. Abortion clinics preparing for more violence, *New York Times*, March 12, 1993, https://www.nytimes.com/1993/03/12/us/abortion-clinics-preparing-for-more-violence.html ?searchResultPosition=21

20 I can't wear a tank

"How do you protect yourself?" Many people have asked me this question. My most frequent answer is: "I talk to journalists who ask me about my work."

The reason I live in the United States instead of Brazil or some other place I like is because here I have the right of free speech, and journalists represent the free press. There are other reasons, of course, but that's the main one. I believe in the free press and believe that democracy can't survive without it. The free press is a candle in the darkness. Tyrants always try to extinguish it, and sometimes they succeed. This allows them to become and remain tyrants.

The other answer I give is: "I can't. I can't wear a tank." For me to be protected all the time, I would have to wear a tank, and it isn't practical. Too many narrow doorways.

I have to assume that someday, someone who wants to be famous for killing an abortion doctor will bump me off when I least expect it. At least, that's the way fanatic anti-abortion assassins operate: by ambush. They're cowards.

It's a one-sided struggle, what military analysts call "asymmetric warfare." One side has all the advantages. Even though I'm a good shot, I don't carry weapons both as a matter of principle and as a matter of convenience. The advantage goes to the assassin who is stalking the target. It isn't fair, and that's the point.

Dr. David Gunn had a gun in his car when he was shot in the back on March 10, 1993, by Michael Griffin, a fundamentalist Christian who was acting "on behalf of God." Dr. Gunn had stepped out of his car and was going into a clinic to help women by performing safe abortions for them.

The assassin gets newspaper headlines, national fame on TV, book contracts, and movie deals, and I get to be dead. It would be very inconvenient for my family and those who work with me, and the patients would go somewhere else until that doctor is killed by the anti-abortion fanatics.

Their message is: Do what we tell you to do or we'll kill you. And they do.

It's called *Killing for Life*.

The assassins are "pro-life," and killing doctors is the policy of the "pro-life" movement. If this seems a little contradictory, check out George Orwell's *1984* and read it. It's called "doublespeak." Black is white. Up is down. War is peace. Freedom is slavery.

But I would really rather not be assassinated by one of these fanatics. Most people die for nothing, and it's better that way. Daniel Schorr once said, "The joys of martyrdom are considerably overrated." My friend and colleague, George Tiller, was assassinated by Scott Roeder, and it hurts. It was a great loss for his family, for all of his friends, and for his patients. George is a martyr to our cause, and that doesn't help anyone. I liked the world better with George in it.

DOI: 10.4324/9781003514961-21

Since I don't want to be assassinated by one of these mindless terrorists, I do things to keep myself as safe as possible, and some of these things warp your life. This has gone on for 50 years, in my case, and that's how it is. I could have been a dermatologist, and nobody would care. But I do this work because it matters and because it's my definition of practicing medicine.

It matters to the women we help, it matters for the health of their families, it matters for the health of our society, and, now, it matters for freedom.

It matters for freedom because a woman making her own decisions about her own life and health means that the individual matters, and that person's identity matters. Does the individual exist to serve the state or does the state exist to serve the individual person and society in general? That's a critical point in political philosophy.

Helping individual women have safe abortions is a blow for freedom because it says that her health, safety, and dignity as a person is more important than the needs of the state to control her life, especially her reproductive life. She is more competent to make those decisions than any government or politician.

Taking away freedom and reproductive choice from women has been a tool of tyrants for a long time. Think of Hitler and the Romanian dictator, Nicolae Ceaușescu. Think of Donald Trump. Think of the fascist, white supremacist Republican Party.

That's why it's dangerous for doctors who do abortions and also for others who perform abortions or help with that work. This defies the notion that the state, represented by, say, Republican legislators and governors, knows what's better for each individual woman than she does. This obviously carries over into other categories of the state's assignment of sex, gender, ethnicity, or other forms of being. Why does it matter to anyone that's not that person? Because under tyranny, any form of individual being or expression is dangerous.

I began learning how dangerous it was to be a doctor who performs abortions when I got an obscene death threat at 3 AM at my isolated house in the mountains during the second week after we opened the first private non-profit abortion clinic in Colorado in November 1973. From that moment until today, I have lived with fear. It's why my attitude of "hypervigilance" was identified for me by a combat medic who barely survived being blown up with her comrades in Iraq, all of whom died. It's part of "post-traumatic stress disorder," or PTSD. As it turns out, I have all the signs and symptoms of PTSD although my TSD is not "post." It is with me every day, 24/7/365 and has been since I got that first phone call. I try not to let it interfere with my life, but it does, and it has. It takes a lot of conscious work to keep it out of sight and not interfere with my work. Whether I am really successful in that is to be judged by other people.

In spite of this, I have enjoyed much of my life, I have loved others and have been loved, I have done many of the things I wanted to do and enjoy, and I have exercised my freedom as much as possible in spite of these continued threats of violence. Much of the time I have been looking over my shoulder and wary. It distorts your life and diminishes your freedom. That is the whole point, of course. That is the point of having a police state where the totalitarian system determines what you can do, say, and think. That is the purpose and goal of the anti-abortion Christian fanatics. It works. I will give some examples.

That first phone call in November 1973 has caused me to worry all the time since then about being ambushed when I arrive at my home or leave it at any time, day or night. Several things have happened to make that worse.

One time in the 1970s, before I really understood the kind of danger I might be in, I decided to go out into the parking lot by my office where the anti-abortion protesters were parking and write down some license numbers. I was in my scrubs and carrying a clipboard. The guy who was the principal fanatic, Zenon Raskowski, came after me in his car and tried to run over me. I got away, but it was a close call. The police did nothing.

When five shots were fired through the front windows of my waiting room in 1988 after I had just walked through, the bullets having just missed a member of my staff, I installed bullet-proof windows in the areas that were most vulnerable. I couldn't afford to put them everywhere, including my own office.

When I finally had to buy a house in Boulder because my practice got more complicated and I couldn't stay at my mountain home as much, I got one where I could park in the back and not be seen going into my front door.

The assassinations of doctors began in 1993, and there were several reports, including from one colleague in another state, of would-be assassins firing shots into a doctor's house. This happened several times, twice to physicians I knew. I installed heavy drapes for privacy and to keep this from happening to me.

On several occasions, I was put under 24-hour protection by armed federal marshals who put me and my house under surveillance 24 hours a day. They went with me at all times, including when I went to a bookstore or to a restaurant with or without a friend. They told me that I must not sit with my back to the window, and the marshals were always either at the next table or sat where they had an unobstructed view of me. It wasn't very good for striking up a new relationship with someone.

In the early 1990s, I taught an anthropology graduate seminar on culture and fertility in the evening. My normal routine was to walk a few blocks from my office to the

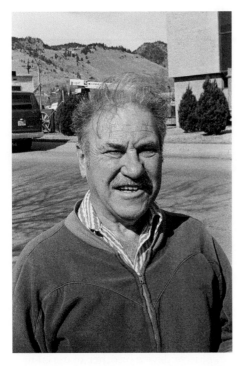

Figure 20.1 Zenon Raskowski, who tried to kill me with his car. Photo © Warren Martin Hern

Alfalfa's market on the other side of downtown Boulder, go in an order a "smoothie" drink of fruit and juice, then walk up the hill to the University of Colorado campus, go to the seminar room to teach my class, and then walk back to my office. This made the marshals nervous. One of them would walk with me on the sidewalk, and the other one would follow close by in a car ready to jump out an help if something happened to me. They had guns. When we got to Alfalfa's, they came in with me so I could buy my "smoothie."

While I was waiting for my smoothie, they would be by me looking around for suspicious people.

Unfortunately, they were from New York, dressed in suits and ties, heavily armed with 9mm Glocks, and everybody with long hair and sandals in this laid-back "natural" food store in Boulder looked suspicious to them. Then I would walk up the hill to the anthropology building. We were joined by the campus cops. The chief of the campus police confessed that the hair raised on the back of his neck as we walked across campus because he realized this was one occasion when he could actually get shot.

That evening, there were more cops in the room than students. After the class, the marshals took me to a fast-food joint where we could all get something else to eat. It was a little strange sitting there with these guys carrying serious heat. I enjoyed their company, but it was bizarre.

On January 22, 1995, the "American Coalition of Life [sic] Activists" (ACLA) held a press conference in Lynchburg, Virginia, announcing their hit list of the first 13 abortion doctors they wanted assassinated. The Mafia has the decency to keep its hit lists private. I was on the list; so was George. They called us the "Deadly Dozen." Since Dr. Elizabeth Newhall was just a woman, she wasn't included in the title of the list.

On that day, a Sunday, I left Boulder to go to my mountain home where I could get dressed for a special event at the Unitarian-Universalist Church in South Denver. I was invited to be present to honor the several physicians who had been assassinated up until then. I was simply to hold a candle.

On arriving at my home, the ACLA press conference was national news, and the phone was ringing off the hook. I had calls from a more than a dozen law enforcement agencies from the local sheriff to the Boulder police to the State Patrol, the FBI, and the U.S. federal marshals. I hadn't heard about the anti-abortion press conference, but all the law enforcement people had, and they knew I was on the hit list. By the time I got to the church, the parking lot was full of police cars, and I was taken into a conference room where a dozen officers and federal marshals were waiting for me. I was told that I would be under close surveillance and immediate protection of the federal marshals and that all law enforcement agencies were alerted for threats to me or suspicious actions.

After the ceremony, which was attended by several hundred people, the marshals drove in front of and behind me all the way to my home in Boulder and staked out the premises. This went on for months. They were at my office and accompanied me everywhere.

In June, the Republicans who had taken control of Congress decided that killing doctors who do abortions was not a crime, so they pulled the Department of Justice funding for protecting doctors, and the personal protection ended.

From that time, I had paid private security guards and consultants who warned me to keep the shades in my Boulder home drawn at night and to be very observant of my surroundings, especially if I saw any cars following me. I was advised to get a locking cap for my car's gas tank so nobody could put an explosive device or other material in it and to try to keep my car out of sight. I was advised to use a different route every day in going to my office. I was given a special radio by the local sheriff's office and a code so I could call the sheriff at any time (obviously before cell phones). All I had to do was press a button and give my code name. I carried it with me all the time. It was heavy and bulky.

I was told not to leave any papers with my name showing in my car when I was not in it. I was advised to get bullet-proof vests to wear at speaking engagements, so I did. I was told always to stand behind a lectern in case somebody started shooting at me. I was told to keep my car locked at all times, no exceptions. I already knew not to receive any mail at my home. All mail at my office was to be inspected for signs of tampering, for oil spots that might be from an explosive substance, and for unaddressed or suspicious packages. Call the bomb squad. Watch for loiterers around my home or office. Get and wear a sidearm (I declined).

I got a letter saying, "Don't bother getting a bullet-proof vest. We're going for a head shot."

On another occasion, I was warned by the FBI that a group of people in Maryland had started driving across the country with a car full of weapons and explosives to attack me and my clinic building. I was put under federal protection until they intercepted this group and neutralized the threat.

On October 24, 1998, I was getting dressed to go to a conference of the National Society of Genetic Counselors (NSGC) in Denver when I saw on the TV news that Dr. Barnett Slepian had been assassinated in Amherst, New York, the previous evening. Dr. Slepian had just returned from his synagogue where he attended a memorial service for his late father. He was fixing soup for his family when he was shot in the back through the kitchen window with a high-powered rifle by James Kopp, a well-known "peaceful" "pro-life" activist. The bullet severed Dr. Slepian's spine and tore his aorta. The exiting bullet almost hit his son.

I watched this announcement in horror. I immediately got a call and was asked to report to the U.S. federal marshals' office in Denver, which I did. I was put under federal protection again. From that point on, it was necessary for me to hire a private security detail each time I was a speaker at the NSGC or other major national conference.

When I went to testify against anti-abortion legislation being considered by the Colorado legislature, I hired my own private security detail and was accompanied by an armed Colorado State Patrol officer until I finished my testimony at the hearing and was ready to leave. By then, my own attorney had helped me to obtain a restraining order to require that a would-be assassin, Ken Scott, stay at least one mile from me at all times. Scott had followed me through the streets of Boulder and had attempted to find my house in the mountains. On one of these occasions, he made the mistake of actually calling the local sheriff to find out where I lived.

Two of Scott's associates attempted to come to my mountain house in the winter while driving a small car with bald tires. The sheriff's office found out about this, and a sheriff's deputy parked his truck on the upward part of a hairpin turn going to my house. He was a tough, wiry guy with an attitude that you would prefer to have on your side in a serious disagreement.

The terrorists had to stop on the turn because the sheriff's truck, with the deputy standing in front of it, blocked their way. "Where are you going?" the deputy asked. "We're going to see Dr. Hern." "He already knows what you think. Don't come up here and don't come back." These guys, wearing city clothes and slick soled city shoes, tried to back down, went off the road, got stuck in the deep snow, and had to shovel out their little car with their hands and a couple of things in the trunk. They didn't come back.

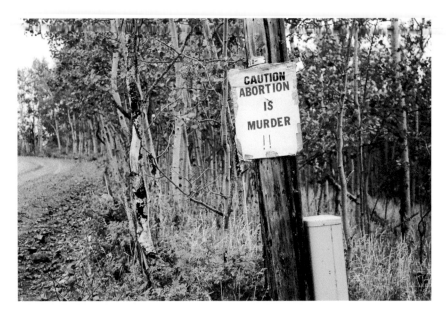

Figure 20.2 Anti-abortion sign on pole by road leading to near author's house. Photo © Warren Martin Hern

On another occasion, there were anti-abortion signs posted on the county road near my house, and there were anti-abortion signs nailed to telephone posts and to a tree at the beginning of my driveway. It was unnerving.

On the morning that my friend George was assassinated in Kansas in 2009, the Attorney General of the United States ordered U.S. federal marshal protection for me and several of my medical colleagues. There were several dozen assigned to protect me on a 24-hour round-the-clock basis. They would not let me drive my car. When I needed to go to my office or anywhere, I rode with them in a bullet-proof SUV with dark windows and several heavily armed marshals. They were stationed in my office and all around my office and home at all times.

That week, I was invited by Rabbi Steve Foster and the heads of several pro-choice organizations to speak at a memorial service for George at the Temple Emanuel in Denver. I was taken there in the bullet-proof SUV and my family couldn't go with me. A visiting journalist gave my wife, our son, and my 92-year-old mother a ride to the synagogue so they could be there. The speech I gave in honor of George is included in Chapter 9 of this book.

George's family asked me to be a pallbearer at his funeral in Wichita. When I flew there, I was surrounded on the plane by U.S. federal marshals, and this arrangement continued through the ceremony and return home. I was informed that there were about 60 federal marshals at the funeral, many of them to protect me and a couple of our medical colleagues and to prevent or deal with any anti-abortion violence that might erupt.

Three weeks after George's assassination, my office got a call from a man in Spokane, Washington, threatening to kill my family. I was in Denver attending a book event for my paleontologist friend Tony Barnosky at the Tattered Cover. I was terrified, beside myself with fear.

Once again, we were protected by federal marshals and given close surveillance by the Boulder Police Department. My wife was terrified. We had just finished building a playground set for our nine-year-old son, and we couldn't let him out of the house to play with his friends on this new treat.

As we were surrounded by police in uniform and armed guards, Fernando asked his mother: "*Mami, somos los malos o los buenos?*" (Mommie, are we the bad ones or the good ones?")

My 92-year-old mother had to leave her apartment and live elsewhere until they apprehended the fanatic who made the threat and took him into custody.

The man who made the threat, Donald Hertz, was indicted, convicted in a federal district court of making threats across state lines and interfering with a reproductive health clinic, and sentenced to five years probation.[1]

Since the modus operandi of the anti-abortion assassins is to kill the doctor between his or her car and the clinic door, we installed, at great expense, a welded steel bar fence at the front of my office with an electrically controlled steel gate and another at the back exit/entrance of my staff parking lot. Then a new construction in the neighborhood resulted in a three-story building two doors from my office with an unobstructed view of my staff parking lot from the third floor. That would obviously serve well for a sniper trying to kill us in my parking lot.

Also at an expense of tens of thousands of dollars, I modified part of the parking lot so I and other doctors who help me could park right by the secondary back entrance to my office to avoid exposure in the open parking lot. I was worried about my staff, but I was the main target. The result was that my parking spot was right at the bottom of a driveway and I could look straight up to the gate by the street. Even though I was right by the door, I got my keys ready as I parked so I could move quickly from my car a few feet to the back door in order to minimize the time for a sniper to get me in the crosshairs before I could duck into the building. I didn't want to take time fumbling with my keys at that moment.

But that didn't stop the anti-abortion demonstrators from coming to stand right by one side of the gate so they could look down at me as I arrived for work. It was alarming, but every Tuesday, one of them would do this. I couldn't help wondering which one would be armed and ready to take me out as I parked my car. This is a problem every day when I come to my office.

It is a bad way to start my day.

I am working on putting up a bullet-proof or steel barrier just ahead of where I park so the stalker can't get a shot at me while I am parking my car.

How many doctors have to do things like this in America? Only those of us who are helping women. Thank the Republicans, but do us all a favor: don't vote for them.

When I had a book event at the St. Julien Hotel in Boulder on January 25, 2023, sponsored by the Boulder Book Store, to present my new book on global ecology, I paid for a large detail of off-duty Boulder police officers to protect all of us, including me and my family, from a possible mass shooting event. The police, including the SWAT team, were highly professional, and we felt safe. But I was just there to talk about my new book on global ecology with people who might be interested. *A book on global ecology. How dangerous is that?*

Why, in the United States of America in the twenty-first century, do people at a gathering to discuss a book of any kind, much less on ecology, have to be protected by heavily armed police officers? Because that's where we are as a society and because the doctor speaking at the event takes care of women in his medical practice. Think about it.

With some exceptions, when I know the security will be good, I now hire private armed guards to be with me at all times day and night, their hotel rooms next to mine, when I have a speaking engagement at a national meeting or one that has my name printed on the schedule available to the public. This caused a problem recently when I was invited by two women surgeons to speak at an annual meeting of the American College of Surgeons (ACS) in Boston.

The two physicians had tried the previous year to have panel discussions of the kinds of problems that surgeons might encounter follow the overturning of *Roe v. Wade* by the U.S. Supreme Court. Their program for this in 2022 was canceled at the last moment by the executive leadership of the ACS without an explanation. For the October 2023 meeting in Boston, I was invited by these same doctors to share my knowledge about these issues on a panel of experts, of which I was the physician engaged in performing abortions and taking care of the complications that women experienced arising from the lack of safe early abortion services in half of the United States.

The doctors called me in May to invite me, we had many discussions of what I needed to do, I prepared my 12-minute slide presentation and discussion, my wife and I made hotel and plane reservations, and we paid over $1,000 each required to register for the conference. The program was ready. My colleagues on the panel were all experts on the abortion issue, including a top attorney for the Center for Reproductive Rights. I arranged for another physician to see my patients that week.

I told my surgical colleagues about my security situation and described the kinds of security measures I needed for such an occasion. I offered and agreed to pay for all the security measures that I needed for the meeting, including my personal security detail.

Two weeks before we were due to arrive in Boston, the doctors called me to inform me, with great anguish and regret, that the executive leadership of the American College of Surgeons canceled my appearance over the strong objections of my hosts. The ACS leadership cited the risks of violence and the "liability" risk concerns for the ACS. My work and contribution was just too controversial to allow me to be present on the program. It was censorship, pure and simple.

We went anyway, and the security appeared to me to be quite adequate except for my personal bodyguard protection, which was no longer necessary since my name had been deleted from the program. It was clear that security wasn't the reason for my participation being canceled. Members of the panel and my hosts made their displeasure known by recognizing my work and the contributions of my late friend, Dr. George Tiller.

It was okay to discuss the frightful and horrifying trauma wounds caused by AR-15 bullets on schoolchildren at the American College of Surgeons meeting, but the catastrophic surgical and medical problems caused for women across the country by the *Dobbs* decision were too tough to handle. They only affected women.

Note

1 Man arrested in threats to Colorado abortion clinic, *New York Times,* August 27, 2009.

21 Keep your paws off my pussy and your laws out of my uterus

Trump: ....*And when you're a star, they let you do it. You can do anything.*
Bush: Whatever you want.
Trump: Grab 'em by the pussy. You can do anything.

Donald Trump has set a new low standard for vile and scabrous behavior toward women and repugnant immorality in general, which reflects his deeply pathological personality disorder.

These horrifying episodes such as the *Access Hollywood* tape are so numbingly frequent that it is difficult to comprehend and process the attack on normal human behavior much less the moral leadership that should reside, at least nominally, in the president of the United States.

Trump's disturbing pathology tends to obscure the much deeper attack on the identity and value of women embodied in the constant legal attacks on the freedom of women to live healthy lives and make their own decisions about how they should live.

These legal attacks on women by the Christian evangelical and Catholic minority began almost immediately after the *Roe v. Wade* decision was handed down and have proliferated into an overwhelming number of state laws restricting women's access to safe abortion services and countervailing legal challenges to these laws.

In 2018–2019 alone, there were 30 states that passed laws restricting abortion in some manner, but from 1973 on, there have been countless state and federal laws and regulations that have been placed on the books. Some have been successfully challenged, but the overwhelmingly anti-abortion majority on the U.S. Supreme Court, but also in many lower federal courts, make it an exhausting challenge for agencies such as the Center for Reproductive Rights and the American Civil Liberties Union to track much less challenge each new ant-abortion legal atrocity in the courts. The purpose here is not to make a catalogue in massive detail of these attacks on women but to identify some of the most egregious.

Federal agencies

Attempts to restrict abortion at the federal level began well before the *Roe v. Wade* decision was announced. The first director of the Office of Economic Opportunity (the "War on Poverty" initiated by President Lyndon Johnson) was Sargent Shriver, the brother-in-law of President Kennedy, who had helped Kennedy start several of the New Frontier programs, such as the Peace Corps. Dr. Gary London was trying to help incorporate family planning programs into OEO Community Health Centers in California, and he

DOI: 10.4324/9781003514961-22

was invited to start up the OEO family planning office in 1967 at the national level. Shriver, who was Catholic, decreed that there would be no abortion or sterilization service included in the OEO family planning programs. Since abortion was still illegal in most states, this was not particularly controversial.

There was considerable confusion and different policies in the federal agencies by the time that I arrived in Washington, D.C., in early 1970 to help run the OEO family planning program with Dr. George Contis, who succeeded Dr. London. The Department of Defense had a policy that permitted abortions to be performed for military service members for medical reasons. Our program at OEO was operating under the restrictive Shriver policy.

An early supporter of family planning services for poor women and their families was President Richard Nixon. He was also concerned about the effect of uncontrolled fertility on population growth in the United States and in the world. In 1969 he wrote to Congress and requested that Congress pass legislation to create the Commission on Population Growth and the American Future. He also requested that Congress create programs that would permit women of all economic circumstances to receive family planning services, saying that poverty should not be a barrier to obtaining these services.

In 1970 Congress passed the "Title X" Family Planning and Population Services Research Act and established the Office of Population Affairs with broad bipartisan support (co-sponsored by, among others, Representative George H.W. Bush from Texas). The act prohibited the use of federal funds in programs in which abortion was used as "a method of family planning." Congress further specified that the funds could not be used for the provision of abortion services.

Although we did not attempt to change the policy prohibiting abortion in the OEO family planning programs, we changed the policy permitting the use of OEO funds for voluntary sterilization services, and I helped the Anderson County Family Planning Program in Oak Ridge, Tennessee, start such a program for poor mining families that were seeking this help. Unfortunately, the official guidelines for voluntary sterilization services that I prepared to help protect poor women from sterilization abuse were suppressed by the Nixon White House. One of the results was the involuntary sterilization of the Relf sisters, ages 12 and 14, in Alabama.

With the changes in state laws permitting abortion, starting with Colorado in 1967 and the 1970 repeal of the New York abortion law, there was increasing pressure to make abortion legal everywhere. There did not seem to be much vocal or public opposition to these changes at any level.

Helms Amendment

In 1973, with the *Roe v. Wade* decision and the entrance of Jesse Helms (R) from North Carolina into the U.S. Senate, serious opposition to abortion services erupted. One of the first signs of this was the 1973 introduction and passage of the Helms Amendment to the Foreign Assistance Act, which prohibited the use of federal funds in foreign aid for abortion services or for any program that included abortion services in its activities. The officials of the U.S. Agency for International Development protested this amendment for several reasons. The first was they felt it was a colonialist attitude for the United States to tell a foreign country what its population and family planning policy should be, and, second, they held that abortion services were an integral part of family planning and fertility control services. But the Helms Amendment carried the day, as it still does.

Danforth

In 1974 the Missouri legislature passed House Bill 1211, which placed restrictions on abortion services in that state. The bill required not only written consent from the woman who had requested the abortion but written consent by her husband as well, if she was married, or written consent by her parents if she were unmarried and under the age of 18. The bill required that the physicians performing the abortion make efforts to save the life of the fetus, and the bill prohibited the use of saline injection for abortions performed after the first trimester. Living fetuses were to be reported to the state as abandoned children. Physicians were required to keep records of all abortions.

The bill was signed into law on June 14, 1974, by Missouri governor Kit Bond. It was immediately challenged in court by Planned Parenthood of Central Missouri and two physicians. John Danforth was the Attorney General of Missouri.

Attorney Frank Susman argued the case before the U.S. District Court for the Eastern District of Missouri in St. Louis. Susman argued that the law's definition of viability would make any abortion illegal. He also argued that the consent requirements in the law exceeded those for other medical and surgical procedures and would be obstacles limiting access to abortion that were unconstitutional under *Roe v. Wade*. And Susman argued that the prohibition against saline abortion interfered with the physician's right to practice medicine. At the time the bill was written, saline abortion was one of the principal techniques in ending a pregnancy after the first trimester.

The district court upheld all sections of the Missouri law except the section requiring the physicians care for a live-born fetus as if it were a fully developed and mature infant born at term. The plaintiffs appealed directly to the U.S. Supreme Court, which heard the case on March 23, 1976. Frank Susman argued the case before the Supreme Court. He pointed out that the Missouri law was the only one that had limited abortion since the Court's decision on *Roe v. Wade*, and that it included restrictions not permitted under *Roe*. Susman pointed out that the number of unsafe abortions had dropped by half since *Roe*, and that maternal mortality ratio had dropped by 80 percent.

The Supreme Court's decision on July 1, 1976, overturned most portions of the Missouri law and thereby strengthened the provision in *Roe* that a woman had a right to have an abortion in the first trimester without unreasonable restrictions, such as requiring consent of her husband. Justice Harry Blackmun wrote the opinion for the majority, but there were several opinions that both agreed and disagreed, showing a wide variety of perceptions among the justices on the meanings of the law and the facts concerning abortion. Issues concerning viability showed great confusion as did the restriction on saline abortion, which, at that moment, was being abandoned by physicians performing abortions in the second trimester of pregnancy. It was a moot point.

The *Danforth* decision played an important role in the *Casey* decision later and contributed to confusion in that case.

The Hyde Amendment

On September 30, 1976, the Hyde Amendment passed the U.S. House of Representatives by a 207–167 vote. It prohibited the use of federal funds for abortion except for the life of the woman or in the cases of rape or incest. The federal funding affected is that of Medicaid funds through the Department of Health and Human Services. Before the Hyde Amendment was passed, it was estimated that approximately 300,000 abortions were paid for with federal funds, ostensibly for poor women who had no other access to abortion services. Medicaid currently serves about 16 million women. Henry Hyde was a Republican congressman from Illinois who was seeking a way to limit abortions in the United States, and the most vulnerable population for these purposes were poor women, who had no other means of having an abortion and no political power.

Hyde's philosophy, embodied in Republican platforms and his law is: "You can have a safe abortion if you can afford it." Hyde's objectives were soon affirmed by two U.S. Supreme Court decisions: *Maher* and *Poelker*.

Maher v. Roe, Poelker v. Doe, *and* Harris v. McRae

In the *Maher v. Roe* and *Poelker v. Doe* cases, both decided by the U.S. Supreme Court in 1977, the Court basically told women, "You can have a safe abortion if you can afford it." The Court reached the same conclusion in *Harris v. McRae* in 1980. These decisions, of course, reflected and sanctified the prevailing Republican philosophy found in the Helms and Hyde Amendments of 1973 and 1974.

The Mexico City "gag" rule of Ronald Reagan

At the 1984 meeting of the United Nations Conference on Population and Development in Mexico City, former U.S. senator James Buckley, Ronald Reagan's ambassador to the United Nations, announced a new policy at limiting abortion services worldwide. From that point on, the policy of the U.S. government required foreign non-governmental organizations (NGOs) to certify that they will not "perform or actively promote abortion as a method of family planning," using funds from *any* source (including non-U.S. funds) as a condition for receiving U.S. government global family planning assistance.

On January 23, 2017, the day after he was inaugurated, President Donald J. Trump extended this to most other forms of U.S. sponsored global assistance. From that point, family planning programs all over the world that were relying on American support for their efforts were denied any if they even spoke to women desperately seeking their assistance about the subject of abortion. There was no right of free speech under these conditions.

"The Trump administration's application of the policy extends to the vast majority of U.S. bilateral global health assistance, including funding for HIV under PEPFAR, maternal and child health, malaria, nutrition, and other programs. This marks a significant expansion of its scope, potentially encompassing $7.4 billion in FY 2018, to the extent that such funding is ultimately provided to foreign NGOs, directly or indirectly (family planning assistance accounts for approximately $600 million of that total)." (From a report by the Kaiser Family Foundation)

Reagan's Mexico City policy was continued under the administration of George H.W. Bush, it was rescinded by President Bill Clinton on the day of his inauguration, it was reinstated by President George W. Bush on the day of his inauguration, it was rescinded again by President Barack Obama on the day of his inauguration, and it was reinstated by President Donald Trump on January 23, 2017. It was rescinded again by President Joe Biden on January 28, 2021.

The Republican Mexico City policy is one of the stupidest, cruelest policies in the history of human government.

Under the Trump extension of the Mexico City policy, the regulation applies not only to all programs of family planning and reproductive health, but also to

- Maternal and child health programs (including household-level water, sanitation and hygiene (WASH).
- Nutrition.
- HIV control & treatment under PEPFAR (President's Emergency Fund for AIDS Relief).
- Tuberculosis.
- Malaria under the Presidents Malaria Initiative (PMI).
- Neglected tropical diseases.
- Global health security (pandemics of infectious diseases).
- Several kinds of critical medical/scientific research on the causes and epidemiology of dangerous diseases.

Both the United States population and the global population are rendered more vulnerable to a wide variety of disease and severe health issues as the result of the Mexico City policy.

A study published in the Bulletin of the World Health Organization showed a direct correlation in the number of unsafe abortions and maternal deaths in sub-Saharan Africa with the application and/or withdrawal of the Mexico City policy. Abortion rates increased in countries which were subjected to the Mexico City policy, and use of modern contraceptives declined. The study results suggested that "the Mexico City Policy is associated with increases in abortion rates in sub-Saharan African countries." Another study showed that "increased access to and use of contraception has been shown to be key to preventing unintended pregnancies and thereby reducing abortion, including unsafe abortion."[1] People working in family planning programs have known this for 50 to 60 years. It is also widely known from direct experience and published studies that limitations on access to safe abortion care results in high maternal mortality rates in all regions where this has been studied.

A study published in the *New England Journal of Medicine* in 2002 estimated that five million unsafe abortions are performed in Africa each year, and that at least 34,000 women die from this cause.

One of the first medical papers I read on this subject, a study of the epidemiology of unsafe abortion in Santiago, Chile, was published in 1962 in the *Revista Medica de Chile* by Drs. Rolando Armijo and Tegualda Monreal. A large proportion of all hospital admissions in Santiago were due to women suffering the complications of unsafe abortion, and a large proportion of all blood transfusions were for treating these women.

The people making and enforcing the Mexico City policy are either ignorant of these widely published studies or they don't care how much suffering is inflicted by its application. There is no excuse for this kind of stupidity and lack of compassion for women. But it has been enshrined in every Republican administration as a matter of course since Ronald Reagan took power in 1980.

James Buckley, a Senator from New York before he was appointed U.N. ambassador by Ronald Reagan, was especially known in the Senate for his fervent opposition to abortion.

Delusional decisions by the U.S. Supreme Court and other legal vexations

Planned Parenthood v. Casey

The *Casey* decision gutted *Roe v. Wade*. Although she joined Justice Harry Blackmun in the majority affirming the "essential holdings" of *Roe*, that a woman's right to choose to have abortion was protected by the Due Process Clause of the Fourteenth Amendment as long as the abortion was to occur before the point of viability, a principal actor in the evisceration of *Roe* was Justice Sandra Day O'Connor, who, with Justice William Rehnquist and Justice Byron White, pressed for a substitution of the test of "undue burden" in examining restrictions on abortion for the "strict scrutiny" and "compelling state interest" standards. This changed the burden of proof from the state to prove that it had a "compelling state interest" that justified the restriction on abortion to the woman, who must now prove that the restriction caused an "undue burden" on her effort to obtain an abortion. This removed a principal protection for women that existed under *Roe*. O'Connor had pressed for this change in *Akron*.

The other major change in *Casey* was the substitution of the test of fetal viability for the trimester system set up under *Roe* by Justice Harry Blackmun. Under the trimester system, the woman's right to have an abortion was inviolate during the first trimester of pregnancy. The test of fetal viability is extremely controversial, difficult to ascertain with any accuracy, subject to a wide variety of confounding factors within the fetus, within the woman's circumstances and health, and with respect to the availability of a top-level Neonatal Intensive Care Unit. A baby born prematurely at home or in a small hospital in a small town in southwestern Colorado has a slimmer chance of survival than a severely premature baby born in the University of Colorado Health Sciences Center in Denver.

The test of fetal viability could be used to challenge the performance of an abortion at virtually any stage, particularly at the end of the second trimester or beyond, which is often when women discover the most catastrophic medical disorders or malformations in the fetus or when the very young adolescent girl is discovered to have become pregnant following sexual abuse by a member of her family. These are tragic situations that occur often and are in danger of unreasonable regulations at that stage of pregnancy under *Casey*.

The capriciousness and uncertainty of the Supreme Court decision was emphasized in this case by the change of heart late in the decision-making process by Justice Anthony Kennedy, who voted finally with the majority to "uphold" the *Roe v. Wade* decision. That was already in doubt by the replacement of two liberal justices, Justice William Brennan and Justice Thurgood Marshal, by two conservative justices, Justice David Souter and Justice Clarence Thomas. At least on this case, Justice Souter proved not to be as conservative as he had been predicted to be.

Gonzalez v. Carhart

Since there was no essential difference in Dr. Lee Carhart's challenge of the federal Partial-Birth Abortion Ban Act and the original Nebraska law, one seeks in vain for a justification for the rabidly anti-abortion language written by Justice Anthony Kennedy in the majority opinion upholding the constitutionality of the federal law. Justice Kennedy's opinion, which appears that it could have been prepared in the offices of the National Right to Life Committee, presents no rational explanation for the decision that the Nebraska law was unconstitutional and that the federal law, which is made based on the same specious assertion, was constitutional.

The surgical procedure being defended by Dr. Carhart is highly controversial among medical colleagues, but the plain fact is that the "Partial Birth Abortion Ban" act of 2003 was the only time in the history of the United States that a particular medical procedure, albeit by a fraudulent name, has been outlawed. There is no such thing as a "Partial

Birth Abortion" described in the medical literature. As previously stated, it is a political propaganda term coined by Douglas Johnson in the offices of the National Right To Life Committee. Since it has not been described in the medical literature, the interpretation of such a law is wide open to discussion. The law obviously appears to be unconstitutional on the basis of vagueness. Neither the Nebraska law nor the federal Partial Birth Abortion Ban Act contain a health exception.

The main difference between the Court that decided in *Stenberg* that the Nebraska law was unconstitutional, however, and the Court that decided in *Gonzalez* that it was constitutional, was that Justice Sandra Day O'Connor had been replaced by Justice Samuel Alito.

That's the difference, and that's why Justice Anthony Kennedy was appointed to write the majority opinion instead of someone who did not have a bias against abortion.

Dobbs v. Jackson Women's Health Organization

The *Dobbs* decision overturning *Roe v. Wade* was not the first legal assault on women's freedom and health care in the United States, but it is arguably the worst and most punitive. It denies that safe abortion is health care for women and defies the arguments of privacy and equal protection under the law articulated by the *Roe* decision. It hands the authority over women's lives to millions of White Republican men in dark suits who have used women's bodies and the abortion issue to gain power. It drops women from second-class to third-class citizens in the United States. Coming as a result of and in the context of Trump's hideous assaults on women and Republican hostility to women and their interests, it is a deadly attack on women, human rights, and democracy itself.

We now know that the *Dobbs* case was used by the anti-abortion fanatics on the Supreme Court, starting with Samuel Alito, to overturn *Roe* through manipulation, political log-rolling, and deliberate frustration of attempts by Chief Justice John Roberts and Justice Stephen Breyer to prevent this by sticking to the narrower decision of upholding the restrictive and punitive Mississippi law. This was not a matter of following the law. It was the brutal use of raw power by the anti-abortion justices, strengthened to an overwhelming 6-3 majority by the last-minute appointment of anti-abortion Justice Amy Comey Barrett, to roll over the liberal justices and impose this draconian decision on hundreds of millions of American women and their families.

Amy Comey Barrett, whose confirmation was pushed through in a few weeks before the 2020 election because of her publicly stated opposition to abortion and Trump's hope that she would hand him the election that he expected to lose, stood on a platform in Kentucky with Mitch McConnell and said, "I am not a political hack."

"*The lady doth protest too much, methinks.*"[2]

Sorry, Justice Barrett, you're a political hack. If you lie down with a dog like Mitch McConnell, you get up with fleas.

The special case of Texas against women and safe abortion

Wendy Davis, who went from living on welfare in small trailer to a graduate of Harvard Law School and election to office as a State Senator in the Texas legislature, made history by successfully challenging a restrictive Texas abortion bill, S.B.5, by conducting a heroic filibuster against the bill standing her pink tennis shoes and speaking continuously for 11 hours on June 25, 2013. Her valiant efforts were overwhelmed when Governor Rick Perry then called a special session of the legislature, got the bill passed, and signed it into law. The guys in black suits, cowboy boots and wearing un-sweat-stained Stetsons won the day.

The terminally regressive Texas legislature went on to pass the notorious S.B. 8, prohibiting abortion after 5 weeks of pregnancy, before most women know they're pregnant, in 2021. The punitive consequences of this law anticipated the catastrophe inflicted on American women by the *Dobbs* decision overturning *Roe v. Wade* the next year.

Molly Ivins once said, speaking of the Texas legislators, "If these guys were any dumber, they'd have to be watered twice a day."

The punitive stupidity of the Texas state government was exemplified by the cruel treatment of Kate Cox, a mother of two with a history of two cesarean deliveries, who was denied an abortion in her own state when her doctors advised her to end a dangerous pregnancy in which the fetus had a lethal abnormality of Trisomy 18. This particular cruelty was administered by the Texas Attorney General, Ken Paxton, who overrode a Texas court decision granting the "exception" to Ms. Cox. She had to leave Texas for the proper health care to save her life.

Women must be punished

The following is an excerpt from Chris Matthews's interview with Donald Trump on March 20, 2016:[3]

Matthews: ... *should the woman be punished for having an abortion?*
Trump: I would -- I am against -- I am pro-life, yes.
Matthews: -- how do you ban abortion? How do you actually do it?
Trump: Well, you know, you go back to a position like they had where people will perhaps go to illegal places –
Matthews: Do you believe in punishment for abortion, yes or no as a principle?
Trump: The answer is that there has to be some form of punishment.
Matthews: For the woman.
Trump: Yeah, there has to be some form.
Matthews: Ten cents? Ten years? What?
Trump: I don't know. That I don't know. That I don't know.
Matthews: Why not?
Trump: I don't know
Matthews: I'm asking you, what should a woman face if she chooses to have an abortion?
Trump: I'm not going to do that.
Matthews: Why not?
Trump: I'm not going to play that game.
Matthews: Game? You said you're pro-life.
Trump: I am pro-life.
Matthews: That means banning abortion.
Trump: With exceptions. I am pro-life. I have not determined what the punishment would be.
Matthews: Why not?
Trump: Because I haven't determined it.

Matthews: When you decide to be pro-life, you should have thought of it. By saying you're pro-life, you mean you want to ban abortion. How do you ban abortion without some kind of sanction? Then you get in that very tricky question of a sanction, a fine on human life, which you call murder?

Trump: It will have to be determined.

Matthews: A fine, imprisonment for a young woman who finds herself pregnant?

Trump: It will have to be determined.

Matthews: What about the guy that gets her pregnant? Is he responsible under the law for these abortions? Or is he not responsible for an abortion?

Trump: Well, it hasn't -- it hasn't -- different feelings, different people. I would say no.

This edited exchange between Chris Matthews in the 2016 presidential campaign showed that Donald Trump is willing to punish women for having abortions, but Matthews's questions were never answered clearly by Trump. Instead, he continued to spout the propaganda cliché and dog-whistle buzzword, "pro-life," pounding that in at every point even if it was nonresponsive to the question. He won over 80 percent of the white Christian anti-abortion Evangelical vote in 2016 and in 2020 even though he represents the antithesis of what the fundamentalists supposedly believe as bedrock principle.

Trump is not the first man to treat women as objects of ridicule, sexual abuse, and punishment for being human beings, but he did a lot to make these offensces acceptable, popular, and politically profitable.

How is this happening in twenty-first-century America?

Trump is also not the first presidential candidate to say he would punish women for abortions. George H.W. Bush's response to a question in his 1988 debate with Michael Dukakis was widely understood as being that women should be punished for having abortions.

Much earlier than that, abortion appeared as a critical issue in federal elections.

In 1974, when he was running for reelection to the U.S. Senate, Bob Dole (R-KS) was trailing his Democratic opponent, Dr. Bill Roy, by six percentage points on Labor Day. Dr. Roy was a Topeka obstetrician/gynecologist with a law degree who had delivered thousands of babies and had done a few abortions for medical reasons. He had served two terms in Congress. At the last moment of a county fair debate a few weeks before the election, Dole asked Dr. Roy how many abortions he had performed. Dole then said that Dr. Roy was for "abortion on demand," a concept that had not occurred to Dr. Roy. Ads appeared throughout the state calling Dr. Roy an "abortioner" that were accepted as in-kind contributions to Dole's campaign. The Right to Life Committee placed 50,000 pictures of dead fetuses on car windows. Dole won the election by 1.7 percent, 13,532 out of 794,437 votes cast. He voted consistently as a senator against abortion rights and reproductive freedom.[4]

From that point, the Republican Party decided to use the abortion issue to win elections. It worked. At the direction of Jesse Helms (R-NC), the Republican Party threw Mary Dent Crisp, leader of the Republican Women for Choice, out of the 1980 Republican National Convention, included an anti-abortion plank in the Republican Party platform, and nominated Ronald Reagan for the presidency. That fall, running against abortion, gun control, school busing, and for prayer in the schools, the Republicans elected Ronald Reagan president.

They threw Frank Church, Birch Bayh, and George McGovern out of the U.S. Senate and took control of that chamber. Being against abortion helped get the fundamentalist Evangelical vote and put the Republicans in charge.

The anti-abortion leaders had seized the high moral ground by claiming to "defend life." It was clear to me that the only way for those of us who were helping women to keep the moral high ground was by placing our own lives on the line by doing our work to help them. It was a frightening and sobering moment of moral clarity. We were facing powerful forces from the president of the United States on down.

We now have the state of Ohio prosecuting a woman as a criminal because she had a miscarriage at 20 weeks with the fetus in the toilet after having gone twice for medical care that was refused her. On her first visit, the proper treatment would have been a D & E abortion performed by a skilled physician experienced in this procedure. She would have been saved from this tragedy and egregious prosecution in a few hours at the first hospital, including pre-op preparations and post-op recovery period. The failure to provide this correct treatment on the first visit is inexcusable.

Every pregnancy has become a potential crime scene.

In Michele Goodwin's book, *Policing the Womb*, she describes the systematic prosecution and persecution of women, especially minority women, for matters that women have dealt with for hundreds of thousands of years.[5] It is madness

The Tuberville tantrum

Of the innumerable examples of madness concerning the abortion issue, one of the most flagrant – which directly harms the nation's security – is the stupid, obstinate obstruction for nine months of the legislative act that would authorize the promotion of over 300 military leaders in the armed services by Senator Tommy Tuberville (R-AL), a retired football coach who clearly played too many football games without a helmet – not that there was ever anything to protect in there. Tuberville's stunt, which left the U.S. Marines without a commandant for the first time in the nation's history, was imposed on the Senate and the U.S. Armed Services because Tuberville objected to the Pentagon's policy of helping with the travel expenses of military women who had to leave their assigned home bases to receive reproductive health care (such as abortions) because of local state restrictions imposed by, of course, Republican legislatures.

The repression of women and denying them essential health care is more important to Tuberville and his followers that defending the country. Forget about the millions of people who have given their lives defending it.

This stunt by Tuberville illustrates the cynicism of Republican leaders and shows the lengths they will go to keep women from having safe abortions, not to mention women's basic health care even if it means sacrificing the security of all 330 million American citizens.

There are hundreds if not thousands of examples of important legislation being stymied or stopped cold by anti-abortion fanatics in Congress by the use of anti-abortion amendments to critical legislation concerning dozens of topics not related at all to the subject of abortion. These are examples of the unbounded fanaticism of opponents of abortion to impose their will on an unwilling society. This will continue until voters expel idiots like Tuberville from public office. Unfortunately, his level of astounding stupidity and self-righteousness appears to be treasured by Alabama voters.

Notes

1 Kaiser Family Foundation. *The Mexico City Policy: An Explainer*. January 28, 2021. https://www.kff.org/global-health-policy/fact-sheet/mexico-city-policy-explainer/#footnote-257134-33

2 Lady Gertrude (Hamlet's mother) in *Hamlet*, Act III, Scene II, by William Shakespeare

3 Kertscher, T. *Politifact Wisconsin*, March 30, 2016. Transcript, Chris Matthews MSNBC interview with Donald Trump on March 30, 2016 at https://www.politifact.com/article/2016/mar/30/context-transcript-donald-trump-punishing-women-ab

4 Kolbert, E. Abortion, Dole's sword in 1974, returns to confront him in '96. *New York Times,* July 8, 1996. https://archive.nytimes.com/www.nytimes.com/library/politics/dole-campaigning.html

5 Goodwin, M. *Policing the Womb: Invisible Women and the Criminalization of Motherhood.* Cambridge, UK: Cambridge University Press, 2020.

3 April 2009
Caro Dr. Hern,
Volevamo ringraziarla per tutto l'aiuto e la comprensione dimostrataci durante quei giorni passati a Boulder.

We know that this is your job, but we have met few doctors so professional, kind and understanding as well, in our life. Those days in Boulder have been so tragic for us, as you know, we have lost a baby we wished to have with all our heart.

The sadness, we feel, was (and is) so great that we had not the bravery to see him, but we think of him every second of our days. Rationally we think that the choice we get was the best as so to avoid him a life full of pain, but the feelings... are different.

It's difficult to say what it is right and what it is wrong...

However, now I feel better, I am still tired but much better every day. S. [husband], my sister C. and my father are very sweet and try to help me in doing everything but I know that I have to find the strength, first of all, in myself and then in the others.

Finally, I have found a new doctor who are going to follow me in the next period. We arranged an appointment on ..... but I already talked with her yesterday and I told her that if she needs more information she can contact you.

After the appointment at the end of April I'll send you the papers with all the information you asked.

Grazie nuovamente sia a lei che al suo staff per l'aiuto, la gentilezza e la dolcezza con cui mi avete trattato.
Un abbraccio di cuore,
A____ e S____
Italia

Letter from T., (U.K.) received in August, 2005
Dear Doctor Hern and all the nurses.
Thank you very much for all the support and care I received during my time at your clinic. I am feeling much better thanks to you.
Love,
T
X

DOI: 10.4324/9781003514961-23

June 2005 from Canada
To: Dr. Hern and his staff,
        "With a world of thanks."
    Thank you for giving us the opportunity to continue to pursue our dreams and achieve our goals. Thank you for your kindness, support and encouragement during the process.
    Sincerely, J_____

July, 2018 from C_____
A todos los integrantes de la clinica:
Muchísimas gracias ¡!!
Por muchas letras que escriba aquí no serare suficientes para demonstrar el nivel de gartitude que esta familia siente...
Jmas ovidaremos lo que han hecho...
Estábamos en una oscuridad total, y ustedes aportaraon la luz
Por ello esta familia los estará eternament agradecida...
Muchísimas Gracias ¡!!
    (Signed) C____

Received in 2014 from M_____ family
Dear clinic doctors, nurses and staff,
    On August ____, my daughter, K_____, was treated at your amazing facility. My daughter's decision to have the procedure was a most difficult one. Yet, the help, support and care you all gave her were exceptional. Though she was very apprehensive about what she would go through, each of you helped to calm her, prepare her, answer her questions, manage her fears, and even make her laugh.
    Not only did you give my daughter excellent care, you gave me kindness and reassurance as well. Your meticulous attention to providing clear information and your efficient, pleasant and compassionate management made our nightmare bearable.
    During the past week, my daughter and I and even her father have talked a great deal about our experience at the clinic. It was an extremely emotional and stressful time for all of us. As she is "getting back to normal" physically, she is gaining a positive perspective on this experience.
    The work you all do is essential. We are forever grateful that your service allowed my daughter to avert a potentially disastrous future.
    You have our sincere appreciation and support always. If we can ever be of help in advocating your cause, please feel free to call upon us.
    With our deepest gratitude,
    The M_____ Family

Received in August, 2018
    Thank you! You saved my life
    Love,
    A___

7 June 2018
Pat Schroeder
Dear Warren,

Thank you for sharing reflections on your amazing life's work and I cheered your letter to Cong. Marsha Blackburn, who is now running for Senate - sigh.

When I volunteered at Planned Parenthood in 1964, if someone said this is where we would be in 2018, I would have howled. I guess we just have to keep on keeping on. Victories were just beach heads they try and wash away.

All my best – Fight on !

Pat

(Pat Schroeder represented Colorado's 1st Congressional District from 1974–1997. She was the first female representative from Colorado, the third-youngest person ever elected to that body. She was the first woman to serve on the House Armed Services Committee. She was a dear friend.)

E___ & S____
California
Dear Dr. Hern and all staff members at Boulder Abortion Clinic,

We were at your clinic last ____ for the difficult decision to end our daughter's life, Y____, at 32 weeks pregnancy. Not a day goes by that we don't think of our sweet Y___. We think of all the love, care, and support you gave us during our week in Colorado. We remember all your kind words, genuine care, and devoted attention. Boulder, Colorado has become a part of us in a way. As Y___'s 1st anniversary approaches on ____, we think of you all and thank you for honoring our daughter, honoring us as parents, and for the hard work you do every day. This is a small donation in appreciation of you all and in loving memory of our little girl, Y____.

With love,
E_____ & S____

To: Dearest Dr. Hern & all staff in Boulder Abortion Clinic

Words cannot express our feeling at the moment. This was the hardest decision in our life and we don't know how we managed to live through this darkest period of our life since we received the bad news. I cannot remember how we made the appointment and how we flew over to Denver. But now I know ____ will be healthy and active again very soon. We will eventually have our own baby/babies thanks to your help and support. I am so sorry I cannot remember most of your names but only D_____. But all of you have been so kind and helpful while we lost in sadness. We are leaving tomorrow and we would like to express our deepest appreciation to all of you. Hopefully you will see ____ back on the stage very soon and we will update her _____ so you will all see her. Anytime you are in _____, please let us know and we will be glad to see you.

Lots of love
J____ & ____
(patient is a professional musician)

C_____

France

Hello Boulder Clinic! It's C____

I'm fine, I started a job in shop of cupcake : the "carelé" (a little specialty cupcake of Bordeaux). Until I go back to school next September. I found a flat in the historic center of Bordeaux. My dad and my mom are fine, and my cats too!

I want to thank you Dr. Hern, for your patience with me. You did what many doctors would never have done in France if he had the choice.

Thank all the nurses present from the depths of my heart. You alleviated the traumatic effects of this experience. You supported me, help when needed, comforted and comforted in the reasons I did what I did.

You defend respect, the rights of woman, their will much more than France does. You can be proud of yourself. France and other have to learn from you, and from your values that translate into action. If in dark moments you doubt yourself or why you work, think that many people would not be in their situation without you. I thank you because in what you do, I could not have chosen. I will have suffered like many women.

But thanks to you, I overcame my apprehensions, y fears, I tried to give the best of myself to have the life that I want. And not to become a mother of a child that didn't want because I was afraid, or full of traumas that would have prevented me from having an abortion. I will become a mother of a child that I have wanted, with a man by my side, when it will be a project full of love and desire.

I promise to be a wonder woman every day of my life. I will not give in to the facility. I will not disappoint you.

I will never forget you.

C_____

C_____

Louisiana

Dr. Hern & staff,

Thank you for hosting me this past December. I learned a great deal about performing abortions from a technical standpoint as well as what it means to dedicate your life to your medical practice. The whole staff was patient & kind with me as well as patients. I'm generally grateful for the work your office does. My favorite part was the close relationship that forms with each patient throughout the week.

Yours,

C_____

Wishing you a Happy New Year !

All our very best wishes to all the staff, especially to Dr. Warren M. Hern, D____ and L_____.

Thank you again for your help and kindness.

Take care,

S___ & A____ (France)

Dear Boulder Abortion Clinic Staff,

On behalf of the Guttmacher Institute and our Abortion Provider Census research team, we want to let you know how much we appreciate all you do – not

just for your invaluable assistance with our research projects – but for all that you do to provide quality, compassionate, life-affirming health care for your patients. We hope you have a wonderful Abortion Provider Appreciation Day, and know how much we respect and value the work you do !
    Best,
        signed
        9 GI staff members
                      31 May 2018

S_____
Pennsylvania

Dear Dr. Hern,
    My name is B_____, and next week I will begin my Ob-Gyn residency. In preparation and for inspiration, today I watched After Tiller for the umpteenth time. I would like to take a moment to thank you for the essential abortion care that you provide to your patients. The work has doubtlessly been arduous & dangerous for you at times, and yet you carry on, so that your patients can stay safe and healthy. I chose the path of medicine, and specifically ob/gyn, to provide abortion care to those who need it most. I am committed to carrying on your work, and I am not the only one. Many of us currently in training will do whatever it takes to continue this work. So, please accept this trainee's heartfelt THANK YOU for all you do, and just hold on – we're coming to help.
        Love and respect,
          B_____

Georgia   October, 2018

Dr. Warren & staff,
    My name is L_____. It has been about a year and a half since I was at your office. I can't put into words my gratitude for your compassion during the hardest time in my life.
    I attached a copy of my reflections from this year. If my story can help others coming to your office, please feel free to share.
    Thank you for all you do !
        L_____

    Accompanying document,
        The Painful Reality of Terminating A Very Wanted Pregnancy
        A personal reflection of a heartbreaking experience.

A_____
Westminster, Colorado
Dr. Hern and Dr. _____,

Thank you both, so much, for coming to speak with our small group of students on Saturday. We were honored to meet our heroes in medicine and discuss such important, intimate aspects of abortion practice. I think we will continue to reflect on your words as we mindfully approach our clinical years. Thank you for the honesty, guidance, and literature you provided us.

Sincerely,
Med Students for Choice, CU

K____
Wisconsin 2018

To the Phenomenal Dr. Hern & Superb Staff
Thank you does not begin to describe how grateful we are for everything all of you did for us!
We are so lucky that you were the ones that took care of us in our time of need. You are all truly the BEST!
Dr. Hern, what you have stood for over the last four decades, and what each of you personally do every single day for women's health is truly inspiring and forever appreciated!

Love,
K____ & A____

Thanksgiving card from the W____s
Dear Dr. Hern & Everyone at the Clinic,
Thank you again for everything you did for us. Your care & compassion was exactly what we needed in order to start our journey towards physical, emotional & spiritual healing. You guys are who we are thankful for this year (heart)
May you and yours be filled with love, community & thanks, not only this season, but all year round!

Love,
K____ & A____
Wisconsin

J_____ New York
THANK YOU!

Dr. Hern,
I recently watched a documentary you were featured in & felt compelled to write you a sincere card of appreciation for your work. It is clear that it has come with great personal sacrifice, and you need to know that you make a tremendous difference in your patients' lives, which has a massive ripple effect. You do God's work. You treat women as adults with dignity, respect, minds of their owns and I have the utmost gratefulness for you and your persistence in the face of adversity. Keep up what you continue to accomplish – we need you.
I will keep you in my thoughts & prayers.
Thank you be well
J____, LMSW

Dear Dr. Hern,

It was an honor to meet you in person, I have read about you before I arrived at the clinic, and I am still reading about you now (*Risus Sardonicus*)/

I want to thank you for having your clinic and helping people like me. I am so glad I found out about your clinic, it is fate and made to be. One of the better choices I made in life so far. Please continue to help and train wonderful doctors like Dr. _____.

In addition to saying: "thank you for giving me back my life" (exact words I also wanted to say), I want to say, thank you for SAVING my life.

Sincerely,

H_____

You will be a part of my life, in a positive way forever

TO EVERYONE AT DR. HERN'S OFFICE,

Just want to express my thanks to everyone I have encountered in the office. From day one, the nurse, the nurses, the lady who does paper work, the gentlemen who changes the lightbulb, I appreciate everyone's kindness and care.

I know some of you have worked many long years there on many long days, but I am grateful for the professionalism and the attention and care every time I step into the office. It was not an easy experience for me and honestly I don't ever wish to be there again, however I acknowledge that you are all doing necessary and meaningful work for women/people. I appreciate you all.

Thanks,

H_____

Postcard from the C family Massachusetts

Happy holidays from the C's! L (5) learned to swim. Loves: unicorns, mermaids, & constructing incredible 3-3 creations out of paper. Hates: putting on cold pant in the morning. E (9) learned to skate. Loves: bees, books, and drawing detailed comics. Hates: loud noise and being hurried. E (36) mashed up 100+ lbs of pears from our trees to brew perry. Loves: blueberries. Hates: attention. K (36), can be found nose-in-the-dirt snapping photos of creepy crawlies and mushrooms. Loves: gentle yoga. Still afraid of spiders.

This year we raised 15 monarchs to adulthood. And for one glorious day, …. 2018 each of us was a perfect square. (4, 9, 36, 36).

What a year.

Postcard

Thank you for all you do.

Marilyn NYC (Brooklyn)

The R____ Family

Seattle, Washington   21 December 2018

Sending you PEACE & LOVE in 2019. Thinking of you lots and so grateful.

Lots of love, Dr. Hern

Love,

The R____s

20 December 2018
Palm Beach, Florida
    Dear Dr. Hern,
    Thank you so very much for all of the good works you have done and the sacrifices you have made. We admire and respect you and just wanted to let you know.
    Jake

LASALLE POLICE DEPARTMENT
745 Second Street – LaSalle IL 61301
(815) 223-2131 - FAX (815) 223-6395

March 31, 2014

Boulder Abortion Clinic, P.C.
Warren M. Hern, M.D., M.P.H., Ph.D.
1130 Alpine Avenue
Boulder, Colorado 80304

Dr. Hern,
I wish to write you to first and foremost thank you and your employees in assisting me. I am working an Aggravated Criminal Sexual Assault case where a 13 year old victim from _____ and their family came to your clinic to terminate the young girl's pregnancy. Knowing the DNA would be a vital part of the successful prosecution of the 43 year old suspect, I contacted your office. I first spoke to your lab manager, C.C. C. was helpful, beyond words, and very reassuring.
    C., I feel, went above and beyond to assist me. This included her having to endure countless pestering telephone conversations. This matter, due to the circumstances, crossed a new career milestone for me and she made it as smooth as possible.
    I also want to thank F.A. for stepping up to make sure the samples were packaged properly and safely handed off to the Boulder Detective.
    Hopefully, the direct result of your employees' professionalism will aid in the arrest and prosecution of a very bad person.

Sincerely,
(signed)
Jason Quinn
Detective
LaSalle Police Department

To the staff of Dr. Hern's office
    May of 2018 was when I was a patient at our clinic. My daughter, E_____, was born an angel under the loving care of Dr. Hern and his staff. You were all with me in the hardest moments of my life. I will always be grateful for the love and compassion I experienced then. Because of the intimate care I received, I felt an urgency to spread the love. When E____ was brought to her dad and I for our viewing, she was wearing a mini beanie hat that I was told someone had made and donated to your clinic. It is one of my most cherished possessions along with a baby blanket

my mom made for her. It was an idea that turned into an action. For the last 9, almost 10 months, I have knitted and crocheted love into every stitch of every blanket I made in this box. My mom contributed a couple as well to support me. These blankets aren't perfect but they were created to provide love, warmth and comfort. I hope with every fiber of my being, that this donation will be accepted in the name of my special girl, E_____. Thank you for your kindness and support. Love.

        Sincerely,

   C_____

P.S. If you need to reach me for any reason, my cell number is _____

Dear Dr. Hern and Staff,

I don't know how often you receive letters of this nature. I know that many in our nation believe that the work you do is wrong and send you awful hate mail thinking they can get you to stop. I was one of your patients three years ago and I know that the work you do is immeasurable. I wanted to take the time to write this letter to you to know how much I and my family appreciate the work you do.

At the beginning of this month I graduated with my master's degree. While sitting waiting to go up on stage I thought of how grateful I am to you and your staff's incredible work. Without it I would not have achieved my degree. I wasn't ready to be a mother and you let me make that choice for myself. I am sure you see a lot of women who have many reasons for being in your office. Your work makes our dreams and futures possible and that is something that the other side doesn't understand. I want you to truly understand that you gave me a second chance at my future and my dreams.

Being in your office is a hard and at times scary place but the people there make it less scary. Words of reassurance and clarification help to make it all a lot clearer. When I first called your office I was numb, unable to really comprehend what was going on with me. The voice on the other end of the line was so kind and reassuring I felt myself able to speak to her, even though I was a bit hysterical. There was a point when I was too overwhelmed and the woman on the other end told me to "take a deep breath. I am not going to hang up on you. When you are ready let me know." I felt like an angel was helping to take care of me in that moment. When my mother and I arrived at the clinic we were greeted kindly and the voice on the phone became a face who hugged me and comforted me. From then on I met people who were there to support me. The nurses were beyond angelic to me. Even when all I could do was lay there and cry, gentle strokes and soft spoken words filled the room. Dr. Hern you are incredibly professional and remarkable in what you do. My mother would wait in the waiting area reading everything she could about what you do and I know she is incredibly grateful for what you did for me.

There is a lot of uncertainty in the country right now and in what your work could end up looking like. I wish I had a magical wand and could wave all of the concerns away. However, I know there are many, many women like me who know that what you and your team do for us is something that should never be taken away. Because of you and your team I have found a voice in fighting for those who were not as fortunate as me and who are currently facing losing their healthcare coverage. I am a strong woman because of your clinic. I am pursuing my life, my passions and my dreams because I was given a second chance.

I cannot imagine you and your staff not being available to women across the nation. You and your staff deserve to know that you are the most remarkable people. I thank you! I know my family thanks you for what you were able to do for me. I know my future life thanks you. So no matter how awful the hate mail, or what the politicians say. Please please remember that there are individuals out there, like me, who are forever grateful !!!!

Love,

A former patient

*If you wish to use this letter for any purpose please feel free to do so :)

USA TODAY February 19, 2019

I had a later abortion because I couldn't give my baby girl both life and peace

Kate Carson, Opinion contributor Published 5:00 a.m. ET Feb. 19, 2019 | Updated 4:08 p.m. ET Feb. 19, 2019

No one loves my baby more than I do. Her death was a gift of mercy. Now, women like me will always be a scapegoat for policies limiting women's rights.

People are talking about me again, loudly, unkindly. Even the president of the United States has had his say about families like mine. I have told this story so many times, but I will tell it again as many times as it takes.

I help run a support group for families who have ended pregnancy after poor prenatal or maternal diagnoses. If you're wondering, "Who are these women who get abortions in the third trimester?" We are. I am. Parents who love our babies with our entire hearts. Desperate acts like an abortion in the 36th week of pregnancy are brought about only by the most desperate circumstances and are only available to those who can come up with a lot of money quickly.

I know. I've been there.

My daughter, Laurel, was diagnosed in May 2012 with catastrophic brain malformations (including Dandy-Walker malformation) that were overlooked until my 35th week of pregnancy. I did not know much about brain disorders at that point. I imagined developmental delay, special education classes, financial pressure, an overhaul of expectations for Laurel's life and my motherhood. Here were the doctors' real expectations for Laurel: a brief life of seizures, full-body muscle cramps, and aspirating her own bodily fluids.

When I heard the list of all the things my beloved daughter would not do — talk, walk, hold her head up, swallow — I grasped for what she would be able to do.

"Do children like mine just sleep all the time?" I asked.

The neurologist winced. Children like yours, he told me — slowly — are not often comfortable enough to sleep.

Our choice was sad — but clear

Let me answer some questions you might be thinking: Yes, we were sure that these problems were severe. No, there is no cure, nor any on the horizon. Yes, we were counseled in-depth on our options, including adoption. Because we wanted to spare our daughter as much suffering as possible, our choice was very sad, but crystal clear: abortion.

I imagined an abortion at eight months would be grisly. But no matter how violent my imagination, it surely could not compare with the suffering Laurel would have endured in her own broken body.

In Massachusetts, my home state, a later abortion can be obtained only if the life or health of the mother is at risk. So I set off on a 2,000-mile journey from Massachusetts to Colorado to access this abortion. I landed, not in the nightmare I had imagined, but in the safest, kindest, most dignified hands I have ever encountered as a patient anywhere. Dr. Warren Hern at his Boulder Abortion Clinic is one of the few doctors in the country performing this procedure. After a single injection and a couple of hours, my baby was laid to rest in my womb, the purest mercy that I knew how to give my Laurel.

As the usual hubbub of hate and misunderstanding around abortion swelled to a roar this month, the president unfairly addressed families like mine in his State of the Union address. He hasn't really listened to women like me or doctors like Dr. Hern. He seems to care nothing for the true stories of heartbreak, loss and extreme medical complexity behind abortion later in pregnancy. Instead, his agenda must inflate fear and horror until every last American thinks of unspeakable violence.

Mercy means something different to each family

This is not about abortion. It is about power. This administration needs the public to be angry at women like me and misinformed about what compels women to seek later abortions, which make up less than 1.5 percent of abortions, according to the Centers for Disease Control and Prevention. But I believe that Americans can hear our story and meet the painful, complicated truth about abortions later in pregnancy with love and understanding.

And most Americans have compassion for a woman's choice when it comes to her reproductive health care. In fact, nearly 70 percent of Americans do not want to see the Supreme Court completely overturn Roe v. Wade, according to the Pew Research Center.

Nobody loves Laurel more than I do. Her death was a gift of mercy. Mercy means different things to different loving families, and that has to be OK. To all the families who faced similar circumstances and made a different choice, I honor you. I trust your wisdom. I celebrate your child's brief and beautiful life.

We must treat each other with love, tenderness and respect. It is horrible, as a parent, to choose between life and peace for our children, especially when we want to give our children both beautiful and precious gifts.

It is devastating to lose a child. But, unlike most bereaved parents, women like me will live out the rest of our lives as scapegoats, fuel for an agenda that seeks to strip women and families of our reproductive freedoms.

When I think of my baby Laurel, I feel love and peace. Unfortunately, I cannot be with that peace because there are fresh wounds in the way, the throbbing pain of being hated and misunderstood.

Kate Carson is a teacher and mother who lives with her family in the Boston area. She is a member of NARAL Pro-Choice America.

Dr. Hern and the team at Boulder Abortion Clinic,
Last week your team cared for my daughter, A.

I'm writing to thank you for our supportive, attentive care – and to let you know I'm praying for you.

I know, I know: "I'm praying for you" is sometimes code for "Here's hoping God strikes you down, evil-doers." But please know that's not at *all* what I have in mind.

What I am praying for is that there be no conflict at your clinic, that you have no cause to fear for your safety. That you can do your work in an environment where you receive the civility and respect you deserve. For your team to be free to continue providing caring, professional support to the women who come to you for help.

You've met your share of conservative Christians who know how to picket, protest, and send condemning letters….and for that I'm sorry. While I'm a part of the tribe – a relatively conservative Christian – I'm not from that particular *branch* of the family.

When my daughter told me about her unplanned pregnancy, I asked her to consider all the options – and she chose abortion. As her father, I had a choice to make: Would I provide support as she sought out a clinic and followed through on her decision…or not? Could I accept her and her decisions without necessarily endorsing them?

I won't lie about it: I wish she'd chosen differently. But I opted to provide support…because I love her. And because this was *her* decision to make – not mine.

And she chose your clinic. She did so on the advice of a referring ob-gyn, but that didn't cinch the selection. After doing more research, we came to Boulder expecting outstanding support on both the medical and emotional fronts.

And I wasn't disappointed.

So, thank you. Thank you for taking such good care of my daughter. For treating her without judgment. For fielding multiple phone calls. For navigating the details with our insurance provider.

I'm grateful – and I wanted you to know it.

(signed)

Patient's father

Loveland, Colorado

November, 2023

Dr. Hern, Dr. W… & staff,

I wanted to reach out and thank you for everything. The decision to end our wanted pregnancy was extremely difficult for my husband and me. At your clinic, I felt so supported and comforted. It was reassuring to have the support, resources, and compassion about our situation.

Thank you to each staff member for being so understanding and caring throughout the entire process and each procedure. I knew I was safe and in the best of hands. Additionally thank you for putting my comfort and consent first – and cheering me when I got scared.

I truly felt love, compassion and cared for by everyone I interacted with. You and your staff made the difficult week easier to handle. Although we are grieving our loss, I can look back and know this was the best and safest decision for my family - and it was provided by the best doctors, nurses, and staff

Again, thank you.

Love,

G.

From a patient whose pregnancy was afflicted by a catastrophic fetal anomaly (December, 2023):

Dr. Hern, Dr.   , A (patient's counselor), RN, & staff:

Exactly two weeks as I write this letter from the date of the procedure. Seems as it if it's a time that I will be unable to process. However, I do know your kindness and warmth will always surround those three days. I'm not sure if there are words to sufficiently portray my gratitude. There aren't enough "thank you's" in this lifetime, to state how thankful I am for you all and the level of work you perform.

My heart goes out for the thousands of other women and families processing their grief. I hope your book, Dr. Hern, will provide a voice for your career and the people you have assisted during a life altering experience. Please consider the $40 as a pre-purchase order for the book, or as a donation to the clinic.

With great respect,

K.

March 7, 2024

Hi, Dr. Hern -

I'm a bit late with this note as January 19th marked 19 years since S___ and I were in your office and you were helping us through our most difficult time in our lives. I can't quite wrap my head around how much has changed between then and now for women in our midst today facing reproductive decisions. (heart) In every new article I read or news story I hear, I am constantly reminded of your gentle spirit and Herculean efforts for women. Thank you from the bottom of my heart for your all you did for our family, Dr. Hern. I hope this note finds you well and not too overworked. In this challenging time you are always in my thoughts and please know I sent you love, peace, and safety. All the family is thriving here in S.....

(heart). Lots of love and care. J___R____ (written on note card "Love and Peace")

---

* * *

These are some of the thousands of letters I have received over 50 years from grateful patients and others who have expressed their support and appreciation. I have not included the hundreds of anti-abortion letters that range from prayers for my lost soul (that will remain lost, thank you) and hate mail of the most vicious kind including one that told me not to bother wearing a bullet proof vest because they were going to go for a head shot.

The most poignant letter I received was from a Black woman inmate who was brought to me in chains from the state prison. An armed guard stood outside the operating room door as I performed her abortion. She was very sweet, we enjoyed taking care of her, and she expressed profound gratitude.

Another young woman wrote a note to me and included her graduation announcement from an elite liberal arts college on the west coast. She said that she found out that she was pregnant after she had been accepted to this college, she had no job and little money, I performed an abortion for her, and she was able to attend the college, graduating with honors. She had been accepted to medical school, and that was the next step. She is now practicing medicine in an important specialty related to the health of women and children in a major teaching hospital on the east coast.

I cannot begin to express my appreciation and gratitude for these letters from patients and their families. Their deeply felt and touching comments sustain me in the difficult times I have experienced in doing this work.

23 After *Dobbs* and post-*Roe*

On January 22, 1973, the world changed for the better, especially for women, but for American society in general. The *Roe v. Wade* decision was a critical and important historical step toward human freedom. It had global significance.

The *Dobbs* decision on June 24, 2022, was the opposite. It was a step backward into time hundreds or thousands of years ago when women had no recourse for medical help in surviving a pregnancy or its life-threatening complications. Even in Mauriceau's seventeenth-century-Paris – 350 years ago – there was no law against helping women survive these problems. Medical care for women was primitive by modern standards, but it was not illegal. It is now illegal in many parts of twenty-first-century America, and we have Donald Trump, the Republican Party, and white Christian Evangelicals to thank for that. The fetus is a fetish object and women's bodies are for stepping on to get political power.

Every single Republican candidate for public office must be held accountable in the voting booth for this catastrophe.

What are the costs for women and their families of keeping women from having abortions?

One place to start is with a classic study of the effects on women – and their children – of being denied an abortion.

What happens to women who are denied an abortion? What happens to their children?

In spite of the fact that pregnancy is a life-threatening condition and there is no justification for denying an abortion to a woman who wants to end a pregnancy, there is a long history of women being denied abortions for many reasons.

One of the most important studies of this problem was carried out in various countries in eastern Europe under the direction of Dr. Henry David, an American psychologist originally from Germany who organized a multicenter study of these women. Over a period of 35 years, Dr. David and his European colleagues followed two cohorts of 220 pair-matched children. In one group, the mothers had twice been denied abortions for an unwanted pregnancy, and the other group of children were all the result of wanted pregnancies. "Differences between the two groups of children widened over time, always to the disadvantage of the unwanted children. In the aggregate, unwantedness in early pregnancy has a detrimental effect on children's psychosocial development. In adulthood, marital partners of the unwanted children were similar to their spouses. Families founded by men or women unwanted in early pregnancy were more problem-prone than

DOI: 10.4324/9781003514961-24

families founded by individuals wanted or accepted in early pregnancy."[1] The authors concluded that "Denial of abortion for unwanted pregnancy entails a risk for negative psychosocial development and mental well-being in adulthood."[2]

The "Turnaway Study," designed and conducted by ANSIRH under the direction of Diane Green Foster, Ph.D., studied a thousand women who had sought abortions.[3] Some obtained the abortions, and some were denied. The research studied the effects of these two outcomes. The investigators found that

> many of the common claims about the detrimental effects on women's health of having an abortion are not supported by evidence. For example, women who have an abortion are not more likely than those denied the procedure to have depression, anxiety, or suicidal ideation. We find that 95% of women report that having the abortion was the right decision for them over five years after the procedure.

The Turnaway Study does find serious consequences of being denied a wanted abortion on women's health and wellbeing. Women denied a wanted abortion who have to carry an unwanted pregnancy to term have four times greater odds of living below the Federal Poverty Level (FPL).

In addition, women denied abortion are:

- More likely to experience serious complications from the end of pregnancy including eclampsia and death;
- More likely to stay tethered to abusive partners;
- More likely to suffer anxiety and loss of self-esteem in the short term after being denied abortion;

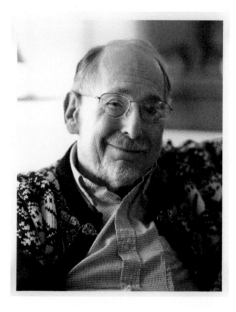

Figure 23.1 Dr. Henry David, director, Transnational Family Research Center, organizer of research study of women denied abortions in eastern Europe, *Born Unwanted: Long-Term Developmental Effects of Denied Abortion.* Photo © Warren Martin Hern

- Less likely to have aspirational life plans for the coming year;
- More likely to experience poor physical health for years after the pregnancy, including chronic pain and gestational hypertension.

The study also finds that being denied abortion has serious implications for the children born of unwanted pregnancy, as well as for the existing children in the family.

Denying a safe abortion to a woman who wants one and needs it damages her, her children, and everyone in her family. It damages her life.

Forced birth is cruel and unusual punishment. It is unconstitutional.

How can anyone defend a law that inflicts this damage on a woman and those around her?

Post-*Dobbs* catastrophes across America

The nationally reported cases are familiar and horrifying. A ten-year-old girl who has been raped has to be taken from Ohio to another state to have an abortion.

A woman with a potentially fatal hydatidiform mole, a rare but true pregnancy that looks like a bunch of white grapes and can become cancerous, but which can be removed safely and quickly with abortion procedures we are using routinely, as in my office, had to be taken from her state to Kansas for the correct life-saving treatment.[4]

Kate Cox, a mother of two with a history of cesarean delivery that compromises her safety in a desired pregnancy has a fetus with catastrophic complications, and the pregnancy is a clear risk to her life.

Texas laws prohibit her abortion _unless_ there is a clear threat to her life – which there is. A judge grants the exception so she can have the pregnancy ended in the safest way possible, but then the Attorney General of Texas, Ken Paxton, who has no medical education, overrules the judge and threatens doctors and hospitals who help Ms. Cox with criminal prosecution. It is utter madness. It is criminal blackmail.

A young woman twice seeks medical attention in Ohio for a threatened miscarriage at 20 weeks, which is lethal for the fetus and potentially lethal for her, is twice denied the correct medical care (which could save her life in a few minutes), delivers the fetus in the toilet instead of the hospital, and then is indicted for abusing a corpse. It is madness. It is medieval stupidity.

Women have experienced these problems for thousands of years, but it is now illegal in much of the twenty-first-century America to give them the correct modern medical care. It is madness. How can we call ourselves a "civilized" country?

A patient of mine, whom we discover on her arrival is suffering from acute pyelonephritis and is in extreme pain, has driven across Texas, Oklahoma, and Colorado in pain to reach my office to end a pregnancy with fetal anomalies that no one in Texas was allowed to help her terminate. She couldn't get treatment for the life-threatening pyelonephritis in Texas because she was several months pregnant.

Another woman calls me from Texas, a person who is a well-educated health professional in her 30s, who has a desired pregnancy, but who has been refused medical care in Texas for ruptured membranes at 16 weeks. This means that she will miscarry with the possibility of fatal hemorrhage from a condition that I could resolve for her in a few minutes in my medical office. She is desperate for help after being told days before that she must leave Texas for this basic medical care. It is the weekend, she has had ruptured membranes for several days, she feels sick, and she must be seen on an emergency basis. I advise her to go to a university hospital emergency care in Colorado near the airport where I know she can be seen immediately. She is admitted to the hospital and gets the correct care, but she is in the intensive care unit for several days and almost dies. It is madness.

Pregnancies resulting from rapes in states restricting abortion following the *Dobbs* decision

In a study just published in the medical journal *JAMA Internal Medicine*, the authors report: "In the 14 states that implemented total abortion bans following the *Dobbs* decision, we estimated that 519, 981 completed rapes were associated with 64, 565 pregnancies during the 4 to 18 months that bans were in effect."[5] Only 21 percent of the victims reported their rape to the police.

Is there a more vivid example of the punishment inflicted on women in Republican-controlled states?

Thousands of women are having these experiences all over the United States. It is because the Republican Party, dominated by the white Christian Evangelicals and Catholic fundamentalists, has made abortion illegal or highly restricted in almost half of the United States. It is incredible.

It has been increasingly hard for women across the country to find safe abortion services during the past 20 years, became severely worse after the Texas law S.B. 8 in 2021, became impossible for many after the *Dobbs* decision, and it is getting more impossible by the minute.

Doctors who have referred patients for decades from Republican-dominated states are afraid to refer patients for fear of prosecution and can give a patient only purposefully vague suggestions. They are afraid to see the same patients who got to my office anyway for follow-up exams in Texas for fear of being prosecuted. Women needing follow-up exams or postoperative care for minor complications are afraid to tell doctors that they had an abortion. That's how it was *a hundred years* ago in this country.

There was an incident in Nevada in which a young woman who had received a medical abortion had complications that were untreated in spite of the fact that she presented herself twice for medical care, was refused, and who died. It is madness.

It is a national catastrophe for women and their families. It is inexcusable, horrifying, and indefensible. But it got a lot of Republicans elected with the help of crazed Christian anti-abortion fanatics.

It is a mass psychosis with casualties. The casualties are the women who can't get medical care.

> **Breaking News:** *On January 26, 2024, a New York jury awarded E. Jean Carroll with a judgment of $83.3 million against Donald J. Trump for violent sexual abuse and defamation of character.*

Going forward after *Dobbs*

If the struggle for reproductive health and freedom is won finally, it will be won by women. If the struggle to preserve freedom and democracy in the United States is won, it will be won by women. If the struggle to save the Earth as a habitable place for future generations of humans and other species, it will be won by women.

How? Why? Because their lives are at stake, they understand this, and they vote (at least, in places where they can vote). For now, they can vote in the United States of America, but it is a struggle to maintain that truth. That is because those in the United States who oppose reproductive freedom and health for women also oppose democracy and freedom in America. They are opposed to voting by those who are not white male Christians. They are called "Republicans," which is an oxymoron because they oppose a constitutional democracy in a republican form of government. In their view, the benefits of American wealth, power, and its Constitution are not for everyone.

The Republican Party has increasingly over the last 50 years become an authoritarian, totalitarian political party and personality cult catering to and empowering a white supremacist movement composed of white Christian Evangelicals and white Christian Nationalists, many of whom hold great power at this time in the American government. Their openly stated goal is the establishment of white Christian fascist theocracy. Trump has a team working on it as we speak. They're hiring. They are fascists.

Women will have completely subservient roles as livestock for producing babies to maintain the fascist state.

Don't believe it? Read this:

> **Breaking News:** *In a first-of-its-kind ruling, Alabama's Supreme Court said frozen embryos are children and those who destroy them can be held liable for wrongful death.*[6]

In this system, people exist to serve the state, not the other way around. As stated in Michelle Goldberg's book, women are forced to be *The Means of Reproduction.*[7] It is the realization of *The Handmaid's Tale.*[8] It is described in Tim Alberta's book, *The Kingdom, The Power, and the Glory*[9] and in speeches by Mike Johnson, the current Republican Speaker of the U.S. House of Representatives.

Now, the Alabama Supreme Court has made the State of Alabama the Supreme Keeper of Women's Fertilized Eggs whether women like it or not and exposes women and their doctors to liability for criminal prosecution if anything goes wrong (what could possibly go wrong … go wrong … go wrong? Except for the person who dropped the container of frozen embryos on the floor, which started this episode. Who woulda thunk?).

The Alabama Supreme Court decision is clear fulfillment of the anti-abortion movement's crusade to establish the sick fantasy that a "person" exists from the moment of conception, and this leaves the Republicans hoist on their own petard.[10]

Having reached their preposterous goal, they are now confronted with the cries and outrage of tens of thousands of people living in the real world who want to have babies and families using in vitro fertilization (IVF), which is now outlawed by the Christian Republican success.

Senator Tommy Tuberville (R-AL), He of "missing football helmet" fame, is flummoxed by trying to answer questions about this inexplicable contradiction and catastrophic consequences for families from NBC reporter Dasha Burns since he is ignorant not only about the issue and basic biology but also the fact that the Alabama Supreme Court issues decisions, not laws.

The hammer and tongs for this fascist fantasy and successful drive to control the American government in whole or in part is the issue of abortion. No matter that a large majority of Americans favor the availability of safe, legal abortion: it has been the goal of the Republican Party and Christians (including both the Catholic Church and Protestant denominations) for 50 years to establish control of the federal judiciary, especially the US Supreme Court, in order to overturn the *Roe v. Wade* decision and to enable the Republican state legislatures to make abortion illegal at the state level. They have accomplished this goal through the *Dobbs* decision. Safe abortion is either completely illegal or severely restricted in almost half of American states, all controlled by the Republican Party.

And now tens of thousands if not hundreds of thousands of families are wrenched into this unfathomable political nightmare because the Alabama Supreme Court has given the "right to run everybody else's life" anti-abortion fanatics and Christian Nationalists exactly what they have wanted and successfully fought for since 1973 with all its *reductio ad absurdum* consequences – a fertilized human ovum the size of a pinhead is now a fully recognized person before the law with civil rights, voting rights, eligibility for passports and drivers' licenses, views on foreign policy, and attitudes toward immigration. The fanatics caught the car and now they don't know what to do with it. The best thing is that all these embryos are Republicans, and it will help at the time of the next election since they can vote.

The families who are suffering from this political monstrosity and are really counting on IVF to have children that they love don't think this is funny. Neither do I, but it is the certain obscene logical consequence of the will to power among the Christian and Republican fascists that the people who are now making national policy are people who talk to God and carry Guns.

The spectacularly lurid presence of Donald Trump on the American political scene as a candidate in 2016, as president for four chaotic years, and an interminable election-denying violence-inciting self-pitying candidate since then, now a convicted felon, has energized, validated, and consolidated the most authoritarian, racist, and violent elements in American society. The Alabama IVF decision followed *Dobbs* as night follows day, and the Republicans have foisted this excruciating dilemma on us. Think about that when you vote.

The demonization of abortion and its political use

Some people wonder why abortion, a private medical/surgical operation to end a life-threatening condition of pregnancy for women who choose or need to do this, has become demonized and so politically useful. People are astonished at the fact that white Evangelical Christians as well as other extremely traditional Christians are so willing to embrace such an ostentatiously depraved, corrupt, racist, dishonest, psychopathic monster and embracing him literally as a gift from God – a Messiah – to save them. Trump is literally regarded as the Second Coming of Christ by Evangelical Christians. The conflict Trump brings will lead to the long-awaited End Times "Rapture" that will take Christians to Heaven and mercilessly and cruelly destroy everyone else. Republican members of Congress openly refer to Trump as "the Orange Jesus." Is that sarcasm or belief? What kind of sadistic person really wants this hideous sequence of imaginary events? What kind of a religion bathes in this fantasy of violent retribution?

It is one of the most terrifying political and cultural upheavals in American history. Why do these Christians believe every one of the thousands of lies that Trump utters?

Do they believe the bizarre, delusional video Trump made of himself, *God Made Trump*, as the "God-Given Caretaker" and "Shepherd to Mankind?" It illustrates an openly psychotic delusion of grandeur and pure pathological narcissism. What about the biblical injunction against "believing in false gods?"

Tim Alberta, in his book, explores this subject in a highly personal way from the inside of Christian Evangelism as the son of an Evangelical pastor. His basic answer is that white Christian Evangelicals and other extremist white Christian sects feel highly threatened by the changes and ethnic diversification in modern American society. The white majority is going to become the white minority. "The barbarians are at the gates, and the Evangelicals need a barbarian to protect them," he said in an interview for *Meet the Press*. Alberta understands this to his core because he is still an integral part of this deeply authoritarian delusional system. "I walk with Jesus," he says.

The preposterous delusional nonsense that Donald Trump tells the Christians reverberates with their delusional system. And Christians are taught to believe absolutely preposterous absolute nonsense from their first waking hours and consciousness about imaginary beings with imaginary behavior and characteristics, magical thinking and the occurrence of imaginary supernatural events.

The white Evangelical Christians have made a Faustian bargain with one of the most malevolent and despicable persons in human history, who openly plans to be a dictator and who has displayed these abnormal behavioral characteristics for decades. He promises the Christians that he will use the coercive power of the state in order to impose their religion's harsh values and beliefs on the rest of their fellow citizens. What does that tell us about Christian values and beliefs? They are intellectually and morally bankrupt.

Christians want Trump to protect them from normal people and society. Looks like he's up to the job.

Trump's demagogic invocation of existential fear in his followers and true believers crystalizes their racism and paranoia about "Others" who are "Different," especially those who are not white. It also makes them obey his delusional instructions.

The New Right in the Republican Party decided to exploit white Christian racism and this special vulnerability 50 years ago, and especially the highly effective issue of abortion, to secure political power.[11] Opposition to abortion is their best organizing issue because it pleases Christians who are fanatically obsessed with eliminating it from women's health care. This suits their patriarchal, misogynist ideology of keeping women subservient, in the kitchen, making cookies, and having babies. Kinder, Küche, Kirche (children, kitchen, church).

This Republican strategy has been an astounding, historic, earth-shaking success. It is a little less indecent, a little more polite and "respectable" than openly advocating violent racism and racial segregation. It worked for the Republicans. It's working for the Christians.

It will destroy America.

At this moment, America is at the mercy of a collective psychosis and organized delusional system called Christianity which controls a fascist Republican political party led by a criminal delusional demagogue with orange hair in place of a black mustache.

Christians regard him as the Messiah, the Second Coming of Christ. Republicans call him the Orange Jesus. Tough to overcome stuff like that at the ballot box in a rational, secular constitutional democracy.

The face of fascism in America

Like the Roman god Janus, fascism has two faces in America: Christianity and the Republican Party. Faux "News" is the voice of fascism in America bent on spreading this rabid ideology. Ratings. Their gullible devotees love it.

The point of fascism is to crush individuals and to crush the meaning of their individual lives in favor of the state. That's one of the reasons why E. Jean Carroll's successful lawsuit against Donald Trump for sexual assault and defamation is so important.

Trump first humiliated and physically violated Carroll and then he tried to crush her, but he did not succeed. She stood up to him, and she stood up for all women who have been abused in this way and survived. She said so, and we celebrate her victory over this vile person.

Women who have safe abortions in spite of the Republican effort to crush them, their bodies, and their lives are standing up to fascism in the same way that E. Jean Carroll stood up to Trump.

The attempt by Trump to crush E. Jean Carroll and the attempts by Christian Nationalists and others to crush women, minorities, and LGBTQ+ people in America is similar to the same efforts to crush Jews, Romas, and LGBTQ+ people in Nazi Germany. They cannot be allowed to choose their own lives and identities.

Each individual who asserts his or her unique identity is a threat to the totalitarian state. Standard personal pronoun, please.

At the courtesy of our white Christian Nationalist Speaker of the House:

> *News item: February 1, 2024*
> **Anti-LGBTQ+ hate pastor gives opening prayer in House of Representatives**[12]

Religion has been a tool of tyrants for thousands of years.

Safe abortion defies fascism in America. That's why the Christians and the Republicans hate it. Safe abortion defies their tyranny. Safe abortion is an intolerable symbol of resistance to their power. It must be eliminated. Then, what's next?

In Florida, under the fascist rule of Ron DeSantis, it's books, sociology, Black history, and free speech.

It is unlikely that Trump can spell the word "fascism" or understand the meaning of the word, but he is a natural fascist. He can't and doesn't have to think about it. An admirer of Hitler, he wants to be the dictator of the new "Reich." We know how that worked out 90 years ago when another guy had this idea.

The danger to democracy

As this is written, the 2024 election poses the most danger to American democracy since the founding of the country in the eighteenth century. If Trump is reelected or reinstalled as president by the congressional Republicans, reproductive health and freedom for women will be road kill and collateral damage on the way to personality-cult dictatorship by Trump and his fanatic minions. Democracy in America will not survive this fascist assault if it happens.

The hope is that women across the country will continue to respond at the polls as they have in numerous recent elections to the threat to reproductive freedom posed not just by ballot measures (as in Ohio and Kansas) but by voting against Republican candidates on the ballot. It's even better if women like Allie Phillips in Tennessee turn their grief and outrage into a political candidacy.[13]

A vote for a Republican candidate is a vote to end reproductive rights for women and access to safe abortion services. It is also a vote to end effective government, constitutional democracy, and personal freedom in America.

Further, it is a vote against necessary measures to protect the environment and stop global warming, which is a towering threat to the continued existence of the human species and millions of other species.

The Republican policy toward the environment since Ronald Reagan has been rape and pillage as distinguished from protection and conservation of the natural environment in which we live and on which we are totally dependent. A strong vote by women to support reproductive rights and safe reproductive health care for all women – which means voting for Democratic candidates under the circumstances – means protecting democracy and freedom in America and protecting the environment everywhere. This is a matter of survival on both the individual and the species level.

The abortion issue: roots of twenty-first-century American fascism

As a physician, I have been looking down the barrels of the guns of the anti-abortion fanatics for decades. They have threatened my life, made violent attacks on my medical practice, and assassinated five of my medical colleagues and many others who help physicians. They have worked closely with the Republican Party and gained enormous political power over the past 50 years.

The fact that the U.S. Supreme Court is now a wholly owned and operated subsidiary of the Republican Party, which has a misogynist, anti-abortion, anti-environmental, antidemocratic agenda that suppresses voting rights, human rights, social justice, and economic justice, is not an accident. The Roberts Court majority is now completely corrupt. The Court is no longer a refuge for justice.

I do not believe it could have arrived at this total success without the vigorous efforts, including electoral support, political violence, and terrorism, of the white supremacist anti-abortion movement.

Beginning in the 1970s, the anti-abortion movement made clinic invasions, fire bombings, arson, vandalism, and obstruction of clinic entrances its modus operandi. The anti-abortion movement's open defiance of law, basic social mores, assaults on the personal, private needs of other people, and willingness to use violence to attain its political goals set the stage for the belligerent, anti-social candidacy of Donald Trump and the violent insurrection against the U.S. Capitol incited by Donald Trump on January 6, 2021. There is a straight-line pattern here.

Symbols of violent Christian nationalism and anti-abortion fervor were visible throughout Trump's mob that stormed the Capitol – our national symbol of democracy and the heart of our working democracy – on January 6, 2021.[14] Nothing accidental about this.

It's a straight line from the anti-abortion fire-bombings of gentle, kind Jim Armstrong's family medical office in Kalispell, Montana, to the violent, fanatic, brutal, bear-spray wielding, shit-throwing democracy-stomping mob of Donald Trump supporters desecrating the citadel of American democracy on January 6, 2021.

The American anti-abortion movement, which is dominated by Christian fundamentalists, has a policy of killing doctors who perform abortions. "Do what we tell you to do or we'll kill you." And they do. They are now threatening to convict women of homicide for having an abortion or even a miscarriage, especially if it's from an IVF pregnancy. That's the plan.

For Christians and Republicans, women are walking incubators, and they should do their duty. First, shut up and get pregnant.

What to do?

Hand-wringing, gnashing of teeth, wailing, eloquent lamentations, prayer, and chest-pounding will not do. Those of us who believe that women should have access to the best reproductive health care available, including abortion, and the right to make decisions about their own lives, health and futures, must win elections. This means finding, encouraging, supporting, and working for political candidates who support women's health and choices. Right now, this means Democratic Party candidates for public office who are unequivocally pro-choice.

This means running for public office yourself if there is no one in your town/county/district/state to carry that flag (*see* Allie Phillips).

Among other things, it means rescinding the tax-exempt status of white Christian Evangelical churches that engage in political activities. They are a danger to the nation.

There was a time that I remember quite well when there were Republican leaders and officeholders who were strongly pro-choice and who supported women's rights. That day is gone. If there are any Republicans like this, they are unable to secure nomination or to win a primary in a party that is now a fanatic fascist personality cult devoted to Donald Trump.

It is essential to remember certain critical points:

- Pregnancy is not a benign condition, and it only affects women.
- Pregnancy, desired or not, can kill you even under the best conditions. The death rate due to pregnancy is called the "maternal mortality ratio," which is the number of deaths due to pregnancy per 100,000 live births. When abortion is illegal, this ratio goes up. Everywhere.
- Every woman who is pregnant is at risk of dying from this cause during the pregnancy and for a period of time after the pregnancy has ended.
- The risk of death from carrying a pregnancy to term and having a baby is at least 14–15 times higher than the risk of dying from an abortion.[15] **Abortion at any stage, properly performed, is many times safer than term delivery.**
- Modern medical care has lowered the maternal mortality ratio, but not enough in the United States. It has been going up, especially in red states run by Republicans (*see* Texas). Texas is one of the most dangerous places in the world for a woman to be pregnant and have a baby, right there with rural Pakistan.
- A woman who is pregnant is entitled to the best medical care available regardless of her desire to continue or end the pregnancy.
- Safe abortion is an essential and fundamental component of women's health care.
- A woman's access to safe abortion should not depend on the results of the last election, her skin color, her zip code, or her income.
- The treatment of choice for the condition of pregnancy is abortion unless the woman wants to be pregnant and have a baby. She should then have access to the safest abortion service available. If she wants to continue the pregnancy, she should have the best medical care available to assure her survival and birth of a healthy baby.

- A woman who is pregnant must not be forced to give birth. This is slavery and human rights abuse. Women are not livestock. It is inhumane and unconstitutional.
- There is no justification of any kind for any law restricting access to abortion (or contraception).
- Every single law proposed that restricts women's access to safe abortion and contraception must be opposed in court and at the ballot box.
- Every single judicial decision that restricts women's access to safe abortion and contraception must be opposed by legal challenge and/or the legislative process.
- Every single candidate for public office who opposes women's access to safe abortion services must be effectively opposed by a pro-choice candidate and banished from elective office.
- People who are against abortion should not have one. And they should leave other people alone.

Abortion as health care or abortion as insurrection?

Along with the advances in modern medicine that saved millions of lives, electronic technology advancing science and communications, the exploration of space and the liberation of women from ancient patriarchy – at least in some places – the discovery of safe and effective contraception and development of safe abortion services are among the most significant advances in the history of human society.

Safe and effective fertility control and medical care for women who are pregnant are equivalent to the domestication of fire at the family hearth in the human evolutionary experience.

For the first time in human experience, women are able to make choices about pregnancy and carry pregnancies to term without sacrificing their lives. They have an excellent probability of surviving pregnancy and childbirth and having a healthy baby, and they can safely choose not to do this. They can choose to have a normal sex life in a loving intimate relationship while carrying out their own personal quest for a creative life with no children or the number they choose to have. If they are raped, they may end the pregnancy and not be forced to carry the rapist's child – unless they live in a Republican-governed state.

This is revolutionary. It assumes a normal, rational human society.

In America, having an abortion has become a political act.

In America, performing an abortion has become a political act.

Both defy the totalitarian ideology that is rampant in America and threatening to destroy all democratic institutions and the rule of law.

Opposition to and psychological warfare against abortion is the principal organizing tool in America for imposing a totalitarian state. That is the objective, and it is no secret:

> *News Flash*
> *"Welcome to the end of democracy. We are here to overthrow it completely."*
> Jack Posobiec, *Conservative Political Action Committee* meeting, February 23, 2024.[16]

Performing one abortion for one woman changes the course of her life, and it may save her life. Performing abortions for tens of millions of women, as we have done over the past half-century, changes the possibilities for those millions of women, and it changes society. It changes power relationships.

Opposition to safe abortion springs from the desire of patriarchal religious and political authorities to maintain a repressive Christian patriarchal society that dictates what women can do with their lives and bodies. Having abortions is a non-violent insurrection by women and those who help them; it is revolutionary.

Both "insurrection" and "revolution" mean opposition to a "governing authority;" each one refers to a *fundamental change in power relationships*. But in this case, the use of violence is caused, carried out and directed by those who oppose the change in power relationships represented by the act of having or performing an abortion.

Nancy Pelosi, the best Speaker of the House of Representatives in history and the most powerful woman in America, represents this change in power relationships, and that is the reason she is hated by the enemies of freedom and choice for women. That's why Trump's January 6 U.S. Capitol mob wanted to kill her.

This is the only explanation for the 50 years of anti-abortion political violence and domestic terrorism, including assassinations, arson, assaults on women who seek abortions, and clinic invasions. The White supremacist Christian anti-abortion movement has shown itself willing to accept and use any level of violence to repress women and to achieve its goals, and it will stop at nothing, including assassination. It has embraced the fascist Republican Party and the orange zombie apparition of Donald Trump to harness the most despicable and unprincipled force in American history to obtain tthis power.

The 2017–2021 Trump administration and Republican control of Congress were the results of this determination to control women and American society. The authoritarian makeup of the U.S. Supreme Court is the result of this movement. Donald Trump, with the indispensable help of Mitch McConnell, reached the goal by completing the appointment of an overwhelming majority of Catholic, anti-abortion, Republican-aligned justices to the U.S. Supreme Court. Mission accomplished.

Because of Trump and McConnell, with the overwhelming support of the Republican Party, the federal judiciary is now heavily anti-abortion at all levels. This makes it almost impossible to overcome abortion restrictions through legislation.

As this is written, the rest of the twenty-first century is before us. Two hundred and 35 years of a democratic, free society trying to live up to its honorable ideals is behind us. The promise and commitment to continue to realize those ideals of humanity, intellectual and personal freedom, and the rule of law are being tested as never before. We are faced with an armed, violent, fascist movement in the United States headed by Donald Trump and the Republican Party that threatens all we have, all freedom, and everyone's lives. If we lose democracy, we will never get it back.

It is up to you, the reader, to take action to protect and expand what we have and treasure in the face of psychopathic tyranny and the threat of extinction.

Notes

1 David, H. P. (ed.). *Born Unwanted: Developmental Effects of Denied Abortion*, Prague: Avicenum, 1988; David, H.P. Born unwanted: Long-term developmental effects of denied abortion. *Journal of Social Issues*, Fall, 1992. https://doi.org/10.1111/j.1540-4560.1992.tb00902.x

2 David, H.P. Born unwanted, 35 years later: the Prague study. *Reproductive Health Matters* 14(27):181–90, 2006. doi: 10.1016/S0968-8080(06)27219-7. ; PMID: 16713893

3 Foster, D.G. *The Turnaway Study: Ten Years, a Thousand Women, and the Consequences of Having—or Being Denied—an Abortion*. New York: Scribner, 2020.

4 Cherry, S.B. Abortion trigger laws compared with the Emergency Medical Treatment and Labor Act. *Obstetrics and Gynecology* 143(3): 366–68, 2024. PMID: 38086056 DOI: 10.1097/AOG.0000000000005483

5 Dickman, S.L., White, K., Himmelstein, D.U., et al. Rape-related pregnancies in the 14 U.S. states with total abortion bans. *Journal of the American Medical Association Internal Medicine*, January 24, 2024. doi:10.1001/jamainternmed.2024.0014 https://jamanetwork.com/journals/jamainternalmedicine/fullarticle/2814274?guestAccessKey=e429b9a8-72ac-42ed-8dbc-599b0f509890&utm_source=For_The_Media&utm_medium=referral&utm_campaign=ftm_links&utm_content=tfl&utm_term=012424

6 Christina Maxouris, In unprecedented decision, Alabama's Supreme Court ruled frozen embryos are children. It could have chilling effects on IVF, critics say, CNN, 20 February 2024 https://www.cnn.com/2024/02/20/us/alabama-embryo-law-ruling-supreme-court/index.html

7 Goldberg, M. *The Means of Reproduction: Sex, Power and the Future of the World.* New York: Penguin Press, 2009.

8 Atwood, M. *The Handmaid's Tale.* New York: McClellan and Steward, 1985.

9 Alberta, T. *The Kingdom, the Power, and the Glory: American Evangelicals in an Age of Extremism.* New York: Harper, 2023.

10 Abcarian, R. How the Alabama IVF ruling unmasks the hypocrisy of antiabortion zealots. *Los Angeles Times.* February 3, 2024. https://www.msn.com/en-us/health/medical/abcarian-how-the-alabama-ivf-ruling-unmasks-the-hypocrisy-of-antiabortion-zealots/ar-BB1jfutx?ocid=hpmsn&cvid=09ed4b32cbb2491799db9d10f5a3d946&ei=26

11 Balmer, R. The real origins of the religious right. They tell you it was abortion. Sorry, the historical record's clear: It was segregation. *Politico Magazine* May 27, 2014. https://www.politico.com/magazine/story/2014/05/religious- right-real-origins-107133 ; Gorski, P.S. and Perry, S.L. *The Flag and the Cross: White Nationalism and the Threat to American Democracy.* Oxford: Oxford Press, 2022. p. 69, p. 145.

12 Alex Bollinger, Anti-LGBTQ+ hate pastor gives opening prayer in House of Representatives, LGBTQ Nation, 31 January 2024, https://www.lgbtqnation.com/2024/01/anti-lgbtq-hate-pastor-gives-opening-prayer-in-house-of-representatives/

13 Hennessey-Fiske, M. An abortion ban turned a grieving Allie Phillips into a candidate. *Washington Post*, January 25, 2024. https://www.washingtonpost.com/nation/2024/01/25/allie-phillips-tennessee-abortion-ban/

14 Andrews, B. Long before the Capitol Riot, Anti-abortion Extremists Showed Us the Dangers of Inflammatory Propaganda. *Mother Jones*, January 14, 2021. https://www.motherjones.com/politics/2021/01/anti-abortion-extremists-capitol-riot-trump-propaganda-abby-johnson/; Winter, J. The link between the Capitol riot and anti-abortion extremism. *The New Yorker*, March 11, 2021. https://www.newyorker.com/news/daily-comment/the-link-between-the-capitol-riot-and-anti-abortion-extremism

15 Raymond, E.G., and Grimes, D.A. The comparative safety of legal induced abortion and childbirth in the United States, *Obstetrics and Gynecology* 119(2 Pt 1):215–19, 2012. DOI: 10.1097/AOG.ob013e31823fe923

16 Ben Goggin, Calls to "fight" and echoes of Jan. 6 embraced by CPAC attendees, NBC News, 23 February 2024, https://www.nbcnews.com/politics/2024-election/jack-posobiec-jan-6-2024-cpac-rcna140225

Selected bibliography

Alberta, T. *The Kingdom, the Power, and the Glory: American Evangelicals in an Age of Extremism.* New York: Harper, 2023.

Atwood, M. *The Handmaid's Tale.* New York: McClellan and Steward, 1985.

Baird-Windle, P. and Bader, E.J. *Targets of Hatred: Anti-Abortion Terrorism.* New York: Palgrave, 2001.

Berger, G.S., Brenner, W.E. and Keith, L.G. (eds.). *Second Trimester Abortion: Perspectives After a Decade of Experience.* Boston: John Wright * PSG, Inc., 1981.

Blanchard, D.A. *The Anti-Abortion Movement and the Rise of the Religious Right: From Polite to Fiery Protest.* Woodridge: Twayne Publishers, 1994.

Blanchard, D.A. and Prewitt, T.J. *Religious Violence and Abortion: The Gideon Project.* Gainesville: The University Press of Florida, 1993.

Bodanis, D. *Passionate Minds: The Great Love Affair of the Enlightenment, Featuring the Scientist Emilie du Chatelet, the Poet Voltaire, Sword Fights Book Burnings, Assorted Kings, Seditious Verse, and the Birth of the Modern World.* New York: Crown, 2006.

Bonavoglia, A. *The Choices We Made: Twenty-Five Women and Men Speak Out about Abortion.* New York: Random House, 1991.

Boonin, D. *A Defense of Abortion.* Cambridge: Cambridge University Press, 2003.

Calderone, M.S. (ed.). *Abortion in the United States: Report of a Conference Sponsored by the Planned Parenthood Federation of America.* New York: Hoeber-Harper, 1958.

Carter, K.C. and Carter, B.R. *Childbed Fever: A Scientific Biography of Ignaz Semmelweis.* Westport, Connecticut: Greenwood Press, 1994.

Chamberlen, H. *The Diseases of Women with Child, and in Child-bed.* Translation of Des Maladies Des Femmes Grosses Et Accouchées by François Mauriceau. London: 1673.

Claire, M. *The Abortion Dilemma: Personal Views on a Public Issue.* New York: Plenum Press, 1995.

Cohen, D.S. and Connon, K. *Living in the Crosshairs: The Untold Stories of Anti-Abortion Terrorism.* Oxford: Oxford University Press, 2015.

Cohen, D.S. and Joffe, C. *Obstacle Course: The Every Day Struggle to Get and Abortion in America.* Berkeley: University of California Press, 2020.

Condit, C.M. *Decoding Abortion Rhetoric: Communicating Social Change.* Urbana: University of Illinois Press, 1990.

Craig, B.H. and O'Brien, D.M. *Abortion and American Politics.* Chatham, NJ: Chatham House Publishers, 1993.

David, H. P. (ed.). *Born Unwanted: Developmental Effects of Denied Abortion.* Prague: Avicenum, 1988.

Devereux, G. *A Study of Abortion in Primitive Societies: A Typological, Distributional, and Dynamic Analysis of the Prevention of Birth in 400 Preindustrial Societies.* New York: Russell Sage Foundation, 1955.

Edelin, K. *Broken Justice: A True Story of Race, Sex and Revenge in a Boston Courtroom.* Science Hill, Kentucky: Pondview Press, 2007.

Everett, C. with Shaw, J. *The Scarlet Lady: Confessions of a Successful Abortionist.* Brentwood, TN: Wolgenmuth & Hyatt, 1991.

Faux, M. *Crusaders: Voices from the Abortion Front.* New York: Carol Publishing Group, 1990.

Finch, A. *Choice Words: Writers on Abortion*. Chicago: Haymarket Books, 2020.

FitzGerald, F. *The Evangelicals: The Struggle to Shape America*. New York: Simon and Schuster, 2017.

Foster, D.G. *The Turnaway Study: Two Years, A Thousand Women, and the Consequences of Having – or Being Denied – an Abortion*. New York: Scribner, 2021.

Freedman, L. *Willing and Unable: Doctors' Constraints in Abortion Care*. Nashville: Vanderbilt University Press, 2010.

Friedman, L. (ed.). *The Supreme Court Confronts Abortion: The Briefs, Argument, and Decision in Planned Parenthood v. Casey*. New York: Farrar, Straus & Giroux, 1993.

Garrow, D.J. *Liberty and Sexuality: The Right to Privacy and the Making of Roe v. Wade*. New York: Macmillan, 1994.

Ginsburg, F.D. *Contested Lives: The Abortion Debate in an American Community*. Berkeley: The University of California Press, 1989.

Goldberg, M. *Kingdom Coming: The Rise of Christian Nationalism*. New York: W.W. Norton Company & Company, Inc, 2006. This book is essential reading !

Goldberg, M. *The Means of Reproduction: Sex, Power and the Future of the World*. New York: Penguin Press, 2009.

Goodwin, M. *Policing the Womb: Invisible Women and the Criminalization of Motherhood*. Cambridge: Cambridge University Press, 2020.

Gorney, C. *Articles of Faith: A Frontline History of the Abortion Wars*. New York: Simon and Schuster, 1998.

Gorsky, P.S. and Perry, S. *The Flag and The Cross: White Christian Nationalism and the Threat to American Democracy*. Oxford: Oxford University Press, 2022.

Greenhouse, L. and Siegel, R.B. *Before Roe v. Wade: Voices That Shaped the Abortion Debate Before the Supreme Court's Ruling*. New York: Kaplan Publishing, 2010.

Grimes, D.A. with Brandon, L.G. *Every Third Woman in America: How Legal Abortion Transformed Our Nation*. Carolina Beach, NC: Daymark Publishing, 2014.

Handwerker, W.P. *Births and Power: Social Change and the Politics of Reproduction*. Boulder: Westview Press, 1990.

Henneberg, C. *Boundless: An Abortion Doctor Becomes a Mother*. San Francisco: University of California, 2022.

Hern, W.M. *Abortion Practice*. Philadelphia: J.B. Lippincott Company, 1984.

Hern, W.M. *Homo Ecophagus: A Deep Diagnosis to Save the Earth*. Routledge Press, 2022.

Hogue, I. and Langford, E. *The Lie That Binds*. Washington, DC: Strong Arm Press, 2020.

Hoffman, M. *Choices: A Post-Roe Abortion Rights Manifesto*. New York: Skyhorse Publishing, 2023.

Holland, J. *Tiny You: A Western History of the Anti-abortion Movement*. Berkeley: University of California Press, 2020.

Howell Lee, N. *The Search for an Abortionist: A Study of 114 Women Who Underwent Abortions – Their Reasons, Their Reactions, and the Ways in Which They Found This "Invisible" Service*. Chicago: University of Chicago Press, 1969.

Jaffe, F., Lindheim, B.L. and Lee, P.R. *Abortion Politics: Private Morality and Public Policy*. New York: McGraw-Hill, 1980.

Jefferis, J. *Armed For Life: The Army of God and Anti-Abortion Terror in the United States*. Santa Barbara, CA: Praeger, 2011.

Joffe, C. *Doctors of Conscience: The Struggle to Provide Abortion Before and After Roe v. Wade*. Boston: Beacon Press, 1995.

Joffe, C. *Dispatches from the Abortion Wars: The Costs of Fanaticism to Doctors, Patients, and the Rest of Us*. Boston: Beacon Press, 2010.

Kobes Du Mez, K. *Jesus and John Wayne: How White Evangelicals Corrupted a Faith and Fractured a Nation*. New York: Liveright Publishing Corporation, 2020.

Kolbert, K. and Kay, J.F. *Controlling Women: What We Must Do Now to Save Reproductive Freedom*. New York: Hachette Books, 2021.

Lader, L. *Abortion*. . Indianapolis, IN: Bobbs-Merrill, 1966.

Lader, L. *Abortion II: Making The Revolution*. Boston: Beacon Press, 1973.

Lerner, M. and Anderson, O.W. *Health Progress in the United States: 1900–1960*. Chicago: University of Chicago Press, 1963.

Lewit, S. (ed.). *Abortion Techniques and Services: Proceedings of the Conference, New York, N.Y., June 3–6 1971*. Amsterdam: Excerpta Medica, 1972.

Luker, K. *Abortion and the Politics of Motherhood*. Berkeley: University of California Press, 1984.

Lyons, E. and Lyons, J. *Life's Been a Blast: The True Story of Birmingham Bomb Survivor Emily Lyons*. Washington, DC: National Abortion Federation, 2005.

Mcfarlane, D.R. and Hansen, W.L. *Regulating Abortion: The Politics of U.S. Abortion Policy*. Baltimore: Johns Hopkins University Press, 2024.

Marty, R. *Handbook for a Post-Roe America: The Complete Guide to Abortion Legality, Access and Practical Support*. New York: Seven Stories Press, 2021.

Mason, C. *Killing for Life: The Apocalyptic Narrative of Pro-Life Politics*. Ithaca: Cornell University Press, 2002.

Mauriceau, F. *Des Maladies des Femmes Grosses et Accouchées*, p 105. Paris: Charles Coignard, 1668. (English translation by Chamberlen H: *The Accomplished Midwife, Treating of the Diseases of Women with Child, and in Child-bed*. London, John Darby, 1673)

McKeegan, M. *Abortion Politics: Mutiny in the Ranks of the Right*. New York: The Free Press, 1992.

Merton, A.H. *Enemies of Choice: The Right-to-Life Movement and Its Threat to Abortion*. Boston: Beacon Press, 1991.

Miller, P.G. *The Worst of Times: Illegal Abortion – Survivors, Practitioners, Coroners, Cops, and Children of Women Who Died Talk About Its Horrors*. New York: Harper-Collins Publishers, 1993.

Mohr, J.C. *Abortion in America: The Origins and Evolution of National Policy*. Oxford: Oxford University Press, 1978.

Neubart, S. and Schulman, H. *Techniques of Abortion*. Boston: Little, Brown and Company, 1972.

Oberman, M. *Her Body, Our Laws: On the Front Lines of the Abortion Wars, From El Salvador to Oklahoma*. Boston: Beacon Press, 2018.

Osofsky, H.J. and Osofsky, J.D. *The Abortion Experience: Psychological and Medical Impact*. Hagerstown, MD: Harper & Row, Publishers, 1973.

Petchesky, R. P. *Abortion and a Woman's Choice: The State, Sexuality, and Reproductive Freedom. The Northeastern Series in Feminist Theory*. Boston: The Northeastern University Press, 1985.

Pollitt, K. *PRO: Reclaiming Abortion Rights*. New York: Picador, 2014.

Rankin, L. *Bodies on the Line: At the Front Lines of the Fight to Protect Abortion in America*. Berkeley: Counterpoint, 2022.

Rapp, R. *Testing Women, Testing the Fetus: The Social Impact of Amniocentesis in America*. New York: Routledge, 1999.

Reagan, L.J. *When Abortion Was A Crime: Women, Medicine and Law in the United States, 1867–1973*. Berkeley: University of California Press, 1997.

Revelle, R., Coale, A.J., Freymann, M., et al. (eds.). *Rapid Population Growth: Consequences and Policy Implications*, Vol II, p. 462. Baltimore: Johns Hopkins Press, 1971.

Risen, J. and Thomas, J.L. *Wrath of Angels: The American Abortion War*. New York: Basic Books, 1991.

Roberts, D. *Killing the Black Body: Race, Reproduction and the Meaning of Liberty*. New York: Vintage, 1998.

Rowland, B. *Medieval Woman's Guide to Health: The First English Gynecological Handbook. Middle English Text, with Introduction and Modern English Translation by B. Rowland*. Kent, Ohio: Kent State University Press, 1981.

Rosen, H. (ed.). *Abortion in America*. Boston: Beacon Press, 1967.

Sanger, C. *About Abortion: Terminating Pregnancy in Twenty-First-Century America*. Cambridge, MA: Belknap Press of Harvard University Press, 2017.

Schoen, J. *Abortion After Roe*. Chapel Hill: University of North Carolina Press, 2015.

Semmelweis, I. *The Etiology, Concept, and Prophylaxis of Childbed Fever*. Translated by K.C. Carter. Madison, WI: University of Wisconsin Press, 1983.

Sexton, J.Y. *The Midnight Kingdom: A History of Power, Paranoia and the Coming Crisis*. New York: Dutton, 2023.

Solinger, R. *Wake Up Little Susie: Single Pregnancy and Race Before Roe v. Wade*. New York: Routledge, 1992.

Solinger, R. *The Abortionist: A Woman Against the Law*. New York: The Free Press, 1994.

Solinger, R. (ed.). *Abortion Wars: A Half-Century of Struggle, 1950–2000*. Berkeley: University of California Press, 1998.

Solinger, R. *Beggars and Choosers: How the Politics of Choice Shapes Adoption, Abortion, and Welfare in the United States*. New York: Hill and Wang, 2001.

Staggenborg, S. *The Pro-Choice Movement: Organization and Activism in the Abortion Conflict*. New York: Oxford University Press, 1991.

Stewart, K. *The Power Worshipers: Inside the Dangerous Rise of Religious Nationalism*. Bloomsbury: Bloomsbury Publishing, 2022.

Taussig, F.J. *Abortion, Spontaneous and Induced: Medical and Social Aspects*. St. Louis: C.V. Mosby, 1936.

Taylor, D. *Undue Burden: A Black Woman Physician on being Christian and Pro-Abortion in the Reproductive Justice Movement*. Advantage Media Group, 2023.

Temkin, O. (translator) *Soranus' Gynecology*. Baltimore: Johns Hopkins Press, 1991.

Tribe, L.H. *Abortion: The Clash of Absolutes*. New York: Norton, 1990.

Tunc, T. *Technologies of Choice: A History of Abortion Techniques in the United States, 1850–1980*. Saasrbrücken: VDM Verlag Dr. Müller, 2008.

Watson, K. *The Scarlet A: The Ethics, Law and Politics of Ordinary Abortion*. Oxford: Oxford University Press, 2019.

Walbert, D.F. and Butler, J.D. (eds.). *Whose Choice Is It? Abortion, Medicine and the Law*, 7th edition. Chicago: American Bar Association, 2021.

Weddington, S. *A Question of Choice*. New York: G.F. Putnam's Sons, 1992.

Wicklund, S. and Kesselheim, A. *This Common Secret: My Journey as an Abortion Doctor*. New York: Public Affairs, 2007.

Ziegler, M. *After Roe: The Lost History of the Abortion Debate*. Cambridge: Harvard University Press, 2015.

Ziegler, M. *Abortion and the Law in America: Roe v. Wade to the Present*. Cambridge: Cambridge University Press, 2020.

Ziegler, M. *Dollars for Life: The Anti-Abortion Movement and the Fall of the Republican Establishment*. New Haven: Yale University Press, 2022.

Ziegler, M. *Roe: The History of a National Obsession*. New Haven: Yale University Press, 2023.

Author bibliography

1961

We must not fear Africa. *The Denver Post*, Voice of Youth column, March 11, 1961.
Turbulence in Nigeria typifies African dilemma. *The Colorado Daily*, March 24, 1961.
"If You're A Good American, Stand Up". Report on a Denver rightwing religious rally.
  Warren Hern and Dan Nickelson. *The Colorado Daily*, May 12, 1961.
Why the Nigerians reacted angrily to girl's criticism. *The Denver Post*, October 20, 1961.

1962

Vignettes of a trip to Nigeria. *Christian Science Monitor*, Monday, July 9, 1962.
Health and economics in West Africa. *Rocky Mountain Medical Journal*, October, 1962.

1963

Sullen silence greets General Somoza. *The Denver Post*, February 6, 1963.

1969

Brazil's rulers crack down on foes: United States' role critical as key S. American country
  jails leaders of opposition. *The Denver Post* Perspective section, January 26, 1969.

1970

Could we have a killer smog in Denver? *The Denver Post* Perspective section, September
  13, 1970.
Family Planning and the Poor. *The New Republic*, November 14, 1970.

1971

Biological Tyranny. *The New Republic*, February 27, 1971.
*Community Health, fertility trends, and ecocultural change in a Peruvian Amazon Indian
  village: 1964-1969.* University of North Carolina School of Public Health, Department
  of Epidemiology, 1971. (Master of Public Health thesis) https://catalog.lib.unc.edu/
  catalog/UNCb4834807.

Is pregnancy really normal? *Family Planning Perspectives*, Vol. 3, No. 1, January 1971. pp. 1-6. Reprinted by the Association for the Study of Abortion; Abstracts published in *Maternity Briefs* and in the 1971 *Yearbook of Obstetrics and Gynecology*. Reprinted in full in *Confronting the Issues: Sex Roles, Marriage, and the Family.* K.C.W. Kammeyer, Ed. Allyn and Bacon, Inc., Boston, 1975. https://doi.org/10.2307/2133950. https://www.jstor.org/stable/2133950.

Contis, G. and Hern, Warren M. *Response to "Slowdown on Family Planning"*. The New York Times: February 20, 1971. Letter to the editor https://www.nytimes.com/1971/02/20/archives/progress-report-on-family-planning.html?searchResultPosition=14.

Contis, G. and Hern, W.M. US Government policy on abortion. *American Journal of Public Health* 61:1038-1041. May, 1971.

1972

The politics of abortion. *The Progressive*, November, 1972.

1973

Abortion: the need for rational policy and safe standards. *The Denver Post*, May 27, 1973.

1975

Abortion issue: The state vs. the individual. *The Denver Post*, March 23, 1975.

Is Pregnancy Really Normal? In *Confronting the Issues: Sex Roles, Marriage, and the Family* K. Kammeyr, Ed.: 1st, 18, 209-222. Boston: Allyn and Bacon, Inc., 1975.

Single pregnancies: are they really accidental? *Denver Singles Guide*, April, 1975.

The illness parameters of pregnancy. *Social Science and Medicine* 9:365372, 1975 (England).

Hern, W.M. *Dr. Hern Responds to Article on Abortion. The Denver Post*: August 10, 1975.

Laminaria in abortion: use in 1368 patients in first trimester. *Rocky Mountain Medical Journal* 72:390395, 1975.

Having an Abortion. Office pamphlet, Boulder Abortion Clinic © 1975, Warren M Hern, MD.

1976

Knowledge and use of herbal contraceptives in a Peruvian Amazon village. *Human Organization* 35:919, 1976. https://doi.org/10.17730/humo.35.1.b7h6706718u56412.

Boulder Abortion Clinic. Office pamphlet © 1976, Warren M Hern MD.

Abortion issue muddles presidential politics. *The Denver Post*, October 31, 1976.

1977

Administrative incongruence and authority conflict in four abortion clinics. WM Hern, M Gold, and A Oakes. *Human Organization* 36:376383, 1977.

Having a Vasectomy. Office pamphlet © 1977, Warren M Hern, MD.

Abortion in the Seventies. Proceedings of the 1976 Western Regional Conference on Abortion. WM Hern and B Andrikopoulos, Eds. National Abortion Federation, New York, 1977.

High fertility in a Peruvian Amazon Indian village. *Human Ecology* 5:355368, 1977. https://doi.org/10.1007/BF00889176.

Multiple laminaria treatment in early midtrimester outpatient suction abortion. W Hern and A Oakes. *Advances in Planned Parenthood* 12:9397, 1977.(first report in American literature of serial multiple laminaria treatment of cervix for dilation for D & E abortion).

New attack on abortion under way in Colorado. *The Denver Post*, February 27, 1977.

1978

Abortion Services Handbook. Interfacia, Chicago, 1978. Available from Boulder Abortion Clinic.

Correlation of sonographic cephalometry with clinical assessment of fetal age following early midtrimester D & E abortion.

WM Hern, WA Miller, L Paine, and KD Moorhead. *Advances in Planned Parenthood* 13:1420, 1978.

The concept of quality care in abortion services. *Advances in Planned Parenthood* 13:6374, 1978. PMID:. 8517. https://pubmed.ncbi.nlm.nih.gov/738517/.

1979

Unique Philosophy Backs Up Boulder Abortion Clinic. *Female Health Topics & Diagnostics Reporter*: 2, 2, 1979.

1980

Program Standards for Abortion Services. Standards Committee, National Abortion Federation. National Abortion Federation, Washington, D.C. 1980.

What about us? Staff reactions to D & E. *Advances in Planned Parenthood* 15:38, 1980.

1981

Helms' abortion amendment unenforceable. *Daily Tar Heel* (University of North Carolina) February 18, 1981.

The human life statute: will it protect life or power? *The Denver Post*, June 21, 1981. https://www.drhern.com/wp-content/uploads/2018/05/human-life-statute.pdf.

Outpatient secondtrimester D & E abortion through 24 menstrual weeks' gestation. *Advances in Planned Parenthood* 16:713, 1981. https://www.drhern.com/wpcontent/uploads/2018/05/outpatient-second-tri-ab.pdf.

Midtrimester abortion. In *Obstetrics and Gynecology Annual*, 1981, Ralph M. Wynn, Ed. New York: Appleton-Century-Crofts, 1981. https://www.amazon.com/Obstetrics -Gynecology-Annual-1981-Ralph/dp/0838571883.

1982

Long term risks of induced abortion. In *Gynecology and Obstetrics*, JJ Sciarra, Ed. Philadelphia, JB Lippincott, 1982, Ch. 63.

First trimester abortion: complications and their management. In *Gynecology and Obstetrics*, JJ Sciarra, Ed. Philadelphia, JB Lippincott, 1982, Ch. 59.

Water sets the limits on exponential growth. *The Denver Post*, January 10, 1982.

"Society" Well reasoned study of resource overexploitation. Book review of *Building a Sustainable Society* by Lester R. Brown. *The Denver Post*, January 31, 1982.

Secretary Schweiker's flawed plan to curb teenage sex. *New York Times*, Editorial page, Friday, February 26, 1982. https://www.nytimes.com/1982/02/26/Guest Opinion/l-secretary-schweiker-s-flawed-plan-to-curb-teen-age-sex-253713.html?searchResultP osition=18.

Dilatation and evacuation abortion. Letter to the editor, *Obstetrics and Gynecology* 60:667, 1982. https://journals.lww.com/greenjournal/citation/1982/11000/dilatation _and_evacuation_abortion.27.aspx.

1983

Discussion remarks. In Shaw MW, Doudera AE (eds): *Defining Human Life: Medical, Legal, and Ethical Implications*. Ann Arbor, AUPHA Press, 1983. Proceedings of the conference *Human Life Symposium: An Interdisciplinary Approach to the Concept of Person*, Houston, Texas, March, 1982.

Holy Cross Wilderness Defense Fund Newsletter, Vol. 1, No.1. 12 pp. WM Hern, Editor. 1983.

First and second trimester abortion techniques. *Current Problems in Obstetrics and Gynecology*, Vol.6, No.11:July 1983.

Alta fecundidad en una comunidad nativa del Río Ucayali. *Ginecologia y Obstetricia* (Lima) 28:2025, 1983.

First and second trimester abortion techniques. *Current Problems in Obstetrics and Gynecology*: 6, 11, 1-50. July 1983.

1984

Correlation of fetal age and measurements between 10 and 26 weeks of gestation. *Obstetrics and Gynecology* 63:26-32, 1984.

Serial multiple laminaria and adjunctive urea in late outpatient dilatation and evacuation abortion. *Obstetrics and Gynecology* 63:543-549, 1984.

Abortion Practice. Philadelphia, JB Lippincott Company, 1984. 368 pages, 59 illustrations, 3 color plates, 16 tables. Reviewed in *Family Planning Perspectives, New England Journal of Medicine, Journal of the American Medical Association*.

Reagan's war on abortion. *The Sunday Camera*, December 9, 1984.

Reagan turning abortion into crime against state. *The Rocky Mountain News*, December 14, 1984.

The antiabortion vigilantes. *The New York Times*, OpEd Page, Friday, December 21, 1984. https://www.nytimes.com/1984/12/21/Guest Opinion/the-antiabortion-vigilantes.html?searchResultPosition=19.

1985

Abortion `compromise' flawed. *The Denver Post*, April 27, 1985.
History shows us how to get it all wrong in Central America. *The Sunday Camera*, May 19, 1985.
Silent Scream' is propaganda. *The Denver Post*, July 6, 1985.
Notes on Peru. National Abortion Federation *Update*, Summer 1985.

1986

Drug won't end abortion dilemma. *The Daily Camera*, April 5,1986 (concerning RU486).
Boulder Abortion Clinic Announces Its New "Pledge A Picket For Choice" Program. The Daily Camera: March 5, 1986.
Must Mr. Reagan tolerate abortion clinic violence? *The New York Times*, Op-Ed page, June 14, 1986.
https://nytimes.com/1986/06/14/Guest Opinion/must-mr-reagan-tolerate-abortion-clinic -violence.html.
Reagan faces anti-abortion terrorists - and winks. *The Rocky Mountain News*, Commentary, June 17, 1986.
Evolution of second trimester abortion techniques. In *Prevention and Treatment of Contraceptive Failure*, U Landy and SS Ratnam, eds. New York: Plenum Press, 1986.
Proceedings of the First Christopher Tietze International Symposium on the Prevention and Treatment of Contraceptive Failure, sponsored by the International Women's Health Coalition, September 21-22, 1985, Berlin, Federal Republic of Germany. https://doi.org/10.1007/978-1-4684-5248-8_19.

1987

Protect Abortion Rights. *New York Times*, Op-Ed page, January 22, 1987. https://www .nytimes.com/1987/01/22/Guest-Opinion/protect-abortion-rights.html?searchResul tPosition=3.
Protect Abortion Rights. *The Rocky Mountain News*, Jan. 23, 1987.
Buffer zone is important. *The Daily Camera* January 5, 1987.
Questions About Homestake II. *The Denver Post*, Op-Ed page, October 24, 1987.
Book review: *Abortion: Medical Progress and Social Implications*. Porter, Ruth, and O'Connor, Maeve, Eds. Ciba Foundation 115, Pitman, London, 1985. In *The Journal of Nervous and Mental Disease* 175:638-639, 1987.

1988

Polygyny and fertility among the Shipibo: An epidemiologic test of an ethnographic hypothesis. University of North Carolina School of Public Health, Department of Epidemiology, 1988. (Ph.D. dissertation, Epidemioogy).

Use of prostaglandins as abortifacients. In *Gynecology and Obstetrics*, JW Sciarra, Ed. Philadelphia, JB Lippincott Co, 1982, Ch. 58. Published in 1988.

Anti-abortion campaign rhetoric prompts attacks on clinics. *Sunday Camera*, September 4, 1988.

Abortion clinics under siege. *The Denver Post*, November 1, 1988.

1989

Population growth: the real reason behind the peril to the planet. Enviroscope column, *Colorado Daily*, February 3, 1989.

Abortion as Insurrection. *The Humanist* 49 (2):18, 1989, March/April issue. https://www.proquest.com/openview/7d8aee2e14d28219b9f4cbc6bbdd02cd/1.pdf?pq-origsite=gscholar&cbl=35529.

1990

Abortion as insurrection. In *Births and Power: Social Change and the Politics of Reproduction*, W. Penn Handwerker, Ed. Boulder, Westview Press, 1990. https://doi.org/10.4324/9780429043116. https://www.taylorfrancis.com/chapters/edit/10.4324/9780429043116-8/politics-choice-abortion-insurrection-warren-hern.

Abortion Practice. Softcover reprint. Alpenglo Graphics, 1990.

Why are there so many of us? Description and diagnosis of a planetary ecopathological process. *Population and Environment* 12(1):1-27. 1990. [News Brief. Holden, C. *Science* 251(4999):1311, March 15, 1991, p 1311 (DOI: 10.1126/science.251.4999.1311); Commentary by Andy Ogle, *The Edmonton Journal*, Oct.14, 1990]. Reprinted in *Carrying Capacity Network Journal*, June, 1992.

Holden, C. *Planetary Malignancy*. News Brief. *Science*: 251, 4999, American Association for the Advancement of Science, 1311. March 15, 1991.

All Latin America will hate the U.S. for invasion of Panama. Guest Opinion, *The Daily Camera*: January 7, 1990.

Values clash over wild waters. *Rocky Mountain News*, Op-Ed, Page, August 22, 1990 (concerning Homestake II project).

The human species is a cancer, and here's what to do about it. [not my headline!]. Op-ed response to editorial in the *Daily Camera* published September 9, 1990. September 16, 1990.

Individual Fertility Rate: A new measure of fertility for small populations. *Social Biology* 37(1-2), 1990. https://www.drhern.com/wp-content/uploads/2019/10/Individual-Fertility-Rate.pdf.

1991

Proxemics in the abortion debate: the use of anthropological theory in conflict arising from antiabortion demonstrations. *Population and Environment* 12(4): 379-388, 1991. https://doi.org/10.1007/BF01566306.

Report on the Epidemic of Cholera on the Pisqui River and Lower Ucayali, Peru: Trip of 8 June to 20 June, 1991. Report prepared for the Special Program of the Campaign Against Cholera, Regional Health Center (Ministry of Health), Pucallpa, Peru. 21 June, 1991. (Translated from the original Spanish).

Effects of cultural change on health and fertility in Amazonian Indian societies: Recent research and projections. *Population and Environment* 13(1):23-43, 1991. https://doi. org/10.1007/BF01256569.

Informe sobre la epidemia del colera en los rios Pisqui y Bajo Ucayali, Peru: 8 a 20 de junio de 1991. *Boletin de Lima* (78):29-31, 1991.

Book review: *The Population Dynamics of the Mucajai Yanomama*, J.Early and J.Peters, San Diego, Academic Press, 1990. *Population Studies* 45:359-360, 1991.

Resolution Concerning Population. Hern, Warren M. and Reining, Priscilla. *Science*: American Association for the Advancement of Science, 1991.

1992

Saúde e demografia de Povos Indígenas Amazônicos: Perspectiva Histórica e Situação Atual / Health and Demography of Native Amazonians: Historical Perspective and Current Status. In *Cadernos de Saúde Pública* (Brazilian Journal of Public Health) 7(4):451-480, 1992. Special edition: South American Indians.

Book review: *Anthropogenic Climatic Change*, M.I. Budyko and Yu A. Izrael, Eds., Tucson, University of Arizona Press, 1990. *National Geographic Research and Exploration* 8(1):125-126, 1992.

Resolution Concerning Population, American Association for the Advancement of Science, February, 1991. Co-author with Priscilla Reining. *Science*. 1991.

Polygyny and fertility among the Shipibo of the Peruvian Amazon. *Population Studies* 46:53-64, 1992 (England) https://doiorg.colorado.idm.oclc.org/10.1080 /0032472031000146006.

Upper Pisqui River, Peruvian Amazon: July to August 1991. *National Geographic Research and Exploration* 8(2):234-236, 1992.

Shipibo polgyny and patrilocality. *American Ethnologist* 19(3):501-522, 1992 (August). https://doi.org/10.1525/ae.1992.19.3.02a00050.

Book review: *In Search of Human Nature: The Decline and Revival of Darwinism in American Social Thought*, Carl N. Degler, New York, Oxford University Press, 1991. *Journal of Nervous and Mental Diseases* 180(11):740, 1992.

Colorado voters sent a clear pro-choice message. *The Daily Camera*, December 18, 1992.

1993

Family planning, Amazon style. *Natural History* 101(12):30-37, 1993. December. (Included in anthologies *Conformity and Conflict*, Eight Edition. Spradley JP and McCurdy DW, eds. New York: HarperCollins, 1994.)

Hern, W.M., Zen, C., Ferguson, K.A., Hart, V., and Haseman, M.V. Outpatient abortion for fetal anomaly and fetal death from 15-34 menstrual weeks' gestation: Techniques and clinical management. *Obstetrics and Gynecology* 81(2):301-306, 1993.

Cervical treatment with Dilapan prior to second trimester dilation and evacuation abortion: A pilot study of 64 patients. *American Journal of Gynecologic Health* 7(1):15-18, 1993.

Hunted by the right, forgotten by the left. *The New York Times*, Op-Ed page, March 13, 1993. https://www.nytimes.com/1993/03/13/Guest Opinion/hunted-by-the-right -forgotten-by-the-left.html?searchResultPosition=26.

Doctors disparaged in abortion debate. *The Daily Camera*, March 19, 1993.

Florida doctor's death resulted from 20 years of inciting violence. *The Denver Post*, March 20, 1993.

The Pope and my right to life. *The New York Times*, Op-Ed Page, August 12, 1993. https://www.nytimes.com/1993/08/12/opinion/the-pope-and-my-right-to-life.html?searchResultPosition=28.

Is human culture carcinogenic for uncontrolled population growth and ecological destruction? *BioScience* 43(11):768-773, 1993 https://doi-org.colorado.idm.oclc.org/10.2307/1312321.

'*Abortionist*' *Carries a Charged Meaning. The New York Times*: September 7, 1993. https://www.nytimes.com/1993/09/07/opinion/l-abortionist-carries-a-charged-meaning-856193.html.

Has the human species become a cancer on the planet? A theoretical view of population growth as a sign of pathology. *Current World Leaders* 36(6):1089-1124, 1993 (Special issue Featuring: World Population Issues). PMID: 12291996. https://pubmed.ncbi.nlm.nih.gov/12291996/.

1994

Anti-abortion movement put weapon in slayer's hand. *Daily Camera*, Guest Opinion, March 20, 1994.

Life on the Front Lines. *Women's Health Issues* 4(1):48-54, 1994. https://dx.doi.org/10.1016/S1049-3867(05)80109-4.   https://www.whijournal.com/article/S1049-3867(05)80109-4/pdf.

Book review: *Environmental Evolution: Effects of The Origin and Evolution of Life on Planet Earth*. Lynn Margulis and Lorraine Olendzenski (eds.). Cambridge, MA: MIT Press. *National Geographic Research and Exploration*. 10(1):132, 1994.

Cultural change, polygyny, and fertility among the Shipibo of the Peruvian Amazon. In *Demography of Lowland South American Indians: Case Studies from Lowland South America*, Kathleen Adams and David Price (Eds.). *South American Indian Studies* 4:77-86, 1994. PMID: 12319069. https://pubmed.ncbi.nlm.nih.gov/12319069/.

The impact of cultural change and population growth on the Shipibo of the Peruvian Amazon. *Latin American Anthropology Review* 4(1):3-8, 1992 (published 5/94).

First trimester abortion: Principles, Techniques, and Clinical Management. In *Fertility Control*, Stephen L. Corson, Richard J. Derman, and Louise B. Tyrer (Eds.). Second edition. London, Ontario, Canada: Goldin Publishers, 1994.

Alta fecundidad en una comunidad nativa de la Amazonia Peruana. *Amazonia Peruana* 24:125-142, 1994. (Special issue of *Amazonia Peruana: La Mujer Amazonica*) https://doi.org/10.52980/revistaamazonaperuana.vi24.113.

Conocimiento y uso de anticonceptivos herbales en una comunidad Shipibo. *Amazonia Peruana* 24:143-160, 1994. (Special issue of *Amazonia Peruana: La Mujer Amazonica*) https://doi.org/10.52980/revistaamazonaperuana.vi24.114.

Poliginía y fecundidad de los Shipibo de la Amazonía Peruana. *Amazonia Peruana* 24:161-184, 1994 (Special issue of *Amazonia Peruana: La Mujer Amazonica*). https://doi.org/10.52980/revistaamazonaperuana.vi24.115.

Laminaria versus Dilapan osmotic cervical dilators for outpatient dilation and evacuation abortion: Randomized cohort comparison of 1001 patients. *American Journal of Obstetrics and Gynecology* 171(5):1324-1328, 1994.https://doi.org/10.1016/0002-9378(94)90155-4.

Anti-abortion zealots' grasp for power. *The Rocky Mountain News*, Guest Opinion ("Speakout") Column. December 19, 1994.

Publisher Fred Praeger fostered freedom. *Daily Camera*, Guest Opinion. June 26, 1994.

Surgical abortion: Management, complications, and long-term risks. In *Gynecology and Obstetrics*, John J. Sciarra (Ed.) and Preston V. Dilts, Jr (Assoc. Ed.) Revised edition, 1994. Philadelphia: J.B. Lippincott Company, 1994. Chapter 59.

Health and demography of Native Amazonians: Historical perspective and current status. In *Amazonian Indians from Prehistory to the Present*, Anna C. Roosevelt (Ed.), Tuscon: University of Arizona Press, 1994. pp. 123-149.

Family Planning, Amazon Style: Amid cultural changes, high fertility imposes new hardships on an Indian people. *Conformity and Conflict*: 8th, New York: Harper Collins, 1994.

1995

Abortion: Medical and Social Aspects. Chapter I in *Encyclopedia of Marriage and the Family*. New York: MacMillan Publishing Company, 1995.

An electronic demon stalks clinic workers. *The Daily Camera*, Commentary. January 9, 1995.

How it feels to be on anti-abortion hit list. Letter to the editor, *The New York Times*, February 4, 1995. https://www.nytimes.com/1995/02/04/opinion/l-how-it-feels-to-be-on-anti-abortion-hit-list-286895.html?searchResultPosition=31.

Parental notice is bad legislation. Commentary, *The Colorado Statesman*, March 10, 1995.

Parental notification law should be rejected. Editorial, *The Rocky Mountain News*, March 19, 1995.

Microethnodemographic techniques for field workers studying small groups. In *The Comparative Analysis of Human Societies*, Emilio Moran (Ed.). Boulder: Lynn Reiner Publishers, 1995.

Is human culture oncogenic for uncontrolled population growth and ecological destruction? *High Plains Applied Anthropologist* Vol 15 No 2 Fall 1995.

'Killing for Life' is senseless. Op-ed piece, *The Denver Post*, April 8, 1995.

Hern. W.M. Population and Peace. *Colorado Peace Mission* 6(5):1-2, 1995.

Who wanted to ban 'partial birth abortion'? *The Daily Camera*, December 16, 1995.

Book Review: *The Evolution of Desire: Strategies of Human Mating,* New York: Basic Books, 1994. *The Journal of Nervous and Mental Disease*: 183, 5, 348. May 1995. https://journals.lww.com/jonmd/citation/1995/05000/the_evolution_of_desire__strategies_of_human.20.aspx.

Statement of Hern, Warren M., M.D., M.P.H., Ph.D. Before the Judiciary Committee of the United States Senate, Concerning S. 939. November 17, 1995.

1996

Statement of Hern, Warren M., M.D., M.P.H., Ph.D. Before the HEWI Committee of the Colorado House of Representatives Concerning H.B. 1298. February 19, 1996.

Abortion: the numbers game. Op-Ed page, *The Washington Post*, October 17, 1996. https://www.drhern.com/wp-content/uploads/2019/05/Abortion-The-Numbers-Game.pdf.

1997

Abortion bill skips the fine print. Op-Ed Page, *The New York Times*, May 24, 1997. https://www.nytimes.com/1997/05/24/Guest Opinion/abortion-bill-skips-the-fine-print.html?searchResultPosition=2.

Is human culture oncogenic for uncontrolled population growth and ecological destruction? *Human Evolution* 12(1-2):97-105, 1997. https://doi.org/10.1007/BF02437385.

Help Save Holy Cross Wilderness. Boulder: *Holy Cross Wilderness Defense Fund*, 1997. (Poster.)

1998

Life on the front lines. In *Abortion Wars: A Half Century Of Struggle, 1950–2000*, by Rickie Solinger (Ed.). Berkeley: Univ. of California Press, 1998. pp. 307-319.

How Roe v. Wade has shaped my life and work. In *Conscience* 18(4): 26, 1998. Special issue on 25th Anniversary of Roe v. Wade. PMID: 12178882. https://pubmed.ncbi.nlm.nih.gov/12178882/.

Statement of Hern, Warren M., M.D., M.P.H., Ph.D. Before the State Veterans and Military Affairs Committee of the Colorado House of Representatives, Concerning H.B. 98-1286. February 10, 1998.

1999

Defeat of SB 80 protected us from anti-abortion violence and terrorism. Commentary, *The Colorado Statesman,* April 9, 1999.

How many times has the human population doubled? Comparisons with cancer. *Population and Environment* 21(1):59-80, 1999. https://doi.org/10.1023/A:1022153110536.

2000

Dodging Bullets in the Abortion War *Anthropology News* Volume 41, Issue 1, pages 7–8, January 2000 https://doi.org/10.1111/an.2000.41.1.7.

Abortion "bubble bill" going before U.S. Supreme Court: Law has origins to buffer zone rule enacted by Boulder City Council. *Sunday Camera*, Guest Opinion, June 11, 2000. https://www.drhern.com/wp-content/uploads/2019/10/abortion-bubble-bill.pdf.

2001

An abortion doctor's fear. Letter to the Editor, *The New York Times* (concerning the Ashcroft nomination). January 10, 2001 (response by J.C. Watts, January 12, 2001).

https://www.nytimes.com/2001/01/31/Guest Opinion/l-a-doctor-s-fear-687693.html ?searchResultPosition=44.

GOP will attack abortion. Guest Opinion, *The Sunday Camera*, January 21, 2001.

Free speech that threatens my life. Op-Ed Page, *The New York Times*, March 31, 2001. (Letter responses 4/6/01) https://www.nytimes.com/2001/03/31/Guest Opinion/free-speech-that-threatens-my-life.html?searchResultPosition=46.

Laminaria, induced fetal demise and misoprostol in late abortion. *International Journal of Gynecology and Obstetrics* 75:279-286, 2001. (*This paper includes the first report in the medical literature of the use of intrauterine misoprostol in late abortion*) https://doi.org/10.1016/S0020-7292(01)00478-7.

2002

Repressive abortion policy of Owens and GOP is similar to Taliban's 9th century attitudes. *The Colorado Statesman*, Commentary, January 23, 2002.

Second-trimester surgical abortion. In *Gynecology and Obstetrics*, John J. Sciarra, M.D., Ph.D., Editor. Philadelphia: J.B. Lippincott Company, 2002. Chapter 125.

2003

Abortion. International Encyclopedia of Marriage and Family: 1, 2nd, 1, 1-7. New York: MacMillan Publishing Company, 2003. https://epdf.pub/international-encyclopedia-of-marriage-and-family19972a777b0985f58aeab8d01508d90f6805.html.

When Legal Abortion Came to Boulder. Guest Opinion, *The Sunday Camera*. November 2, 2003.

Did I violate the Partial-Birth Abortion Ban? *Slate*, October 22, 2003. https://slate.com/technology/2003/10/did-i-violate-the-partial-birth-abortion-ban.html.

HB 1022 is delusional and preposterous. *The Colorado Statesman*: January 31, 2003.

Who Gets to Speak in Abortion Debate? *The New York Times*: December 2, 2003. https://www.nytimes.com/2003/12/02/Guest Opinion/l-who-gets-to-speak-in-abortion-debate-382086.html?searchResultPosition=54.

Book Review: Kayapo Ethnoecology and Culture. Tipiti - Journal of the Society for the Anthropology of Lowland South America: 1, 2, 7, 83-94. 2003. https://digitalcommons.trinity.edu/tipiti/vol1/iss2/7/.

2004

Surgical abortion in the second trimester. In Beëindiging van de zwangerschap: abortus, inductie en bijstimulatie. S.A. Scherjon, W. Beekhuizen, and H.H.H. Kanhai, Editors. Leiden: Boerhaave Commissie voor Postacademisch Onderwijs in de Geneeskund, Leids Universitair medisch Centrum, 2004. Proceedings of Postgraduate Symposium on Abortion, University of Leiden, May 8-9, 2003 ISBN: 90-6767-524-5 p. 299-317. The same material was presented at an international conference on reproductive health in Barcelona in October, 2003.

Selective termination for fetal anomaly/genetic disorder in twin pregnancy at 32+ menstrual weeks: Report of four cases. *Fetal Diagnosis and Therapy* 19(3):292-295, 2004 https://doi.org/10.1159/000076714.

Abortion. Chapter I in *International Encyclopedia of Marriage and Family, Second Edition*, MacMillan Publishing Company, New York, 2003. J. J. Ponzetti, Jr. (Ed.) Vol. 1 pp 1-7.

Shipibo. In *Encyclopedia of Sex and Gender : Men and Women in the World's Cultures* Edited by Carol R. Ember, Melvin Ember. New York: Kluwer Academic/Plenum Publishers, 2004 Vol 2 pp 806-815 (invited chapter).

Shipibo. In *Encyclopedia of Medical Anthropology: Health and Illness in the World's Cultures*. Ed by Carol R Ember and Melvin Ember. New York: Kluwer Academic/Plenum Publishers, 2004 Vol. 2 (Cultures) pp 947- 956 (invited chapter).

What's intelligent about this design? *The Daily Camera*, December 21, 2004 (about George W. Bush).

https://www.drhern.com/wp-content/uploads/2019/10/whats-intelligent-about-this-design.pdf.

Ronald Reagan and abortion. *The Colorado Statesman*, July 30, 2004. https://www.drhern.com/wp-content/uploads/2018/06/regan-tolerate-abortion-violence.pdf.

2005

Misoprostol as an adjunctive medication in late surgical abortion. *International Journal of Gynecology and Obstetrics* 88:327-328, 2005. (*1040* patients in non-blinded controlled clinical trial with sequential treatment allocation, 18 through 38 weeks) https://doi.org/10.1016/j.ijgo.2004.12.008. (First report of use of intrauterine misoprostol in late abortion.)

Anthropologists, abortion and the cultural war in America. *Anthropology Newsletter* 46(2):16-18, 2005.

Obituary: Darrell A. Posey (1947-2001) *Tipiti - Journal of the Society for the Anthropology of Lowland South America* 2(1):83–94, 2005. https://digitalcommons.trinity.edu/tipiti/vol2/iss1/9.

Cover photograph, Darrel A. Posey. *Tipiti - Journal of the Society for the Anthropology of Lowland South America* 2(1):83-94, 2005. https://digitalcommons.trinity.edu/tipiti/vol2/iss1/9.

Book Review: *Kayapó Ethnoecology and Culture*. DARREL A. POSEY (Kristina Plenderleith, editor). New York: Routledge, 2002. Xviii + 285 pp., figures, tables, foreword, glossary, index. *Tipiti, Journal of the Society for the Anthropology of Lowland South America* (SALSA) 2(1):83–94, 2005 © 2003 *SALSA*.

Bi-ignorant in Brazil. Guest Opinion, *The Sunday Camera*, November 27, 2005. (Dubya's trip to Brazil) https://www.drhern.com/wp-content/uploads/2018/05/bi-ignorant-in-brazil.pdf.

Burial of ashes an unethical spectacle. *Daily Camera*, March 6, 2005.

2006

Bill Ritter and Abortion. *The Colorado Statesman*, 2006.

Having an abortion: A guide for my patients. 6th, 2006.

The following letters were sent to Bill Ritter on May 16, Sept. 1, and Oct. 25, 2005 concerning the issues of Abortion in Public Policy. *The Colorado Statesman:* January 2006.

Election of an anti-abortion Democrat for governor would set us back to 19th century. *The Colorado Statesman*: January 20, 2006.

Ritter unacceptable for many women today. *Rocky Mountain News*: February 7, 2006.

A Resolution for Reproductive Freedom and Protection of the Health and Safety of Women by the Colorado Democratic Party. *The Colorado Statesman*: March 31, 2006.

Latin American Immigration & Trade. March 31, 2006. (Memo to U.S Representative John Salazar (D-CO).

2007

Happy birthday, Edna! *Daily Camera*, 7 April 2007.

The doctor's dilemma: Truly delusional decisions from the Supreme Court. Guest opinion, *The Colorado Statesman* 108(18):6. May 4, 2007. https://www.drhern.com/wp-content/uploads/2018/05/doctors-dilemma.pdf.

When is an egg not an egg? Guest opinion, *The Colorado Statesman*, July 27, 2007.

2008

Urban malignancy: Similarity in the fractal dimensions of urban morphology and malignant neoplasms. *International Journal of Anthropology* 23(1-2):1-19, 2008. https://www.drhern.com/wp-content/uploads/2018/05/IJA-urban-malignancy-2008.pdf.

Thirty-five years in a whirlwind. Guest Opinion, *The Daily Camera*, 8 November 2008. https://www.dailycamera.com/2009/08/14/warren-m-hern-thirty-five-years-in-a-whirlwind/.

This...Is A Person. No! It's a Chicken! The Colorado Statesman: January 18, 2008. (Photo of an egg).

Second-trimester surgical abortion. In *Global Library of Women's Medicine*. Hern, W, *Glob. Libr. Women's med.*, *(ISSN: 1756-2228)* 2009; DOI 10.3843/GLOWM.10442.

2009

Shipibo Hunting and the Overkill Hypothesis. *Tipiti - Journal of the Society for the Anthropology of Lowland South America*: 5, 2, 1, 123-136. December 2007. (published in 2009) https://digitalcommons.trinity.edu/tipiti/vol5/iss2/1?utm_source=digitalcommons.trinity.edu%2Ftipiti%2Fvol5%2Fiss2%2F1&utm_medium=PDF&utm_campaign=PDFCoverPages.

Risus Sardonicus Boulder: Alpenglo Graphics, 2009. 224 pages, 77 photographs. Original poems, essays, anecdotes, by Warren Martin Hern. First place, Non-Fiction Experience category, 2010 Colorado Independent Publishers Association "EVVY" Awards; Second place, Memoirs category, 2010 CIPA "EVVY"Awards; Special award, Poetry category, 2010 CIPA "EVVY" Awards; Bronze Prize, Best Use of Environmental Printing Materials, 2010 PubWest Book Design competition. *New York Times* "Worst Seller List" every year (15) since publication.

Dr. George Tiller's political assassination is result of rabid anti-abortion harassment. *The Colorado Statesman*, June 19, 2009 (Text of invited speech at Temple Emanuel, June 4, 2009). https://www.drhern.com/wp-content/uploads/2018/05/statesmen-tiller-assasination.pdf.

The evidence-based review of second-trimester abortion missed some important evidence. Letter to the editor. *American Journal of Obstetrics & Gynecology* at www .AJOG.org, December, 2009 e7-8. https://doi.org/10.1016/j.ajog.2009.06.052.

Are we safe in our own country? The Daily Camera: August 14, 2009. https://www.dailycamera.com/2009/08/14/letters-to-the-editor-dec-27-2/.

2010

Thirty-five years of local support. *The Daily Camera*: January 20, 2010. https://www .dailycamera.com/2010/01/20/letters-to-the-editor-jan-21-2/.

2011

Frances Kissling's call for restrictions on late-term abortions as a strategy for the pro-choice movement is like offering the crocodile your arm so he won't eat the rest of you. Letter to the editor, *The Washington Post*. February 24, 2011.

Population 7 Billion Guest Opinion, *Daily Camera*, November 6, 2011 https://www.dailycamera.com/2011/11/04/guest-opinion-population-7-billion/.

Book highlights response to threats. *The Daily Camera*, Letters to the Editor. June 10, 2011. https://www.dailycamera.com/2011/06/10/letters-to-the-editor-june-12/.

Second-trimester surgical abortion. In *Global Library of Women's Medicine*, 2nd edition. Hern, W, *Glob. libr.women's med.*, *(ISSN: 1756-2228)* 2011; DOI 10.3843/ GLOWM.10442.

2012

Choose between candidates who understand global ecological realities and those who don't. Guest Opinion, *The Colorado Statesman* 2 March 2012 Editorial criticism by Vincent Carroll, columnist, The Denver Post: Hern and the "malignancy" of mankind, 17 March 2012. WMH response to Carroll, Letter to the editor, *The Denver Post*, 25 March 2012.

2013

An appreciation: Remembering Al Bartlett. Guest opinion, *Daily Camera*, November 2, 2013. https://www.dailycamera.com/2013/11/01/an-appreciation-remembering -al-bartlett/.

2014

Fetal diagnostic indications for second and third trimester outpatient pregnancy termination. *Prenatal Diagnosis* 34(5):438-444, 2014. https://obgyn.onlinelibrary.wiley.com /doi/10.1002/pd.4324.

Abortion clinic ruling: Freedom to harrass, intimidate, and humiliate. *The Daily Camera*: June 29, 2014. https://www.dailycamera.com/2014/06/27/abortion-clinic-ruling-freedom-to-harass-intimidate-and-humiliate/.

Your vote is critical. *The Daily Camera*: October 28, 2014. https://www.dailycamera
.com/2014/10/27/dr-warren-m-hern-your-vote-is-critical/.

2015

Performing abortions is my life's work. Terrorism won't stop me. *STAT*, December 4,
2015; *The Boston Globe* online at http://www.statnews.com/2015/12/04/abortion-
doctor-violence/.
Cynical exploitation. *The Daily Camera*: February 8, 2015. https://www.dailycamera.
com/2015/02/08/warren-m-hern-cynical-exploitation/.

2016

Yushin Huemena: Visions of the Spirit World, Art, Design, Medicine and Protective
Spirits in Shipibo Ritual. *Tipití: Journal of the Society for the Anthropology of
Lowland South America*: Vol. 14: Iss. 1, Article 1, 1-14. May, 2016. Available at:
http://digitalcommons.trinity.edu/tipiti/vol14/iss1/1.
Segundina and John. In *The Human Touch* The Journal of Poetry, Prose and Visual Art,
University of Colorado Anschutz Medical Campus, Vol. 9, 2016 pp 22,23.
Risus sardonicus (poem) In *The Human Touch* The Journal of Poetry, Prose and Visual
Art, University of Colorado Anschutz Medical Campus, Vol. 9, 2016 pp 14,15.
Second-trimester surgical abortion. In *Global Library of Women's Medicine*, 2nd edi-
tion. Hern,W, *Glob.libr.women's med.*, (ISSN: 1756-2228) 2011; DOI 10.3843/
GLOWM.10442 Revised August, 2016 At https://www.glowm.com/section_view/
item/441.
An abortion doctor on Trump's win: 'I fear for my life. I fear for my patients.' *STAT*,
November 11, 2016; *The Boston Globe* online at https://www.statnews.com/2016/11/
11/trump-abortion-doctor-fear/.
Pushing Back on the House's Abortion Provider 'Witch Hunt'. *Ms. Magazine*: November
22, 2016.
https://msmagazine.com/2016/11/22/pushing-back-houses-abortion-provider-witch-
hunt/.

2017

Mr. Foo. In *The Human Touch* The Journal of Poetry, Prose and Visual Art, University
of Colorado Anschutz Medical Campus, Vol. 10, 2017 p.96 http://www.ucdenver.
edu/academics/colleges/medicalschool/centers/BioethicsHumanities/ArtsHumanities/
Documents/HumanTouch_2017_BookWeb%20final.pdf.

2018

Book review: *Culturing Bioscience: A Case Study in the Anthropology of Science*.
Udo Krautwurst. Toronto: University of Toronto Press, 2014. 224 pp. *American
Ethnologist* 12 Feburary 2018. https://doi.org/10.1111/amet.12612.
Religion, power and reproductive freedom: A checkered history of conflict. 3 May, 2018,
speech on receipt of the Faith and Freedom Award. *Newsletter*, May, 2018, Colorado

Religious Coalition for Reproductive Choice. https://www.drhern.com/wp-content/uploads/2023/06/religion-power-and-reproductive-freedom-warren-hern-md.pdf.

Experience, not money, should matter most. *The Daily Camera*: June 21, 2018. https://www.dailycamera.com/2018/06/21/dr-warren-m-hern-experience-not-money-should-matter-most/.

2019

Pregnancy kills. Abortion saves lives. Op-ed article, *The New York Times*, May 21, 2019. https://www.nytimes.com/2019/05/21/opinion/alabama-law-abortion.html.

New abortion restrictions are madness. Guest Opinion, *The Daily Camera*, June 1, 2019. https://www.dailycamera.com/2019/06/01/warren-hern-abortion-restrictions-madness/.

Dilation and evacuation of thoracopagus conjoined twins per vagina at 26 weeks. Hern, Warren M. MD, MPH, PhD; Landgren, Benedict MD. *Obstetrics & Gynecology*: May 2019 - Volume 133 - Issue - p 100S doi: 10.1097/01.AOG.0000558797.18208.0f At https://journals.lww.com/greenjournal/Abstract/2019/05001/Dilation_and_Evacuation_of_Thoracopagus_Conjoined.350.aspx.

2020

Testing must be priority in historic public health emergency. Guest Opinion, *The Daily Camera*, May 19, 2020. At https://www.dailycamera.com/2020/05/19/guest-opinion-warren-m-hern-testing-must-be-priority-in- historic-public-health-emergency/.

A doctor's perspective: Trump's calamitous incompetence leaves us imperiled. Op-Ed page, *The San Francisco Chronicle*, May 27, 2020. https://www.sfchronicle.com/opinion/openforum/article/A-doctor-s-perspective-Trump-s-calamitous-15296525.php.

A Supreme Court packed with anti-abortion justices puts my patients at risk. Op-Ed page, *The San Francisco Chronicle*, October 6, 2020. https://www.sfchronicle.com/opinion/openforum/article/A-Supreme-Court-packed-with-anti-abortion-15623582.php.

Tyranny is the brand of the Republican Party. Op-Ed page, *The San Francisco Chronicle*, December 15, 2020. https://www.sfchronicle.com/Guest Opinion/article/Tyrrany-is-the-brand-of-the-Republican-Party-15801811.php.

A message to my cousins, kin and neighbors in Kansas. Abilene Reflector Chronicle: October 9, 2020.

A message to my cousins, kin and neighbors in Kansas. Salina Journal: October 11, 2020.

Another Message to My Neighbors in Kansas. Abilene Reflector Chronicle: October 23, 2020.

Another Message to My Neighbors in Kansas. Salina Journal: October 25, 2020.

2021

Helping women who are having the worst moment of their lives should not be controversial, *The Colorado Sun*, July 5, 2021. https://coloradosun.com/2021/07/05/abortion-late-term-Guest Opinion/.

Late abortion: Clinical and ethical issues. *In Whose Choice Is It? Abortion, Medicine and the Law*, 7th edition (David F. Walbert and J. Douglas Butler, Eds.). Chicago: American Bar Association. July, 2021.

Sarah Weddington and her legacy from Roe v. Wade. *Daily Camera Guest Opinion* December 30, 2021. https://www.dailycamera.com/2021/12/30/guest-opinion-warren -m-hern-sarah-weddington-and-her-legacy-from-roe-v-wade/.

2022

Anticipated abolition of Roe v. Wade after 49 years takes away freedom and health for many American women. *Daily Camera Guest Opinion* January 22, 2022. https:// www.dailycamera.com/2022/01/22/warren-m-hern/.

Homo Ecophagus: A Deep Diagnosis to Save the Earth. Routledge Press, September 30, 2022. 336 pages. Hardback, paperback, e-book editions.

'Wake Up, America': Remembering Dr. George Tiller, Assassinated Abortion Practitioner. By Warren M. Hern. *Ms. Magazine*, May 1, 2022. https://msmagazine.com/2022/05 /01/dr-george-tiller-assassinated-abortion-provider-violence/.

2023

A person of Conscience and a force for consciousness. A tribute to Dave Foreman by Warren M. Hern. In *Wildeor: The Wild Life and living Legacy of Dave Foreman*. Essex, NY: Essex Editions, 2023. https://rewilding.org/purchase-wildeor-the-wild-life -and-living-legacy-of-dave-foreman/.

2024

Performing abortions after *Roe*. In *Fighting Mad: Resisting the End of Roe v. Wade*. Krystale E. Littlejohn and Rickie Solinger (Eds.). Oakland: University of California Press, 2024.

Testimony given by the author

Congressional testimony

Testimony before the US Senate Health Subcommittee (Chairman: Edward Kennedy) regarding suppression of OEO Sterilization Guidelines and Relf sterilization case in Alabama. July 10, 1973. Part 4, Hearings before the Subcommittee on Health of the Committee on Labor and Public Welfare, U.S. Senate, 93rd Congress, First session. U.S. Government Printing Office, Washington, D.C. 1973. pp. 1503–33.

Submitted testimony before the US Senate Subcommittee on Separation of Powers of the Committee on the Judiciary, 97th Congress, First session, on S. 158. Serial No. J9716. Appendix, PP 443458. US Gov.Printing Off., Washington, D.C., 1982.

Testimony, as Chairman of the Holy Cross Wilderness Defense Fund, before the Public Lands Subcommittee of the U.S. House of Representatives Committee on Interior and Insular Affairs, Oversight Hearing, Vail, Colorado, 11/12/82 concerning the proposed Homestake Phase II water diversion project.

Submitted testimony before the U.S. Senate Judiciary Committee on the "Partial Birth Abortion Act of 1995," November 17, 1995. Cite volume of Congressional Record.

Government documents

OEO Guidelines for the Provision of Voluntary Sterilization Services (OEO Instruction 61302). Suppressed by White House in February, 1972 (See Medical World News cover story, 11/12/73).

Anti-Abortion Activity at Boulder Abortion Clinic 1975–1995 in a National Context. Warren M. Hern, M.D., M.P.H., Ph.D. Director, Boulder Abortion Clinic. Special Report prepared for JoAnn Harris, Director, Criminal Division, U.S. Department of Justice, Washington, D.C., January 6, 1995.

Suppressed publications

Voluntary sterilization in the Office of Economic Opportunity Family Planning Programs. *American Journal of Public Health* 63–150, 1973. Deleted at press time by the editors of the journal at the request of the Executive Office of the President of the United States (galley proofs available on request).

Federal trial testimony

Reproductive Health Services v. William L. Webster (heard in Kansas City Federal District Court, 1986). Expert witness for plaintiffs challenging Missouri statute restricting abortion. District and appellate court decisions for plaintiff overruled by U.S. Supreme Court on July 3, 1989 in *Webster v. Reproductive Health Services.*

Richard M. Ragsdale v. Bernard J. Turnock (heard in Chicago Federal District Court, 1986). Sole expert witness for plaintiff challenging Illinois regulations restricting abortion clinics. Decision for plaintiff upheld at appellate court, settled out of court by defendant Attorney General of Illinois on plaintiff's terms after hearing scheduled by U.S. Supreme Court.

Catherine Buchanan et al. v. Linda Jorgensen et al. (heard in Denver Federal District Court, 1987). Expert witness for defendant City of Boulder in hearing to deny permanent injunction of Boulder "Buffer Zone" ordinance designed to protect abortion patients from harassment by demonstrators.Injunction denied by district court, upheld on appeal.

Hern et al. v. Beye (heard in Denver Federal District Court, April 6, 1994). Witness as plaintiff in suit filed by Center for Reproductive Law and Policy requesting temporary restraining order permitting use of Colorado state Medicaid funds to pay for an abortion for patient Jane Courage, a rape victim, on grounds that Colorado statute was more stringent than federal standard. Per curium ruling from bench throwing out 1984 Colorado Constitutional Amendment prohibiting use of state funds for abortion. Colorado Medicaid funds may and must be used to pay for abortions for poor women.

Planned Parenthood of Oregon et al. v. American Coalition of Life Activists, et al. (heard in Portland Federal District Court, January 15 - February 10, 1999. Witness as co-plaintiff in private suit filed by Paul Weiss Rifkind for Planned Parenthood of Oregon, Portland Feminist Clinic, and four physician plaintiffs against Michael Bray, ACLA, and 11 other anti-abortion activists who conspired to threaten plaintiffs by publication of "Wanted" posters and hit lists. Civil judgment of $109 million against defendants after concluding defendants had conspired to threaten to harm plaintiffs for performing abortions. Overturned by three-judge panel, Ninth Circuit Court of Appeals, San Francisco, April 4, 2001. Court decision upheld on appeal.

Awards and recognition received by the author

National Organization for Women Denver Chapter, Special recognition award for work in abortion rights, 1974

National Organization for Women, "Unsung Hero Award", June 14, 1986. NOW 20th Anniversary Annual Meeting, National March for Women's Lives, Colorado State Capitol, Denver

Colorado Women's Political Caucus "Good Guys" Award, May 11, 1991, Denver, Colorado

Colorado Chapter, National Abortion Rights Action League, "Local Heroes" Award, May 11, 1991, Boulder, Colorado

Colorado Coalition for Choice, Special Recognition Award, June 3, 1993

Ortho Prize for Best Scientific Paper, National Abortion Federation Annual Meeting, 27 April 1993

Ortho Prize for Best Scientific Paper, Association of Reproductive Health Professionals Annual Meeting, October 8, 1994

Christopher Tietze Humanitarian Award, National Abortion Federation, April 19, 2002

Carl S. Schultz Award, American Public Health Association; Population, Family Planning, and Reproductive Health Section, November 11, 2002

Lifetime Achievement Award, NARAL Pro-Choice Colorado, April, 2010

Faith and Freedom Award, Colorado Religious Coalition for Reproductive Choice. At the Temple Emanuel in Denver, May 3, 2018 http://corcrc.org/sermon/religion-power-and-reproductive-freedom-a-checkered-history-of-conflict/

The Senate of the Colorado Legislature

Hereby extends heartiest congratulations and commendations to

Dr. WARREN HERN

for

Celebrating the Twentieth Anniversary of his private medical practice in Boulder.

Without his work as Director of the Boulder Abortion Clinic, the twenty-second anniversary of the landmark *Roe v. Wade* Supreme Court decision would have little meaning for Boulder and Colorado. One of only three physicians to perform late-term abortions, Dr. Hern has been a target of adversity for more than two decades. We applaud him for his years of personal sacrifice and courage in upholding his beliefs.

On request of SENATORS DOROTHY RUPERT, PAUL WEISSMAN, LLOYD CASEY,

LINDA POWERS, MICHAEL FEELEY, BILL THEIBAUT,

DONALD MARES, SALLY HOPPER, and DOTTIE WHAM

Given this 3rd day of February, 1995, State Capitol, Denver

(signed) Tom Norton

President of the Senate

Author biography

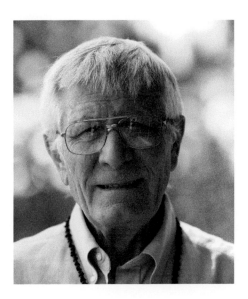

Photo by Odalys Muñoz Gonzalez

Warren M. Hern is a physician and epidemiologist whose principal professional activity since 1975 has been Director of the Boulder Abortion Clinic, his private medical practice in Boulder, Colorado. In 1973, he was the founding medical director of the first private, nonprofit outpatient abortion clinic in Colorado. From 1970 to 1972, Dr. Hern served as Chief, Program Development and Evaluation Branch, Family Planning Division, Office of Health Affairs, Office of Economic Opportunity ("War on Poverty") in the Executive Office of the President in Washington, DC. In that capacity, he helped administer a federal family planning program in OEO Community Health Centers across the nation. Prior to that (1966–1968), he served as a Peace Corps physician in Brazil on assignment from the US Public Health Service. He graduated from the University of Colorado School of Medicine in 1965, completed his internship at Gorgas Hospital in the Canal Zone in 1966, received his Master of Public Health degree from the University of North Carolina School of Public Health in 1971, and his PhD in epidemiology from the same institution in 1988.

Dr. Hern is Professor Adjunct, Department of Anthropology, University of Colorado at Boulder and Associate Clinical Professor, Department of Obstetrics and Gynecology, University of Colorado Anschutz Medical Campus. He has conducted epidemiologic, ethnographic, and demographic research among the Shipibo of the Peruvian Amazon since 1964. His medical and anthropological research has been published in numerous professional scientific and medical journals, and he is the author of a medical textbook, *Abortion Practice* (J.B. Lippincott, 1984). Dr. Hern is a Fellow of the American Association for the Advancement of Science and also Fellow of the American College of Preventive Medicine.

Dr. Hern is also a photographer whose natural history and other photographs have appeared in Sierra Club calendars and magazine, *National Geographic Research and Exploration, Defenders of Wildlife, Americas, Natural History* magazine, *Time* magazine, *The New York Times*, and other books and publications. He is the co-founder and chairman of the Holy Cross Wilderness Defense Fund, which has successfully opposed a massive water diversion project in Colorado's Holy Cross Wilderness.

Dr. Hern is the author of *Risus Sardonicus*, a collection of his poems, essays, and photographs (Alpenglo Graphics, 2009). He lives in Colorado with his wife and son.

Dr. Hern's views presented in this book are his own and do not reflect the views of any institution with which he is associated.

Want to help low-income women have abortions at Dr. Hern's office?

Most of the women who come to Dr. Hern's office, Boulder Abortion Clinic, have insufficient funds for lodging, transportation, food, and other expenses in addition to cost of the abortion procedure. While some patients are eligible for assistance from national funds, many are not and need help. We have a pantry for patients with no food. If you would like to help these women, you may make a tax-exempt contribution to Boulder Abortion Fund, a 501(c)(3) charitable fund. All contributions received by this fund are tax-exempt, fully deductible and are used to assist specific patients. These are especially critical problems for women from Red states where abortion services are illegal or extremely limited.

Contributions may be sent to:
Boulder Abortion Fund
PO Box 4626
Boulder, Colorado 80306
www.BoulderAbortionFund.org

Index

Page numbers in *italics* indicate figures or photographs.